Essentials of Clinical Informatics

Essentials of Clinical Informatics

EDITED BY

MARK E. FRISSE, MD, MS, MBA

ACCENTURE PROFESSOR OF BIOMEDICAL INFORMATICS

VICE CHAIR FOR BUSINESS DEVELOPMENT

VANDERBILT UNIVERSITY SCHOOL OF MEDICINE

NASHVILLE, TENNESSEE

KARL E. MISULIS, MD, PHD

PROFESSOR OF CLINICAL NEUROLOGY

PROFESSOR OF CLINICAL BIOMEDICAL INFORMATICS

VANDERBILT UNIVERSITY SCHOOL OF MEDICINE

NASHVILLE, TENNESSEE

OXFORD
UNIVERSITY PRESS

OXFORD
UNIVERSITY PRESS

Oxford University Press is a department of the University of Oxford. It furthers
the University's objective of excellence in research, scholarship, and education
by publishing worldwide. Oxford is a registered trade mark of Oxford University
Press in the UK and certain other countries.

Published in the United States of America by Oxford University Press
198 Madison Avenue, New York, NY 10016, United States of America.

Library of Congress Cataloging-in-Publication Data
Names: Frisse, Mark E., editor. | Misulis, Karl E., editor.
Title: Essentials of clinical informatics / edited by Mark E. Frisse, Karl E. Misulis.
Description: New York, NY : Oxford University Press, [2019] |
Includes bibliographical references and index.
Identifiers: LCCN 2018049155 | ISBN 9780190855574 (alk. paper)
Subjects: | MESH: Medical Informatics | Health Information Systems
Classification: LCC R858 | NLM W 26.5 | DDC 610.285—dc23
LC record available at https://lccn.loc.gov/2018049155

CONTENTS

Douglas J. Dickey, MD
Chief Medical Officer of Physician Strategy
Cerner Corporation
Kanas City, MO (Missouri)

Jeffrey G. Frieling, MBA, FACHE
Vice President and Chief Information Officer
West Tennessee Healthcare
Jackson, TN (Tennessee)

Christoph U. Lehmann, MD, FAAP, FACMI, FIAHSI
Professor of Biomedical Informatics and Pediatrics
Vanderbilt University Medical Center
Nashville, TN

Paul Weaver
Vice President, User Experience and Human Factors
Cerner Corporation
Kanas City, MO (Missouri)

Part I

Introduction

Areas of Focus

The Healthcare System

MARK E. FRISSE AND KARL E. MISULIS ∎

OVERVIEW

This chapter focuses on people, processes, policies, and technologies aimed at improving the health and well-being of individuals, their families, and their communities.

The US healthcare system is impressive in so many ways, yet it fails to deliver reliable, consistent, and affordable high-quality care to every individual. From the perspective of patients and providers, the system is a complex and opaque labyrinth of processes driven by misaligned incentives and a failure to appreciate the critical role of culture, behavior, human thought, and problem-solving processes.[1] Although the United States is the most expensive (per capita) healthcare system in the world, it ranks among the lowest in patient access and health outcomes among Organization for Economic Cooperation and Development (OECD) countries.[2] It is a system overburdened with excessive complexity, number of payers, administrative requirements, regulatory impositions, and hidden costs. In the future, an aging population, complex comorbidities, family financial distress, changing cultural expectations, and unsustainable healthcare prices will necessitate a radically broader view of clinical care. Things must change and clinical informatics must be up to the task.

ROLE OF INFORMATICS PROFESSIONALS

Clinical informatics professionals historically have concentrated on improving care through more effective use of *electronic medical records* (EMRs). Often, these EMRs were localized to large hospitals and clinics and were entirely disconnected from mobile devices, consumer products, and a range of other technologies. Often, they were only clumsily associated with operational, administrative, and billing systems essential for payment and administration. Over the last decade, federal *electronic health record* (EHR) certification requirements, health plan changes, and federal payment regulations have focused the attention of many clinicians on the administrative aspects of care, at the expense of time with their patients. There was a time when physicians did not do anything that did not require a medical degree. Now, clinicians have become clerical workers.[3]

Our central challenge is to ensure that clinical informatics professionals understand the forces that drive our healthcare system and employ their understanding to address the most pressing needs of clinical practice. From this perspective, a mastery of healthcare delivery in hospitals and clinics is necessary but not sufficient. One heavily cited analysis claimed that clinical care accounts for only 20% of overall health status. According to this analysis, health behaviors account for 30%, physical environment (e.g., air, water, housing, transit) accounts for 10%, and social and economic factors account for a full 40% (e.g., social support, financial status, education).[4] To fix hospitals and clinics, one must look outward and address these other factors.

ROLE OF ADMINISTRATION AND FINANCE

Payment and oversight for clinical services drive much of the day-to-day work of clinicians. Societal expectations, legislation, payment trends, financial constraints, and many other factors drive the ultimate design of our healthcare delivery system and the people, processes, data, and technologies used to support this system. Knowledge of the nuances of mainstream biomedical informatics—clinical systems—simply will not be sufficient to advance healthcare systems increasingly dominated by financial imperatives. To excel, one must interpret clinical informatics through the lens of details of federal programs (e.g., Medicare, Medicaid, disability services, Veterans Affairs [VA], Department of Defense [DoD], Indian Health Service); state programs (e.g., Medicaid, public health); private insurers (both employer-sponsored health plans and pharmacy benefits managers); accrediting bodies; quality improvement organizations; and certification initiatives. Every clinical informatics professional must understand how participation in management, support, and delivery can collectively deliver more effective care, improve quality of care, and support research.

THE CUSTOMER: ROLE OF PATIENTS AND FAMILIES

Patients and their families are central. Every individual patient is supported by an often-hidden network where many family members, friends, and others work in collaboration to assist with a full range of care activities, including shopping or transportation, household tasks, finances, personal care and nursing, and indoor ambulation. The overall composition of these informal patient-centered care teams and the roles individuals play are generally not known to providers. To provide effective care, providers must be aware of both formal and informal caregivers, their tasks, available devices and technologies in the home, and the broader physical and cultural environment in which patients live. Clinical informatics professionals must find means of collecting this information and making it available to improve care delivery.

The patient perspective is that care is often highly fragmented. Studies showed that the average elderly patient sees seven doctors across four practices, and that the average elderly surgery patient is seen by 27 different healthcare providers.[5] Providers pay the consequences of this care fragmentation; they sometimes do not even know who a patient's other providers are. One study found that the typical primary care physician must coordinate with 229 other physicians working in 117 practices.[6] Hence, in most instances, for a single patient, different individuals will have different roles reliant on different data sets collected and presented through multiple technical systems. The EHR of the past must continue to evolve to accommodate these realities.

The care fragmentation experienced by patients and providers alike demonstrates that the EHR would likely best be served by evolving from a database of orders, result, and documents toward a platform supporting true communication and collaboration. Presently, steps are incremental, care quality is uneven, and coordination is limited.

ROLE OF TECHNOLOGY

Technology's rapid advancement has not yet led to a mature healthcare technology infrastructure. Indeed, the rapid evolution of technologies often overwhelm our capacity to grasp their potential and to incorporate them into our healthcare system. As a result, some consumers are taking commercial technologies into their own hands to maintain and monitor health, to monitor chronic disease status, and to communicate with one another. Data collected through these technologies are seldom incorporated into the EHR. Informatics professionals must understand technology trends and make decisions today that will prepare them for future developments.

ROLE OF ANALYTICS

Providers are faced with a growing and increasingly complex array of quality and financial metrics and are increasingly reliant on analytics technologies for their compensation. Researchers, armed with advanced machine learning methods applied to large data sets, are adding insights to relationships between genetics, behaviors, and phenotypes derived from EHR and medical claims data. The vast majority of these more complex analytic approaches are not yet applicable to healthcare delivery and payment; a focus on fundamental, simple techniques is more cost effective. One must always remember that new innovations often take several years before their use and value are widely realized.

Every clinical informatics professional must remain knowledgeable about innovative technologies, yet be advised not to adopt expensive and unstable technologies while more pressing clinical and financial issues are already apparent.

CLINICAL INFORMATICS PROFESSIONAL SKILL SETS

Clinicians who seek to practice informatics within complex care delivery settings must be particularly aware of the techniques and skills required to translate their clinical aspirations into meaningful organizational actions. Informatics is practiced in the context of teams and organizations united toward common goals. Success often depends far more on organizational capabilities and immediate needs than on one's own knowledge and capabilities. One's organizational fit is a major determinant of career success.

Mastery of traditional clinical informatics approaches is only the starting point for a lifetime of effective clinical informatics practice. Much work lies ahead.

KEY POINTS

- Clinical care is only one determinant of health; behavior, social and economic circumstance, and physical environment play vital roles. Clinical care requires deep understanding of patients, families, policies, behaviors, and many other factors.
- Healthcare is delivered by both formal and informal teams composed of individuals pursuing common goals but playing different roles and performing different tasks.
- Understanding roles, tasks, and goals is critical both to traditional care delivery teams and to the informal support care network supporting patients in their homes.
- Because of demographic trends, care fragmentation, technology acceleration, and payment methods, EHRs will increasingly be incorporated into a larger network of systems supporting care communication, coordination, and accountability.
- New technologies and data sources have the long-term potential of transforming clinical care to a dramatic extent but will take time to mature into actionable programs.

Healthcare and the Electronic Health Record

KARL E. MISULIS AND MARK E. FRISSE ■

OVERVIEW OF THE ELECTRONIC HEALTH RECORD IN THE TWENTY-FIRST CENTURY

The *electronic health record* (EHR) is the present preferred term for the digital systems that coordinate healthcare information. The term *electronic medical record* (EMR) was used more prominently in the past and has largely been replaced by current terminology. These terms are not interchangeable. We tend to think of the EMR as the record an individual facility or provider would use to accomplish what they previously accomplished with paper records. We think of EHRs as more of a continuum of records, extending beyond one provider or group of providers and even beyond the enterprise. Ideally, the EHR would be able to access all medical information for a particular patient and be able to execute orders across the spectrum of healthcare services. We aspire to that functional level, but we are not there yet.

Looking to the future, the next step is the personal health record (PHR), for which healthcare data are governed not by the healthcare institutions but rather by the patient. As providers, we will interact with the patient's records using our electronic tools.

The importance of these conceptual and functional transitions cannot be underestimated. As authors of this book, we have clinical responsibilities in oncology (M.F.) and hospital neurology (K.M.) in addition to our Biomedical Informatics appointments. These specialties, or almost any other, practiced with incomplete information results in life-and-death decisions that are difficult and dangerous.

BASICS OF EHR TECHNOLOGY

There are many functions of the modern EHR, but some key core elements include

- Data storage
- Clinical documentation
- Orders
- Results

Some additional expected functions of a modern EHR include

- Patient list management
- Communication with other providers
- Results inbox with check-off
- Decision support

These functions are detailed further in this chapter as well as elsewhere in this book.

The beginnings of EHRs included individual applications that performed orders, provided results, or archived documents. Ultimately, the EHR evolved into a system that could perform most or all of these tasks.

Presently, the EHR is pervasive in hospitals and most clinics. Estimates are that more than 95% of hospitals use certified EHR technologies and have achieved some level of Meaningful Use qualification.[1] As of August 2018, the proportion of hospitals meeting Meaningful Use levels 1 or 2 were as follows[2]:

- Large hospitals = 99%
- Medium hospitals = 98%
- Small rural hospitals = 98%
- Small urban hospitals = 84%
- Critical access hospitals = 96%
- Children's hospitals = 78%

Proportions of EHR use by outpatient clinics are somewhat lower, but still substantial. The Centers for Disease Control and Prevention estimated that 87% of outpatient physicians use an EHR in their practice.[3]

Children's hospitals were quick to begin the journey to EHR adoption, but in recent years, they have lagged behind adult hospitals and behind children's hospitals that are part of adult hospital facilities.[4] As a result, they have lagged in Meaningful Use achievement.[5] Among the reasons implicated in this disparity is the greater inefficiencies of EHRs for pediatric workflow and the challenging finances of many children's hospitals.

Similarly, EHR adoption is less in the outpatient than inpatient arenas. Part of this is functionality; not all EHRs are equally facile at acute and ambulatory workflows. Some EHRs are better in outpatient space and some in inpatient space. Part of the reason for lower adoption is also because, in the ambulatory market, the decision-makers for resource utilization are usually the physicians, and they are less likely to make a substantial investment for a modest incentive payment return.

There are multiple EHR vendors, but there are fewer major players in the market than there were years ago. Part of this contraction is due to consolidation from mergers and acquisitions. Part is from sunset of applications that could not keep up with demands for functionality by users or regulatory agencies. The Office of the National Coordinator for Health Information Technology (ONC) expects certified EHRs to have specified functionality, and many vendors without significant market share have abandoned their segment of the market, not expecting revenues to meet development costs.

Because of the sunset of some applications, healthcare systems have had to re-place them with current applications, with the hope that the new apps will not themselves be sunset. Also, some healthcare systems replace working EHR systems or subsystems because of hospital or clinic mergers and acquisitions, so that most or all units of a healthcare system use the same EHR.

Most healthcare systems have more than one functioning EHR, often because of lags in conversion to an enterprise-wide EHR. Also, some specialties prefer their niche information system. Until a comprehensive EHR can perform the essentials of the niche systems, the specialty systems will be slow to be replaced. Examples of where niche systems have significant market penetrance include radiology's picture archiving and communication system (PACS) and radi-ology information system (RIS); oncology EHR (for chemotherapy and radia-tion therapy); cardiology EHR; and gastroenterology EHR. These systems are particularly image and procedure based, with complex and unique workflows. The niche systems accommodate this complexity by generally well-designed scripting and workflows, automating many of the tasks required for orders, doc-umentation, and billing.

Future directions of the EHR will likely be the following:

- Further consolidation of the EHR vendor market
- Transition of enterprises to use fewer and, it is hoped, one principal EHR
- Improved interoperability as part of core functionality
- Transition from niche specialty apps to functionality embedded in comprehensive system-wide EHRs
- Focus on user efficiency and productivity
- Connection of EHRs with other EHRs to facilitate point-of-care information exchange and care coordination
- Improvement of clinical decision support function to improve quality of care, reduce gaps, and control costs
- Improved use of patient-entered information and facilitation of the move to the PHR

Advantages of EHRs over paper records include legible notes and orders, access from multiple locations, and automation of some previously manual processes, such as order execution. However, composing a note in the EHR is often slower than writing a note by hand and much slower than straight dictation. So, while almost no one advocates returning to paper records, we should understand that efficiency is affected by use of the EHR. Dealing with that inefficiency is discussed in Chapter 4.

In the future, our goal should be a single health record that spans all service locations, incorporates patient data entry, and provides decision support not only to the providers but also to the patient. Quality of care would be better. Costs would be less.

CLINICAL NEEDS

Clinical needs can be divided into the following general categories:

- Point-of-care data
- Decision support
- Analytics
- Billing
- Communication

Point-of-care data management is the principal core function of the EHR. This function not only consists of creation, storage, and manipulation of local data but also extends to include data sharing with other systems.

Decision support is the growing role of the EHR in improving quality of care and reducing costs. This is discussed in detail in Chapter 17. Some of the components include disorder-specific order sets, alerts, and reminders.

Analytics is manifest in a broad spectrum of methods, as detailed in Chapter 16. Among the analytics arenas are both clinical and business performance. Reports are generated at almost every level of the healthcare system.

Billing requires access to clinical data for justification and authorization of appropriate charges and for creation of claims. This includes functions that are dependent on financial arrangements with individual patients, payer contract management, and regulatory requirements.

Communication includes messaging from within the EHR in regard to patients; sending reports and other documents to other providers via exchanges, direct messaging, or electronic fax functions; and secure messaging. Not all of these communication tasks are widely functioning.

CLINICAL APPLICATIONS

Let us explore some of the user-facing functions of a core EHR system. The minimal functions are

- Clinical documentation
- Orders
- Results of laboratory and radiological studies

We focus mainly on these with mention of some of the additional functions that are becoming pervasive but are not yet standard equipment:

- PACS for radiological image viewing
- Secure messaging for provider communication
- Assistance with coding and billing
- Electronic prescribing of medications for outpatient care
- Health information exchange data query and viewing
- Viewing/editing of data from interfaced applications, especially procedural applications

These functions may be illustrated by a use case. Consider a patient who is in our emergency department (ED) with fever and delirium. We assess the patient and review the record. We discover that the patient has a high fever, appears pale, and is hypotensive (has low blood pressure). A general medical examination shows that the patient had previous lower abdominal surgery and bilateral mastectomy.

Our interaction with information systems is as follows:

- Vital signs have already been entered, and the fever and hypotension are noted.
- Review of a discharge summary from an admission 3 months ago shows the patient had a bilateral mastectomy. Pathology shows high-grade adenocarcinoma. There are no other records in the EHR.
- Query of the regional health information exchange identifies documents from a freestanding cancer center. These documents reveal aggressive chemotherapy with neutropenia appropriately treated, with the last documented chemotherapy 2 days prior to this ED visit.
- The ED physician electronically orders laboratory tests, including a comprehensive metabolic panel (CMP), complete blood cell count (CBC), and blood cultures to check for infection. The physician selects *Stat* as the priority of the studies.
- Soon, the EHR displays laboratory results showing the patient is severely anemic, with a very low white blood cell (WBC) count.
- The ED physician electronically orders antibiotics using an order set for *Febrile Neutropenia*; the order set includes typical weight-adjusted doses of medications and the antibiotics most commonly used in this clinical scenario. The order set also has a section for transfusion, but the ED doctor does not believe the patient requires transfusion at this time, so this order is not selected. The ED doctor orders a CBC to be drawn in the morning.
- The ED physician uses secure messaging to notify the internal medicine hospitalist and on-call oncologist about the admission.

- The ED physician uses the documentation module to create the ED note and then clicks the links to send the document by direct messaging to the patient's outpatient oncologist and primary care provider.
- The admitting hospitalist arrives and places an admission order set, which includes entries for level of service, admitting provider identification, admitting diagnosis, resuscitation status, and basic orders.
- As providers complete their notes, they are forwarded to administrative personnel for coding and billing.
- As the patient has tests performed and interpreted, the results are sent to the EHR inbox of the providers for review.
- As the patient receives treatments, details are sent to administration to create the bills and for ordering replacement supplies for inventory.

The patient is admitted to the floor, and the orders are executed. Among these orders are parameters for administering certain medications as needed and instructions regarding notification of the hospitalist of important events.

- Overnight, the patient becomes hypotensive. The nurse calls the hospitalist because of the patient's sudden loss of consciousness and hypotension. The hospitalist gives a verbal order for fluids and medications to increase blood pressure.
- The hospitalist soon arrives at the bedside, assesses the patient, then places an intensive care unit admit order set, with selections tailored to this clinical scenario. The hospitalist also looks at the early morning CBC results and orders a blood transfusion. The hospitalist then electronically signs the verbal orders that he had given on the phone.

A few aspects deserve comment. First, whether an ED doctor has time to review the chart prior to evaluating the patient depends on whether the identity of the patient is known before arrival and the acuteness of the presentation: A patient who is in cardiorespiratory distress and is not known to be arriving will be evaluated emergently, with historical information reviewed later. It is hoped there will be a computer in the room so that the data can be reviewed in the presence of the patient.

When the patient was in acute distress, the hospitalist did not take the time to go to a computer but rather gave verbal orders, which would be executed as fast as the nurse and pharmacist could do them. We strive for efficient use of the EHR by providers, but we do not slow down management when verbal orders can be faster in times of emergency.

OVERVIEW OF CLINICAL INFORMATICS

The remainder of this book presents our visions of where applied clinical informatics is and should be in the healthcare system. We discuss the framework of healthcare information systems from hardware to applications and to policies and regulations.

We discuss how the infrastructure and tools are used to foster better healthcare and reduced costs, thereby improving value.

There have been many criticisms of modern clinical informatics in that the EHRs have not resulted in the improved outcomes and reduced costs anticipated. We believe we are transitioning to the next stage of informatics, which has the potential to produce these results. But, this potential will only be realized with appropriate and focused work.

KEY POINTS

- We are migrating from the EMR to the EHR with a goal of the PHR.
- Electronic methods are a crucial tool but not a replacement for personal interaction between providers and between the patient and providers.
- The functionality of EHRs is expanding rapidly as demands for better outcomes and better value insist on advancements of our technology.
- The role of the clinical informatics professional is to leverage the people and processes as well as the technology to provide the best possible care.

Part II

The Framework

Data, Information, and Knowledge

KARL E. MISULIS AND MARK E. FRISSE ■

OVERVIEW

Data, information, and *knowledge* (DIKW) are fundamental concepts that have been described in a variety of ways. Among the most common is the DIKW pyramid. We prefer a nonpyramidal diagram, adding wisdom and understanding at the top because these are not ensured steps and are not always acquired either sequentially or simultaneously. The reason for abandoning the pyramid structure is because the amount or importance of the level does not necessarily narrow at successively higher levels.

The lowest three layers of our diagram are most relevant to healthcare informatics (Figure 3.1). While the exact structure can be debated, the layered concept is valuable.

- *Data* are values, and a datum is one of these. A creatinine of 3.71 mg/dL is a datum.
- *Information* is data combined to allow for meaningful interpretation. A creatinine of 3.7 mg/dL in a patient with previously normal renal function is cause for urgent action, whereas the same data in a patient with known renal failure on dialysis would be expected. Context of data is important.
- *Knowledge* is a bit more difficult to define. In the context of healthcare, knowledge is a structured compilation of information that can be used

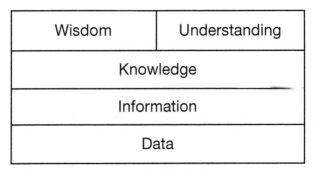

Figure 3.1 Knowledge layers. Elements of the knowledge framework, starting from the bottom with Data and being combined in context to produce Information. When this is used to create guidelines, Knowledge is created. Wisdom and Understanding are more difficult to define and represent higher levels dependent on judgment and comprehension.

    to guide decision-making. International guidelines (Kidney Disease Improving Global Outcomes [KDIGO][1]) for management of renal disease are knowledge.

- *Wisdom* is difficult to define, but most agree that judgment is a key part of this layer. Computers are not able to have wisdom presently. We do not understand the algorithms our brains use to be wise, and we are unable to program our computers to be so.
- *Understanding* is sometimes interjected as a layer between knowledge and wisdom, but we have it parallel. Developing understanding of any complex clinical situation does not lead to development of good judgment and wisdom regarding the issue. Similarly, it is possible to use good judgment and make wise decisions without completely understanding the conceptual framework.

For the remainder of this chapter and the remainder of this book, we focus on data, information, and knowledge and leave understanding and wisdom to others to debate.

DATA

Among the types of data stored and used in healthcare, the most common are numeric, string, and Boolean.

    Numeric data are measurable by a number in one form or another. The number can be an integer, floating point, or fixed point. An integer has no decimal point; it is a whole number. The floating point and fixed point numbers have digits to the right of the decimal point, with either an indeterminate or fixed number of digits, respectively. However, many fixed-point numbers are really represented in the databases as floating points but with a fixed-point display. We are generally interested in three significant digits. I may be interested in knowing that the creatinine was 3.71, but providing me with a number of 3.7147234 does not change my clinical decision-making.

Strings are composed of characters, termed *alphanumeric*, meaning that both alphabetic and numeric components can comprise the string. Text data are represented as strings.

Boolean data are true or false and can be represented by the elemental bits of 1 or 0, where 1 would represent true and 0 would represent false. If the question is asked whether a particular patient is currently an inpatient, the status is either *yes* or *no*; there is no middle ground. Not all apparent binary data are actually binary, however. Gender can be male or female, but it also can be unknown, unspecified, patient refuses to answer, or transgender. A Boolean data point cannot encode this.

Arrays are used to represent complex data. Arrays are series of data elements, usually numeric, where the positions of the data in the array have meaning. For example, images are stored as numeric arrays where the numbers can represent color and intensity for each pixel. The computer keeps track of where on the screen the pixel color for each datum belongs.

Data representation and storage are discussed in depth in Chapter 7. Our databases store all of these types in an organized format, which becomes extremely complex.

Healthcare Data

Healthcare data are of multiple types. Some of these are as follows:

- Provider documentation
- Nursing documentation
- Hospital ancillary staff records (e.g., for physical therapy [PT], occupational therapy [OT], case management)
- Laboratory and pathology data
- Radiology images and reports
- Business information

The applications handling these data include the

- EHR
- Laboratory information system (LIS)
- Radiology information system (RIS)
- Picture archiving and communication system (PACS)
- Business/financial information system

The applications can be part of the same application suite or independent. Suites of programs typically have data connections as part of the suite architecture. Independent programs must be interfaced.

Data Problems

Data can be corrupted in a variety of ways. Some of the issues are as follows:

- Error in data entry
- Misunderstanding the patient
- Incorrect information from the patient
- Data entered in the wrong field
- Delay in data entry
- Inaccurate data association

An error in data entry can be from simple mistyping. If the data are string, surrounding characters can resolve the error. "Never soked" is likely to be interpreted as "Never smoked." However, if the year field in a date-of-birth entry is in error, "2016" rather than "2006" can have implications in decision support for antibiotic selection, dose recommendations, and even patient matching for a health information exchange.

Misunderstanding the patient is common. Considering the amount of data a medical assistant, nurse, or provider acquires from the patient in an encounter, errors in understanding are expected.

Incorrect information from the patient is common and can be unintentional (e.g., misspeaking) or intentional, to hide sensitive or embarrassing information or sometimes to protect personal details the patient does not wish to share.[2]

Entering data in the wrong field is common at every level of the encounter because forms are so commonly used. Fields are designed to recognize some data entry errors, but this does not identify all errors. For example, a patient's weight of 206 entered into the field for birth year would easily be flagged for the user as an error because it is out of bounds.

Delay in data entry is a crucial and usually avoidable cause of error with great patient safety implications. Some providers delay documentation until hours or perhaps even days after an encounter. A busy clinician is incapable of recalling the same level of detail after a significant time interval, and confusing data from different patients becomes a more significant issue. Enterprise regulations or incentives should promote documentation and orders to be completed in a timely fashion; merely encouraging timeliness is usually not successful.

Inaccurate data association is linking of data incorrectly. For example, two patients with nearly identical names and addresses may be assumed by an information exchange to be a single individual, so that the healthcare and financial data are blended. The converse is more common, where a patient has multiple records in the same information system because of variations in how they registered through shifting personal preferences or change in name due to marital status.

INFORMATION

Data are made useful by context. What we typically consider *data* in clinical practice are really *information*. We consider a laboratory value in the context of the normals for age and comorbid conditions. We consider a laboratory value as part of a trend for that particular patient. A digital image is *information* by definition: The pixels are data, but the displayed image and interpretation are information. Information is data presented in a useful form.

Information is created by association of data with norms or expected values. A computed tomographic scan of a 90-year-old patient may be normal for age, but the same appearance in a 40-year-old would be interpreted as premature atrophy.

Information is inaccurate if the data are incorrect for any reason, whether artifactual, wrong data entry, or incomplete. Incorrect information is often propagated, so when a datum is corrected, that fix may not correct the downstream copied datum and may not reach the decision-maker to alter the clinical plan.

KNOWLEDGE

Knowledge is organization of the data and information in way that can be helpful for future decision-making. The decisions we make on the basis of information are guided by our knowledge, whether acquired in school, continuing education, reading, or personal clinical experience. Among the knowledge sources are

- Basic clinical training
- Continuing education from speakers, publications, and colleagues
- Published guidelines for specific presentations or disorders
- Personal clinical experience
- Embedded knowledge base in our workflow

Knowledge Management

Knowledge management is a large academic field, with real-world implications. Ideally, the best knowledge sources would consider all of the data sources mentioned plus local data, such as a local antibiogram.

We recommend that knowledge management in the healthcare arena consist of the following components:

- Online knowledge resources (e.g., UpToDate)
- Context-sensitive information on demand (e.g., drug or laboratory details on hover or click of an orderable)
- Order sets for specific diagnoses designed to adhere to best practices and evidence-based medicine (EBM) principles
- Templated notes to guide complete evaluation and documentation, adhering to best practices and regulatory requirements
- Analytics to determine site-specific factors in management
- Analytics to determine the practice and educational needs for providers and staff

An embedded knowledge base is a principal focus of this book.

Online knowledge resources are commonly subscription services or links to a hospital's online library. The days of physically going to a library have ended. For medical care, we generally favor availability of both book (physical or e-book) and Internet-based access (e.g., PubMed, UpToDate). Many providers have preferred texts that they consult for specific cases. The Internet-based reference material is generally easier to search, partly because the search engine is more robust than a book index and because of more extensive tagging of information with online data. Also, the online reference material is more likely to be updated than that in books, especially the print versions.

Knowledge management has multiple potential pitfalls. Errant and obsolete data are the most common issues. Guidelines change, and for a busy clinician, it is hard to keep track of the new changes. New indications for medications and procedures may be found. This new knowledge ultimately triggers changes to protocols and order sets, and these changes have to be made with appropriate speed as well as caution. During build and review of our order sets, there will undoubtedly be errors, and with each update and review, we repair many, but we are unlikely to be totally free from inaccuracies. We make every decision on the basis of the best and most accurate information we have at the time. In knowledge management, we need to keep up.

KEY POINTS

- Data are values, and a datum is one of these.
- Information is data in combination and context for meaningful interpretation.
- Knowledge is a structured compilation of information that can be used to guide decision-making.
- Data types are multiple, but most include numeric, string, or Boolean data.
- Errors in data entry are common, and our systems must be able to deal with missing and conflicting data and perform reconciliation of errant data.
- Knowledge management is a principal task of the applied clinical informatics professional.

People

MARK E. FRISSE AND KARL E. MISULIS ■

OVERVIEW

The patient is the central focus of health care. The range of individuals employing clinical systems to support the care of patients is vast. Effective clinical support requires sophisticated care coordination and technology skills. Introduction of poorly-designed systems and processes has consequences. Inefficiencies cost money. Errors cost lives.

In this chapter, we review the involvement of a spectrum of people in clinical informatics, with a focus on some of the pivotal roles in healthcare systems.

PATIENTS AND FAMILIES

Family members and other caregivers are reliant on informatics because they are central to care coordination and patient support. The individuals playing supporting roles vary significantly in their capabilities, health literacy skills, formal training, finances, and ability to manage social resources. They need assistance. Each caregiver bears a personal burden of medical and social issues. For example, a deteriorating elderly patient may in turn be cared for by an elderly spouse who is also deteriorating. These behavioral capabilities are often far more important than technology. Often on-site visits or virtual visits through a range of technologies can ease the burden. Similarly, investing in a technology to document medication adherence is not sufficient unless documentation can lead to behaviors leading to better adherence. Information alone will not magically make people act more effectively to address problems they already know they face.

Challenges faced by patients and families that pertain to informatics include

- lack of a clear plan shared by all parties involved in care;
- variance in how providers are contacted;
- lack of communication between providers; and
- difficulty accessing clinical reports, and when accessed, the med-speak descriptions are difficult to understand and sometimes easy to misunderstand.

Providers and healthcare systems do not "connect" effectively. Often they rely on different technical platforms, have varying degrees of technical maturity, and different workflows. For example, one provider may offer a patient portal, but not use the portal effectively for communication, relying instead on the telephone. Another provider may rely on primarily portal messages and not receive updates via telephones. Each provider may have a different approach. To receive the care they need, patients and their families are forced to adapt to inconsistent communication methods.

Patients generally believe providers communicate with one another far more than what really takes place. Patients may arrive for a clinic appointment after a prolonged hospitalization only to discover that his or her trusted provider was not aware of the hospitalization. Even if discharge summary is present in the electronic health record (EHR), the trusted provider may not be aware of it and hence is unprepared for the post-discharge visit. Clinical informatics professionals cannot ensure that all busy providers "close the loop," but they can and should seek to improve notification and communication. Improvements may be as simple as having an up-to-date directory of phone numbers electronically distributed to providers. It may be having secure messaging for all providers in a healthcare system (whether employed or not) and ensure that inbound messages reach the attention of designated providers. The quality of communication must be adequate for clinical care. It often is not.

Patients must understand what portal communications mean. Healthcare systems often include laboratory and radiology reports in their portals. The implications of these numbers must be clear. For example, serum sodium levels of 134 mEq/dL and 135 mEq/dL are not significantly different, but portal user will observe that one value is "abnormal" and the other is not. Similarly, inconsequential abnormalities on a magnetic resonance imaging (MRI) report may create anxiety. Providers must address potential anxiety through simple notes. The patient seeing a report with inconsequential results will be relieved to have the personal note: "You have some small abnormalities on your studies that do not indicate any serious disease. We will discuss further when we meet again, but if you want to chat with us earlier, message us back."

CLINICAL STAFF

Clinicians, staff, and teams performing direct care in hospitals and clinics and at home are formal care providers equally affected by the quality of clinical informatics work. The ability of clinical systems to provide timely information and decision support within effective workflows impacts quality and cost of care.

Besides direct patient providers, there are others in the healthcare system with immediate or long-term dependence on informatics. Clinical actions drive logistics tasks, including patient scheduling, supply procurement, medication management, medical billing, quality reporting, patient/family communication, and care coordination. The quality and efficiency with which these tasks are enabled by data, process, and technology have a significant long-term impact.

Among the pain points for providers pertaining to clinical informatics, some of principal concern are

- Time required to create documents
- Burden of transmitting documents to appropriate individuals
- Medicine reconciliation
- Decision support alert fatigue
- Diagnosis and problem management

The amount of time needed to create clinical documents has increased. Part of this is that entering data in the EHR is not as fast as dictation, but a significant component is new requirements for documentation. We need to make providers as efficient as possible, and streamlining document creation is a priority.

Now that we have these shiny new technical tools and providers can do a lot of the clerical work themselves, we ask them to do so. One of us spent 12 minutes ordering an MRI and doing all of the computer work required to schedule an appointment with a specific surgeon. This is not a good use of our time. We need to have users work at the height of their licenses and capabilities.

Medicine reconciliation is the process of comparing medicine lists, usually at an office visit or a transition of care, such as a discharge or a move to a long-term care facility. This is time intensive and often cumbersome, and we need to improve this process.

Decision support is discussed at length in Chapter 17 and is a process of using stored information and algorithms to remind providers of gaps in care or potential errors. These algorithms are imperfect and may aggravate the user to the point that they ignore important notifications.

Diagnosis and problem lists need to be updated and reconciled, just as medication lists are. This is time consuming and sometimes clumsy. Some patients will end up with a lengthy list of redundant and sometimes errant entries, and with so much information to review, the next user may review none of it. We must help the users with maintenance of these lists.

THE INFORMATICS TEAM

We often refer to an "informatics team" and their work. Who, exactly, is on this team and who leads the team? In this chapter, we describe team members of pivotal importance. We describe leadership further in Chapter 12.

Chief Medical Informatics Officer

The chief medical informatics officer (CMIO; an alternative is chief medical *information* officer) usually has an MD, DO, MBBS, or equivalent degree. Some highly effective CMIOs carry other clinical credentials. Most are trained and experienced clinicians, but many have surrendered some or all direct clinical responsibilities to focus on their informatics. Many CMIOs in academic medical centers also have a doctoral (PhD) degree in informatics. In non-academic settings, many CMIOs have a master's degree in informatics, but some have less formal informatics training. Many CMIOs also have an MBA degree or managerial experience.

Most enterprises of any size have a CMIO with one or more associate CMIOs with fewer formal credentials. Many are generalists, but specialists in surgery, cardiology, or other clinical areas are often found in larger organizations. Many associate CMIOs advance to CMIO positions.

Nothing is more satisfying to clinicians than to know that their CMIO performs clinical work in their own system. Clinicians become alienated by leaders who emphasize promises, present informatics only through demos, and do not actually "eat what they cook." At the same time, CMIOs—especially those in primary care—cannot be effective if their informatics work is continually interrupted by care responsibilities. We recommend that CMIOs pursue balanced clinical activities for a host of reasons, including:

- Ongoing direct interaction with patients, families, and other caregivers.
- Strengthened credibility with other clinicians.
- Hands-on regular experience using the organization's clinical systems

Whether one remains clinically active or not, CMIOs must retain and develop their clinical mindset as they oversee their wide range of responsibilities that include:

- Working with senior enterprise leaders on issues facing information systems and providers involving informatics and enterprise strategy.
- Maintaining effective knowledge management by ensuring order sets incorporate best practice guidelines.
- Providing leadership for decision support efforts for providers.
- Coordinating provider education programs.
- Working closely with nursing, pharmacy, medical specialties and other groups ensure that needs are being met.

- Collaborating closely with the chief information officer (CIO) and other information systems leadership to coordinate enhancements, updates, upgrades, new clinical systems' needs, and information systems strategy.
- Participating in and directing analytics efforts in both clinical and financial domains.

Chief Nursing Informatics Officer

The chief nursing informatics officer (CNIO) may also be called a chief nursing *information* officer. In hospitals, nurses spend more time on direct patient care than physicians. Often, an overemphasis on physician needs comes at the expense of nursing support that can have tremendous impact on care efficiency, care quality, and clinical morale. The CNIO works closely with the chief nursing officer, CMIO, and other leadership as needed to ensure the most efficient and error-free nursing practice, issue identification, and coordination with providers.

The CNIO typically has a nursing degree and additional education leading to a master's degree or other significant training in informatics or management.

Nurse Informaticists

Healthcare systems have nurse informaticists who are responsible for a wide range of tasks, from assistance with design decisions and rollout to education and optimization. Backgrounds are varied, with some having BSN, master's, or even DNP degrees and others having associate degrees as registered nurses (RNs). Most of these individuals learned informatics on the job.

Specialty Informaticists

Large facilities usually have select specialty informaticists. These informaticists can include those practicing in pharmacy, radiology, emergency services, operating room/anesthesia, cardiology, ambulatory clinic, and other specialty operations. Individual healthcare systems will differ in needs in this regard. These informaticians are usually practitioners or administrators in these areas who are familiar with their needs, workflows, and challenges.

ROLE OF THE INFORMATICS TEAM

When seeking solutions, clinical informatics professionals must consider the needs of each of the stakeholder groups and understand how informatics decisions can affect both immediate care and long-term administrative, public health, policy, and research needs. Needs and priorities among these efforts will not always align. Teams working on these projects must respect one another as equals; simply giving orders will not work. Balance requires effective communication, cooperation, and collaboration. The importance of team-building, management, and communication skills cannot be overemphasized.

KEY POINTS

- Individuals may differ in their needs, their values, their ability to understand and communicate, and their incentives to change their behavior.
- Groups of individuals, working together as members of formal or informal teams united by a common purpose, differ in their ability to communicate, coordinate, and effect desired change.
- Organizations have different roles that may include service delivery, administration and payment, regulation, public health, research, advocacy, and governance. Their needs differ, and often benefits accrued to one organization may come at the expense of another organization; incentives among organizations are not aligned.
- Few individuals or organizations have the time and resources to address and reconcile all needs. These struggles are often played out in clinical settings and come at the expense of clinicians providing care.

Policies, Laws, Regulations, Contracts, and Procedures

MARK E. FRISSE AND KARL E. MISULIS ■

OVERVIEW

The adoption and use of clinical systems are driven and constrained by laws, regulations, contracts, and operational procedures. Often, the creation of institutional procedures is influenced by differences in how leaders within an institution interpret the laws, policies, and contracts governing healthcare delivery.

POLICIES

Policies are explicit combinations of decisions, plans, and expected actions. Policies are created to realize specific economic or healthcare goals. According to the World Health Organization, an explicit health policy can achieve several goals:

- Define a vision for the future that helps to establish targets and points of reference for the short and medium terms
- Outline priorities and the expected roles of different groups
- Build consensus and inform people[1]

Because of the breadth of society's health issues; the diversity of personal, religious, philosophical, or societal goals; and the conflicts that arise among concerned stakeholders, policies or their execution through procedures are almost always controversial.

Policies are positions, statements, and courses of action that reflect an organization's goals and values.[2] Policies are the products of government, business, or other authorities. Policies can be expressed as high-level aims or with granular specificity. When simply expressed through position papers or other media, they seek to develop a consensus for action. When expressed through legislation and regulations, they lead to mandates. Policies describe what must be done. Policies are not laws but often are the byproduct of legislation or regulatory action. At both the state and federal levels, laws provide directives to government agencies, which in turn, often through a process called rule-making, create policies that articulate detailed and specific actions a healthcare organization must take to comply with the law or directive.

LAWS

Laws impacting clinical informatics are created at all levels of government. Most of the most important laws are products of federal legislation, but states have a consti-tutional right to create laws that complement or modify federal legislation. States play significant roles in privacy, public health, and the financing of federal programs like Medicare.

At the federal level, some of the most important legislation includes the following:

- **HIPAA.** The Health Insurance Portability and Accountability Act of 1996 (HIPAA)[3] has become the legislative basis for healthcare transaction code sets, privacy rules, security rules, and a national provider identifier system. Some of these rules have been modified in other legislation, but HIPAA is the foundational element.
- **HITECH.** The Health Information Technology for Economic and Clinical Health (HITECH)[4] Act of 2009 established a number of offices and processes to enhance the adoption and effective use of electronic health records. HITECH was enacted as part of the American Recovery and Reinvestment Act of 2009. It was not part of later healthcare reform acts. As part of broad economic stimulus legislation, HITECH was required to move quickly and, critics say, led to the imposition of the current generation of electronic health record (EHR) implementations without adequate understanding of healthcare workflow and future needs.
- **Stark Law.** The Stark law is actually a number of separate legislative elements established in the early 1990s.[5] Their goal was to prohibit physician self-referrals and kickbacks: referring patients for specific tests to facilities in which the physician received additional financial compensation. As collaboration requirements necessitated shared health information systems and data, hospitals sought to expand clinical technologies to referring physicians, which could have been construed as

a violation of Stark laws. These concerns were alleviated when most uses were granted *safe harbor*[6] status from regulatory agencies.

- **Antitrust**. Section 1 of the Sherman Act[7] prohibits actions that unreasonably restrain competition. This issue is raised when provider groups or health plans merge or when collusion on pricing is alleged. Antitrust concerns are often raised when price information is shared in the course of broader clinical data-sharing initiatives. Antitrust is also raised when dominant providers or payers create contracts that exclusively prohibit physicians from referring patients to out-of-network specialists.

- **FDASIA**. The Food and Drug Administration Safety and Innovation Act[8] (FDASIA) Act of 2012 expanded the Food and Drug Administration's (FDA's) authority to regulate medical devices and software. In collaboration with the Federal Communications Commission (FCC) and FDA, advisory panels recommended a risk-based framework for regulating software. EHRs, decision support, mobile devices, and health information exchange may all be subject to some regulation. Established EHRs and other clinical systems are considered relatively low risk and have largely avoided FDASIA scrutiny.[9]

- **ACA**. The Patient Protection and Affordable Care Act[10] (ACA) of 2010 was created to correct inadequacies in healthcare delivery and payment. Although most attention is given to Medicaid expansions, it included removal of preexisting illness coverage exclusions and initiated incentives or penalties to require every adult to have healthcare coverage with certain minimal criteria. The ACA also had mechanisms to study the cost-benefit value of various treatments and to establish a Patient-Centered Outcomes Research Institute (PCORI). PCORI's Patient-Centered Clinical Research Network (PCORNet) is a shared data network of healthcare institutions supporting comparative effectiveness research using routine healthcare translated to meet a PCORNet common data model. Electoral changes and judicial decisions since the Act's passage have eliminated mandatory coverage and weakened other key provisions, but public sentiment, changing demographics, and financial constraints suggest that many of technology and payment approaches stimulated by the Act will continue. In particular, care management across a continuum of care, greater exchange of healthcare information among providers and patients, and value-based reimbursement will remain a primary focus for new clinical informatics initiatives.

- **21st Century Cures Act**.[11] This bipartisan 2016 law builds on prior legislation and requires federal agencies to promote greater patient and provider access to biomedical data for care and for research. It has fostered significant new data interoperability efforts and standardized application program interfaces (APIs) to EHRs. This more open and accessible data infrastructure in turn necessitated new regulations granting additional safe harbor status for many clinical initiatives.

REGULATIONS

Laws at the federal or state level mandate one or more executive agencies to act on the laws by specific times. Laws often issue directives at relatively high levels and require agencies to translate legislative intent into actionable conduct. In response to legislation, agencies must engage in what is called the *rule-making process*. When tasked by Congress, agencies are required to issue one or more *notices of proposed rule-making* (NPRM) to inform the public of the proposed rules before they take effect. The public rule-making record must include the data and analyses supporting the proposed rule.

The public can then comment on the proposed rules and provide additional data. The issuing agency must respond to public comments. In some instances, agencies may publish a second draft proposed rule for an additional cycle of commentary. Ultimately, the agency publishes a final rule that establishes policy; these are the regulations. These rules often are modified over time through the same rule-making process.

CONTRACTS

Contracts are required if organizations work together to accomplish a policy goal. Contracts designate the responsibilities of participating parties and set metrics and penalties if obligations are not met. Most contracts have significant financial implications. Often, failing to read the fine print or not communicating with others under similar contractual relationships can be very costly. Medicare Advantage Plan contracts, for example, define relationships among providers and payers; these contracts often define what quality metrics must be collected and how quality metrics will influence payment.

Information technology vendor contracts define obligations and penalties associated with installation and operation. These contracts are complex and usually involve many different parties.

HIPAA's business associate agreement (BAA) establishes a relationship between a provider, health plan, or claims clearinghouse (*covered entities*) and any vendor that works with a covered entity. BAAs both state what the business associate can do with personal health information and obligate the business associate to comply with all other relevant HIPAA requirements. This is discussed further in Chapter 18.

PROCEDURES

Procedures form a bridge between both policy and contractual requirements and specific actions at the organizational level. At the local level, procedures define the series of actions and actors necessary to ensure the requirements of a policy or contract are met. Some procedures become routinely embedded into care processes (e.g., medication administration, patient registration, granting access rights to personal health information). Other procedures more resemble *fire drills* in that they are only invoked in extraordinary circumstances (e.g., adverse event reporting, mass casualty management, data breaches). These must be kept available and periodically reviewed and rehearsed so that every individual in the organization is aware of their role.

Effective local procedures derived from clear local policies can mean the difference between success and failure. The introduction of EHRs required organizations to formalize procedure statements that described exactly how an organization would incorporate EHRs into clinical workflow and how it would ensure that data were managed effectively. Where HITECH was concerned, the *why* of the legislation and the *what* of the policies were uniform. The success or failure of an EHR implementation was due largely to the extent to which they clearly conceived and executed procedures. Success was about the *how*.

The difference between successful and failed implementations can be explained by how organizations chose their technologies, developed their teams, and redesigned their workflows. The right procedures, when combined with effective execution and ongoing oversight, had significant financial consequences to healthcare delivery organizations. As is the case in every policy, successful outcomes require organizational procedures that are clear, actionable, and managed.

Many procedures arise from policies that do not originate from government but instead come through contractual relationships between and among healthcare providers, plans, regulatory agencies, and other groups. These contracts may restrict or expand coverage and services, may specify mandatory quality metric reports, and may employ different rules for care reimbursement. This may include how a health plan will reimburse clinical work or how delivery organizations must collect and report data on the quality of care. Medicare Advantage programs are an example; these are private health plans approved by the Centers for Medicare and Medicaid Services (CMS) that charge additional premiums but offer additional services, such as vision, hearing, dental, and wellness programs. Most plans also have prescription drug coverage (Medicare Part D). Over a third of Medicare beneficiaries are enrolled in Medicare Advantage plans.[12]

Medicare Advantage plans and other payer contracts invoke procedures that often alter network referral patterns, therapy options, prior authorization practices, and quality reporting requirements. These plans are growing in popularity and may be a model for more aggressive Medicare changes in the future. Coding requirements may also differ from traditional Medicare. Health plans offering Medicare Advantage are revising their client-facing and administrative process to create comprehensive plan-branded consumer engagement platforms that simplify enrollment, increase customer services support, and support clinical care management. From the provider perspective, Medicare Advantage contracts primarily accelerate emerging trends: tighter integration with health plan systems, clinical and administrative decision support addressing both medical and financial issues, and more patient-oriented care management supporting teams working both in institutions and in the home. Provider service administrators must also rely on various analytics methods to understand risk under capitation models. For example, the CMS Hierarchical Condition Categories[13] (CMS-HCC) model is used to adjust capitation payments to Medicare Advantage plans.

CONSEQUENCES OF POLICIES, LAWS,
AND CONTRACTS

Policies, laws, and contracts have many consequences on clinical practice. Minimizing complexity and mitigating administrative time require a thoughtful review of clinical workflows and of the design and use of clinical information systems.

Several issues are particularly relevant to clinical informatics:

Cost. Even in an ideal world, great costs are incurred in creating or interpreting policies, on disseminating policies, on creating subsequent procedures that aid in uniform policy compliance, on measuring policy compliance, and on enforcing compliance. At the federal level, HIPAA and subsequent health information exchange policies often are associated with *regulatory impact statements* created when the policy is put in place. For example, agencies must assess "all costs and benefits of available regulatory alternatives" if a law is expected to impact the economy by over $100 million a year. Unfortunately, these statements are often gross simplifications and tend to underestimate the enormous burdens placed on healthcare professionals and organizations. In the original HIPAA regulatory impact statement,[14] Health and Human Services (HHS) stated that a regulatory impact statement was not necessary because the "aggregate economic impact of this final rule is minimal and will have no effect of the economy," and that the law would not have a "significant impact on a substantial number of small entities."[15] But, the true costs are much higher because of the enormous efforts every hospital had to make to understand the regulation, change workflows, train their personnel, and enforce compliance to avoid costly penalties. More realistic estimates suggested that costs to hospitals alone would range from $670,000 to $3.7 million per hospital. HITECH and subsequent expansions of health information exchange requirements also suggested rosy outcomes that have never been realized. When combining direct institutional costs with the productivity impact of these regulations, the costs are much higher and represent a major administrative challenge to this very day.

Policy Variation. Many health plans have different metrics and policies for reporting clinical activity and quality metrics. These wide variations have enormous consequences on clinical information systems vendors and on providers. System designers must model each complex requirement and providers must spend inordinate amounts of time addressing these requirements in the course of care. For example, providers are confronted with a dizzying array of formularies, each with minor differences in covered drugs and patient payments. Collectively these changes place enormous cognitive as well as financial burdens on patients and clinicians.

Policy Requirement Growth and Complexity. Quality metrics exemplify how regulations and contractual requirements are increasing in number and complexity. When combined with other administrative tasks, these requirements place additional burdens on clinicians and threaten to smother their clinical patient care. In turn, this shift from clinical to administrative work contributes to growing provider dissatisfaction. Vendors have other concerns. Faced with widespread provider backlash, regulatory groups often give the provider a choice of metrics to collect and report. A provider may be required only to address any one of three items: A or B or C. But, the vendor must design its systems for all of the three items: A and B and C. These complexities drive up costs to vendors and, arguably, impede vendor abilities to create EHR environments more conducive to clinical practice and knowledge management.

Rationale. Controversy arises over the extent that cumbersome reporting metrics actually measure care quality. Legitimate arguments can be made about the efficacy of quality metrics with respect to both their sheer number and large variation. A broader national discussion on the validity of metrics would be beneficial. Much is spoken about *evidence-based medicine*. Where is the dialogue about *evidence-based administration*? Along the same lines, in complex areas such as risk-adjustment metrics, it is possible that discrepancies between the provider calculations and payer calculations are the result of payer error, not provider error. Where analytics and implementation of complex algorithms are concerned, no organization is infallible.

Certification. Certification is the process of ensuring that an individual, process, technology, or professional service can do the job it was designed to do. The HITECH Act is an example of a law that created numerous and highly complex certification policies.[16] Its overall goal was to create a nationwide, standardized healthcare technology infrastructure to ensure safer and more effective care in a manner aligned with the spirit of the broader economic stimulus legislation. This is the *why* of HITECH. The authors of HITECH specified in great detail the *what* through a number of specific measures. For example, HITECH authorized the secretary of HHS to create a set of data standards that would ensure effective deployment and interoperable use of EHRs in most American hospitals and ambulatory care settings. The policies were created by the Office of the National Coordinator for Health Information Technology (ONC) and, true to the legislative intent, came with both financial incentives and, later, possible financial penalties. These policies expressed in detail what measures had to be taken by healthcare organizations to receive incentives and avoid penalties. Overall, the legislative ambition was to see that EHR technologies were used in meaningful ways. This intent was converted via policies into three stages of *Meaningful Use*. Initial phases required only that an institution seeking financial incentives demonstrated the capability of performing a number of specific tasks, including selected clinical decision support and transmission of prescriptions and other reports in digital format.

WHAT CLINICAL INFORMATICS PROFESSIONALS SHOULD DO

Clinical informatics professionals must be aware and informed of the process of creating legislation, deriving policies, and execution through procedures. Understanding the context helps a clinical informatics professional explain the rationale behind a procedure when practiced at the local level. Individuals are often less motivated to conform to procedures if they do not understand the context and consequences.

Often, professional groups, technology firms, and others strive to simplify procedures before they are formalized. This occurs typically with notification through an *NPRM*, as discussed previously in this chapter.[17] Each party has a separate agenda in seeking to modify policies. Although some agents seek obfuscation and self-interest, most agents seek to create simpler policies that are easier to implement and reinforce. Despite the complexity and confusion, the public is at least theoretically aware of new policies as they emerge.

One's influence is greatest when focusing on organization policies and procedures. Informatics professionals play a critical role on the ground. At the institutional level, the process is often far more complex for many reasons:

- **First**, policies often originate from relatively isolated management groups, and the clinical informatics professional must ensure that all legitimate concerns of those affected by the policies are incorporated.
- **Second**, policy and procedure creation efforts are often inadequately governed. At times, leaders fail to establish clear project governance, convene a sequential series of meetings leading to a goal, and ultimately state explicitly responsible parties for each task. When in a large meeting, statements like "we will do this" may sometimes translate into "no one will do this."
- **Third**, institutional processes are often inefficient. Rather than establish clear project governance and convene a sequential series of meetings, organizations often wander in circles and incorporate people in meetings whose interest and trust can be more efficiently gained through individual dialogue and constant communication.
- **Fourth**, meetings can be expensive. Value is realized through the impact of policies and procedures; frequent and ineffective meetings merely add to the cost. Time spent by colleagues in meetings necessarily comes at the expense of other tasks. Often, people participate in meetings because they are concerned they will not be informed of the process otherwise; this is a failure of leadership and communication.
- **Fifth**, legal counsel and external consultants, while often essential, may be invoked prematurely. At times, meeting with stakeholders and clearly understanding their needs will minimize legal and consulting costs. The more stakeholders understand the intended purposes of policies and procedures, the easier it will be for leaders to lower costs by providing legal and consulting professionals with clear guidance. One common and

very expensive example concerns creation of policies and procedures around protection of personal health information. Even the experts in an organization often have different interpretations of what is required. Gaining a consensus internally then draws focus onto legal support. One cannot expect counsel to sort it out if key parties disagree. The clinical informatics professional, with an awareness of the impact on most stakeholders, must play a vital role.

KEY POINTS

- We should understand the intent of legislation and the policymaking process.
- We should understand the *why* or the context motivating a policy, contract, or procedure.
- We need to set priorities and focus on the important policies and procedures first.
- We should gain a clear understanding of stakeholder needs and concerns as early as possible so that we can understand the impact on individuals responsible for carrying out required tasks.
- We focus on solving the problem, and to do this we maximize communication but minimize the number of individuals assigned to any task or meeting.
- Within the meeting group, we seek a consensus early so that one can be assured that everyone seeks to solve the same problem.
- We strive for simplicity. Remember that positive consequences only emerge if everyone knows what to do. The simpler the message and the fewer the moving parts, the more effective will be the outcomes.
- We should develop a simple message. No matter how complex the policy or procedure is, we work with our colleagues to develop a simple pitch that can explain to everyone in the organization the *why, who, what,* and *how.*

Process

The Learning Health System

KARL E. MISULIS AND MARK E. FRISSE ■

HISTORY AND THEORY OF THE LEARNING
HEALTH SYSTEM

Scientific research has been performed for hundreds of years, but much of medical care has been guided mainly by the personal experience of the providers and their professors. This was challenged especially in the past 25 years: Study after study have refuted processes that had become accepted medical practice. Also, there has been a cultural change among many providers. We came to appreciate that each of us is not the single source of truth for best practices for our patients. Yet, even today, some clinicians cling tenaciously to their archaic methods of medical and surgical practice. This indicates a serious flaw in knowledge management. When some of us finish training, we stop learning.

The Institute of Medicine (IOM) released *To Err Is Human* in 2000; it reported that as many as 98,000 deaths in the United States can be attributed to medical errors.[1] Subsequent work has emphasized the need for development and practice of *evidence-based medicine* (EBM).

The *learning health system* (LHS) is a logical extension of EBM in the context of our advances in electronic health record (EHR) technology.[2] The LHS is an iterative approach to healthcare improvement: The data in our EHRs is combined with data from other sources and known knowledge bases to produce improvement.

The LHS tries to break the closed circuit of provider and patient interaction and connect to local and regional data sources. These data sources would be used to engage patients, providers, administration, and all knowledge holders in the improvement of care.

Connected partners in the LHS are

- Providers
- Patients
- Local EHR data, including warehoused data for analytics
- Regional and state reporting agencies
- Knowledge bases, including the National Library of Medicine (NLM), universities, medical societies, and other sources

The culture of the providers and patients must be amenable to assessing information from these connections. In some of our facilities, certain providers are not participatory in quality improvement, let alone helping to facilitate an LHS. Moving the culture may be among the most challenging aspects of development and use of the LHS.

Data elements of the LHS are voluminous; some of these are

- Patient demographic information
- Clinical history
- Clinical events
- Laboratory results
- Imaging
- Genomics
- Published knowledge base data
- Repositories of study data
- Evidence-based guidelines
- Received data from clinical practice

Charles Friedman described a cycle that consists of the following steps[3]:

- Decide to study an issue
- Assemble the relevant data
- Analyze the data
- Interpret the results
- Deliver a tailored message
- Take action to change practice
- Assess outcome
- Restart the process

This is similar to the iterative cycles discussed in business school for almost every project, and the take-home lessons are similar. We do not assume we know the reason for an event; we perform careful analysis. We design an intervention that is likely to solve the problem. We implement the intervention. We assess the outcome to ensure that the anticipated improvement is obtained, and if not, we assess potential reasons for the failure. Similarly, we watch for adverse unintended consequences of our changes.

The LHS is needed because there is more new medical information published than a clinician can be expected to digest. One of us (K.M.) is a hospital neurologist. On the NLM PubMed database, there are more than 60 new publications every day in this field. In addition, there will be many other important publications that would not be captured by a search of "hospital neurology." We rely on experts and thought leaders for development of best practice guidelines.

The LHS will take into account local data. For example, in a local affiliate system of seven hospitals, the EHR has embedded the antibiogram[4] of each hospital. When we treat a specific infection, antibiotic selection is guided by the antibiogram for that hospital.

LEARNING HEALTH SYSTEM DESIGN

The LHS is not an application that can be purchased from a vendor. It is a collaborative project engaging a broad range of participants in the healthcare system in the setting of a technical infrastructure that can support the design and operation of the learning objectives. At a minimum, the system needs

- business and clinical leaders who enable the system through adequate financial and personnel resources;
- providers who participate in the development, design, analysis, action, and follow-through on interventions;
- mature EHRs with the ability to assemble and process the key internal and external information required for the design;
- interface and interoperability with other systems from which information is needed and to which information must go;
- a knowledge base for establishment of best practices and for creation of expectations for improvement; and
- analytic power to identify relationships between data and events.

The LHS begins with engagement from clinical and administrative leadership, with information systems leadership being part of both of these silos.

The following steps are included in design and implementation:

- Identify problems and their implications.
- Prioritize problems.
- Establish goals.
- Establish governance structure.
- Design the evaluation.
- Analyze the results of the evaluation.
- Design an intervention.
- Implement the intervention.
- Collect data and analyze results of the intervention.

- Close the loop—assess whether the problem has been solved or progress has been made and whether additional study is needed.

Business transformation is described as the triangle of *people, process,* and *technology.* In the LHS, a modification is the addition of *data.* People, data, process, and technology are engaged to produce system improvement.

APPLICATION OF THE LEARNING HEALTH SYSTEM

There are numerous examples of applications of the LHS. The Comprehensive Unit-Based Safety Program (CUSP) was developed by Johns Hopkins with support of the Agency for Healthcare Research and Quality (AHRQ) to lower the incidence of healthcare-associated infections. Among these are reductions in central line–associated bloodstream infections (CLABSIs) and catheter-associated urinary tract infections (CAUTIs). This was accomplished by a combination of informatics interventions, education, and policy and procedure changes. In addition, there are projects under way in CUSP to promote best practices in surgical care to reduce surgical site infections, and there are initiatives in antibiotic stewardship that it is hoped will reduce cost of care, reduce antibiotic resistance, and improve outcomes. The structure of this program can be applied to other healthcare-associated complications, not just infections.

Geisinger Health uses predictive modeling to identify patients at risk for readmission or patients who are likely not to come for appointments. These patients are targeted for intervention at hopefully a lower cost than the ultimate costs of a delay in care.

FUTURE DIRECTIONS

Early LHSs were developed in academic and large progressive nonacademic enterprises for deployment in their own facilities. This has evolved to learning healthcare projects that can be deployed with modest local resource demands. We expect this will continue. The migration of EHRs and associated applications to greater interoperability through standards will help this development.

The learning healthcare system will continue to develop, not mandated by regulatory agencies but rather because of pressures to remain competitive in the healthcare marketplace by improving outcomes and reducing costs.

KEY POINTS

- The LHS is part of the expected evolution of our EHR and clinical medicine knowledge base.

- The LHS is not an application that is purchased, but a collaborative project involving business and clinical leaders.
- There have been examples of effective quality improvements with LHS initiatives, but we have only scratched the surface of possibilities.
- Leveraging the power of the LHS will be crucial to obtaining the improved outcomes and reduced costs of healthcare, thereby improving the value that we expect.

Part III

The Foundation

Representation and Organization of Health Information

KARL E. MISULIS AND MARK E. FRISSE ■

DATA TYPES

Data in the healthcare operating system (HOS) are classified as *structured* or *unstructured*. *Structured data* refer to data that fits into a defined data structure and often has a value. The value can be numeric, Boolean, or character. A *numeric* variable example would be number of children or potassium level. A *Boolean* variable example would be either the person is married or not, or deceased or not; there are no other values. A *character* value would usually be a single character that has some special significance, such as M for male, F for female, or U for unknown; there are no other possibilities under this simplified classification scheme that might otherwise include gender identity options. Numerical variables can be integer or floating point. Number of children is an integer, and 2.3 is not a valid entry. On the other hand, a potassium value of 3.5893485 is a floating point value, although on the display the result would usually be rounded to 3.59.

Unstructured data do not have the organization of structured data. The best example of unstructured data is the *history of present illness* (HPI) in a patient's medical record. This is usually a series of sentences that tell the story of the patient's presentation. In this case, the data are in string variables, which are chains of characters. Generally, a *history and physical* (H&P) document contains the HPI as well as other sections, including those for *past medical history, family history, social history, review of systems*, and *physical examination*, and is concluded by an *assessment* and *plan*. The review of systems and details of the physical examination can be unstructured or structured, in that the provider might type in a symptom or examination finding, or there may be a menu of possible responses to choose. The past medical history may be structured if the data were entered using standard *ontologies*: organizational structures of medical terms. A common one would be ICD-10 (*International Classification of Diseases, Tenth Revision*), although there are others used in our clinical records, especially IMO (the Intelligent Medical Objects company) and SNOMED CT.[1]

Structured data are relatively easy to search. A query looks for specific values of variables in the database and returns a list of unique identifiers for patients that fulfill the query requirements. For example, a search for male patients with a history of type 2 diabetes mellitus would be performed by selecting Male in the gender field and an *ICD-10* code for diabetes type 2, such as *E11*.[2]

Unstructured data are much more difficult to search. If the patient does not have an *ICD-10* code for type 2 diabetes mellitus entered, then we would have to search for "type 2 diabetes mellitus" in the entire chart. That would eliminate many patients who would otherwise meet criteria because clinicians often do not use that exact wording. Searching for "diabetes" would be problematic because it would capture patients who had type 1 diabetes and patients in whom the documentation indicated "no diabetes."

DATA SOURCES

There are innumerable potential data sources, but we discuss some of the most important data sources for healthcare. *Clinical data* include all of the locally stored, clinically relevant data. These include demographics as well as actual medical data. Clinician-generated data include H&P notes, consult notes, progress notes, discharge summaries, operative reports, among other documents. Also stored are records of orders placed. In addition, the fact that the clinician accesses the chart is recorded as well; this is part of an *audit log*. The sequence of data showing what a user did while in the chart is an *audit trail*.

Clinical data include those from laboratory systems, radiology information systems, other specialty systems such as cardiology and gastroenterology, as well as information from affiliate medical facilities and pharmacies.

If a health information exchange (HIE) is functioning, then data from that exchange may be included to a variable extent. Some exchanges only fetch data on demand and do not store it locally; others do have the capability of downloading and storing outside data. Details of handling of HIE data are important because if a clinician makes a clinical decision based on data from the exchange, a copy of the data better be retained locally so that if the exchange no longer functions or the data source ceases to share data, the clinician has a copy of the pivotal data to rely on. HIE is discussed in detail in Chapter 25.

DATA REPRESENTATION

Data representation is turning the data into a format the computer understands. This process is invisible to the user. While we have discussed various types of data, all the computer can understand is one of two states for a specific *bit*. A *bit* is a binary digit meant to represent a value, which can be 0 or 1. No other values are possible, and a blank or null value is not possible. To represent the 26 letters of the alphabet, 10 single digits (0 through 9), punctuation, and special characters, we need to use a *byte*, which is a series of usually 8 bits. Because each bit has two possible values, a byte has 2^8 or 256 different possibilities. This is still not enough to cover the range of possible data values to be represented. A *word* is an array of bits, usually greater than 8, and can encode a much larger number of possible values. In the recent past, we have seen computers described as having 32-bit or 64-bit processors. This means that this is the standard size of the bit arrays that the processor instruction set is designed to handle. A 32-bit word has 4,294,967,296 possible values. A 64-bit word has 18,446,744,073,709,600,000 possible values. Because dealing with 18 quintillion is a big challenge, let us go back to an 8-bit word.

A single word or byte might be 00001101. If this were considered as a simple binary number, the value in base 10 would be 13.[3] If this word were in a field or array where it was intended to indicate a letter of the alphabet, the 13th letter is M, but that does not indicate case; we would have to represent upper- and lowercases of the alphabet with different words. Last, the word might be an instruction, such as "following is a string array." Then, there would be another instruction to indicate when the string array ended and more instructions to indicate what variable this string is, such as history of present illness.

DATA MODELING

Data modeling is the design of the data organization that we use for the enterprise. The *conceptual* model depends on the purpose, data formats, and interrelationships of the data. This is similar for most healthcare organizations, although not identical.

Conceptual Model

The highest level modeling is *conceptual*. This is establishing the areas we want to record and the relationships between these areas. For example, our healthcare system treats multiple patients from multiple regions with multiple disorders, often in combination. Each patient has multiple encounters. Each patient sees multiple providers, and each provider sees multiple patients. The database has to focus on specific patients, specific providers, encounters for each, facilities where each encounter occurred, disorders and procedures and tests and medications for patients and disorders, and so on. Our conceptual framework will result in our ability to look at the data from the focus on a patient, a provider, an encounter, a diagnosis, etc. We have not decided exactly which data is recorded and how, but we have the concept.

The conceptual model is dynamic. We have to be willing to modify this organization as needed for enterprise planning, metrics, or other analytics.

CONSTRAINTS

Part of the model is the constraints placed on the data. Selected pieces of data have specific allowable values. For example, sex is traditionally male or female. But, this is not a Boolean variable because until the information is provided, the value is *unknown*; Boolean entries cannot be empty. Other options had not been considered until relatively recently, when transgender and other gender identity issues have complicated this category. The conceptual framework and the constraints had to change to accommodate changes in the required data structure. Associations between data are considered in development. For example, if a patient is listed with sex female, then data elements regarding previous pregnancies are considered a routine part of the medical history. Data are usually limited regarding what the range of values can be. Number of children of –4 (negative 4) is an integer but cannot be correct.

DATA TYPES

Part of the conceptual model is types of data, meaning the computer's view of the data elements, introduced at the beginning of this chapter but discussed in greater detail here.

String: The HPI is a string variable, which is a chain of characters that are numbers, letters, and select special characters. Some characters are not allowed in strings because they may be used by the system for control commands. There are typically constraints on the length of the strings. If an entry exceeds this string length, then another string is created, and our data model keeps track of the additional strings, or we get a limit notification.

Boolean: This is a variable that has only one of two possible values, as a bit in computer function. This can be called 0 or 1. What this means depends on the organization of the data model. Does the patient have a provider encounter at our healthcare system? The answer is Yes or No. You might wonder why a patient might be in the database at all if they have not had an encounter. There are a couple of scenarios, the most common is that the patient had laboratory work done at an outside facility, and because our laboratory is a large regional reference laboratory, the patient has a record in the chart without an encounter. Another possibility is that the patient has an upcoming appointment or had an appointment and either missed it or canceled it.

Floating point: A potassium level is usually displayed as 3.61, although the number was rounded from 3.6085434 in the laboratory information system. This is a floating point number, but only three significant digits need be displayed for the provider.

Integer: The number of children that a patient has had would be an integer: 2.3 is not a valid number. The letter *K* is not a valid entry. Invalid entries are not allowed. Integers are often used not only for indicating an integer number, but also for categorical data. When a marital status is entered, among the options are Married, Divorced, Separated, Widowed, Unknown, Decline to answer. There are other possibilities; hence, there is an Other selection option. These words do not end up written as strings in the database. Rather, when the appropriate selection is made, an integer 1 through 7 is entered. If 7 is entered, then our data model may provide a string box to enter the Other specifications, and in this case, the allowable string size is much shorter than what is allowed for the HPI.

Logical Model

The next step in modeling is *logical*. This is the determination of what the database looks like as we create the space. We could place all of our patients' information into a simple spreadsheet, with each row a unique patient and each column one feature, such as last name, first name, date of birth, medical record number, and so on. Farther to the right would be a column for documents and even farther right would be a column for potassium levels. But, most patients have more than one encounter, so when was that encounter? Which data are associated with which encounter?

HIERARCHICAL DATABASE

Because we cannot use a single spreadsheet, we have to have a separate spreadsheet for each patient and then rows of encounters and the data associated with them. But then, the number of columns for each encounter would be huge, so how about we have a series of subsheets for each encounter for each patient? Then, to make things easier to chart, let us create subsheets of those encounters for different kinds of data such as laboratory, radiology, clinical documents, and orders. This is how a hierarchical database works.

The hierarchical database is a tree-like structure with each node having dependent nodes, termed a *parent-child* relationship; each parent can have multiple children, but each child has only one parent. At the top is a specific facility, and there are branches to specific patients; from there are branches to specific encounters, then to specific aspects, including laboratory results, radiology results, clinical notes, and so on. A conceptual diagram of this is shown in Figure 7.1. In some illustrative drawings of a hierarchical database, there is only one data element at each node, but that is not true in practice. The patient node will include other data, such as demographics or medical record number.

In the example in Figure 7.1, the shaded cells are what we are looking for. Starting at the top, we are looking at the database of the Healthcare System. We want the discharge medications for *Patient A* from his admission last month, termed *Encounter 2*. So, we start at the top, go to *Patient A*, then *Encounter 2*, then *Meds*, then *Discharge*.

RELATIONAL DATABASE

A *relational database* is the major alternative and is used more commonly than the hierarchical database. This is where data are stored on a series of tables, which we display as two-dimensional. The computer does not have that constraint; a computer can handle data with multiple dimensions, but this is computationally intensive as well as difficult to visualize, so we stick to two dimensions.

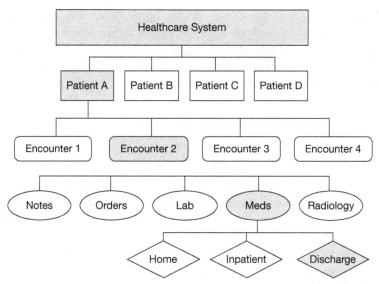

Figure 7.1 Hierarchical database. The elements are in a parent-child relationship, starting at the top and progressing from Patient to Encounter to Medication list to Discharge medication list.

Figure 7.2 shows a data table that lists patients in our database on the top and a second table of laboratory data below. Note that neither the table names nor the column names have spaces, so that neither computers nor humans confuse break points between element names. Underscore can be a bridge (as with our table names), or we just mush the parts of the name together (as with our column names).

Of course, there are millions of patients in our primary database; this is just an illustration, and the names and details are fictitious. At the top is the most important table in our database; we call it the *Patient_Identification* table. The patient names were added to the identity table in the order in which they were registered into the system. They are not rearranged in alphabetical order even though you can do a report that places them as such. Each row is a unique patient, and the first column in each row is a unique identifier. This first column is called the *primary key*. This is the index key for this table. The subsequent columns are demographics and other data.

The second part of this figure is a table called *Laboratory_Tests*; it is a log of laboratory tests in the order in which they were requested. A unique identifier for each test sample is the *primary key* for this table and is *LabOrder*. The second column in the Laboratory_Test table is the patient identifier for each sample. This is the *foreign key*, in that it points back to the Patient_Identification table, so that the name and other details of the patient can be associated with the laboratory test.

The Patient ID numbers are not changeable and are not duplicated. The database controls do not allow for this number to be edited or for a number to be used that was used before. If an entry is in error, a flag is written in one of the columns of the table to tell the database engine to ignore that row.

To find all the laboratory tests associated with a specific person, look at the Patient_Identification table and find the Patient ID number. Then, go to the

Patient_Identification

PatientID	LastName	FirstName	DateOfBirth	City	State
1001	Alpha	Ann	1/30/86	Knoxville	TN
1002	Beta	Betty	2/12/90	Nashville	TN
1003	Gamma	George	3/13/72	Huntsville	AL
1004	Delta	Donna	4/23/56	Nashville	TN
1005	Epsilon	Edward	5/14/92	Lexington	KY

Laboratory_Tests

LabOrder	PatientID	Order	Date	Status	Result
20001	1001	Sodium	9/1/18	Final	150
20002	1002	Calcium	9/2/18	Collected	
20003	1003	Potassium	9/4/18	Canceled	
20004	1004	Donna	9/15/18	Future	
20005	1005	Creatinine	9/3/18	Final	0.61

Figure 7.2 Relational database. A series of tables is created, with connections between tables being the keys. For each table, the primary key is the first column. The foreign key refers to another table, and the second table is in the second column.

Laboratory_Tests table and search for all tests where the Patient ID number is equal to that of the desired patient. If we are looking for laboratory tests on Betty Beta, we look at the top table to discover her unique identifier is 1002. So we then look to the lower table and report the results where column 2 (PatientID) equals 1002.

Or:

```
WHERE Laboratory_Tests.PatientID = 1002
```

If we wanted to ensure that we only reported lab tests that had a result, we would add a qualifier to the search:

```
WHERE Laboratory_Tests.Status = Final
```

This lists all of the laboratory results for that patient where there is a result.

The concepts of primary key and foreign key are fundamental to table creation. There are many tables in a relational database.

COMPARISON OF HIERARCHICAL AND RELATIONAL STRUCTURES
What are the advantages and disadvantages of using the hierarchical versus relational database structures? The hierarchical database works well for looking up the data on a specific patient at a specific facility. We do not have to look in different

tables but rather follow the logical tree to see the data we want for routine medical practice. A problem arises when we want to look for data that are not stored in the routine fashion for clinical care. What if we want to look for all the patients who had a diagnosis of breast cancer and are between the ages of 50 and 65 years? The search algorithm has to follow the trees of all patients in that age range, and not just females, because males can get breast cancer. The search routine looks in every record for a diagnosis of breast cancer, gathers the information you need, and returns it in a spreadsheet.

The relational database makes the second scenario a bit easier. For example, if we want to find breast cancer patients between 50 and 65 years old, we could select all patients between the ages of 50 and 65 from the identity table and then search the diagnosis table for those unique identifiers to see which ones had a diagnosis of breast cancer. An even more efficient way to perform the search would be to go to the table where diagnoses are listed and search the diagnosis column, return unique identifiers of all patients coded for breast cancer, and then go to the identity table to see which ones are between ages of 50 and 65. This is more efficient because a smaller proportion of patients have breast cancer than are between the ages of 50 and 65.

Considering these examples, historically, hierarchical databases were considered to be superior for direct patient care and relational databases were superior for data extraction. But, functionally for the user, this generalization is no longer true. Computers are so fast and search algorithms so efficient that the user would not find a significant difference in response time for most clinical tasks.

To foster ease of searching, hierarchical databases usually create a series of tables for data that they know needs to be looked at, essentially creating a relational database to be used for common queries. But, this is not unique to hierarchical databases. We create subordinate databases from our relational database for queries and analytics so that our data searching does not affect performance of the system while it is being used. This is a data warehouse, discussed further in Chapter 10.

KEY POINTS

- Data representation is organization of our data into a form that can be electronically stored, retrieved, and manipulated.
- Healthcare data are of multiple types, with the most common including numeric, string, and Boolean.[4]
- Healthcare data are from multiple sources, and these might not all represent the data in the same way.[5]
- The hierarchical database structure uses a tree-like structure with parent-child relationships.
- The relational database structure uses tables with index keys, where different tables have different purposes.
  - A primary key is the principal identifier for each table and is unique to each row.
  - The foreign key usually points to a different table to aid in associating data from the different tables.

Basics of Computers

KARL E. MISULIS AND MARK E. FRISSE ■

COMPUTER DESIGN BASICS

Informatics professionals need basic familiarity with computer structure and function to have an understanding of the strengths and limitations of the devices. Also, understanding programming and aspects of computer control and query language gives foundational knowledge of what is doable and what is not doable.

We consider computers to be composed of *hardware* and *software*. Hardware is the physical devices, such as the central processing unit (CPU), display, keyboard, mouse, or printer. Software is the operating instructions, with some of the software being the operating system of the computer and others being applications with specific responsibilities, both to the user (e.g., electronic health records [EHRs], picture archiving and communication systems [PACSs]) and to the system (e.g., network communications, security).

Computer as a Concept

Computers perform calculations on binary numbers. Whenever we ask a computer to calculate creatinine clearance, check the spelling of a clinical document, or draw a radiology image on the screen, the foundation is binary calculation. This is performed by the CPU. In addition, there is memory where data are stored for calculation.

Basic elements of a computer include the

- CPU
- Memory
- Input
- Output

Figure 8.1 shows a simple diagram of a computer. Computers all have inputs and outputs and are connected to users and devices; in this diagram, the user inputs/outputs are separated from those of peripherals, such as databases and other equipment, for conceptual purposes.

The CPU is composed of two major components, the *control unit* and *logic unit*. The control unit is responsible for reading instructions and interpreting them for execution. It reads the instructions one at a time, acts on them, then reads the next instruction. Therefore, some memory is used to keep track of instructions and where the bookmark (pointer) is in the stack of instructions. The control unit also is responsible for returning the results of the instruction execution to memory or to a device. The logic unit is often called the *arithmetic logic unit* (ALU) because it has two principal functions: 1) to perform calculations and 2) to determine whether certain statements are true. For the first, the numbers are turned into binary; then, calculations are performed and then turned into the format instructed for export. This is the arithmetic part. For the logic part, the ALU determines whether statements are true or false depending on logical operators (e.g., whether the result received—perhaps 42—is greater than 73). The response is False or the binary equivalent of that. But, in reality, even the logic task of the ALU is a calculation, so it is all arithmetic. In fact, everything a computer does is mathematical, even spellchecking of a word-processing program boils down to calculating

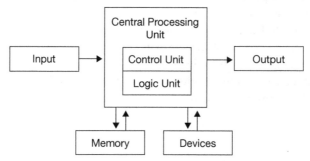

Figure 8.1 Computer schematic. Concise diagram of a computer, with the CPU being at the center comprising a control unit and a logic unit, often called the arithmetic/logic unit. Memory is shown as a connection, but strictly speaking, there are several types of memory involved, including registers integral to the CPU.

values for every word and letter and determining whether it is in the binary library of words.

Next, we consider computer binary operation in a little more detail.

BITS, BYTES, AND WORDS

Because all of the data handled by the computer are 1s and 0s, we talk of bits, bytes, and words. These are discussed in detail in Chapter 7. Briefly, all complex data are reduced to bits, and all computations are performed by manipulations of bits, whether calculating a laboratory value or formatting a clinical document.

MEMORY AND COMPUTATION

The data that are going to be computed have to be stored somewhere so the computation can be performed. Data are stored in memory where they can be read. Most of this is *main memory*, but the CPU has a smaller amount of very fast working memory referred to as a *register*.

The first data read by the CPU are the instruction set. The sequence of events that occurs is as follows:

- Load the instruction set into the register.
- Read the first instruction from the instruction set.
- Read the data to be handled, which can be attached to the instruction or from another location.
- Perform the tasks of the instruction.
- Push the results to the main memory.
- Read the next instruction.

There is a pointer to keep track of which instruction is next to be executed.

Instruction sets will be more complex than our minds can easily handle, but the processes may be illustrated by the following examples:
To calculate the answer to this formula

```
1+9=?
```

the computer uses the binary version of these numbers

```
00000001+00001001=00001010
```

Converting back to base 10 we have

```
1+9=10
```

A more complex task might be

```
Make "a" uppercase-to "A"
```

On our word processor this involves a single keystroke, to toggle case (ChangeCase is the command in Word). But for the computer, *A* and *a* are represented by different binary numbers.

```
a=01100001 in binary
A=01000001 in binary
```

So, the CPU has to take the input and subtract 00100000 from it to get the uppercase character. This is true for every character A–Z and a–z.

Special characters have special functions. For example, 00001101, which would be 13 in base 10, is actually a special character that means to press the Enter or Return key.

This is a very brief introduction to how CPUs working on binary data can perform not only mathematical tasks but also nonmathematical tasks by translating them into numbers.

INPUTS AND OUTPUTS

Inputs and outputs are more than just connections to the CPU. There is usually translation of data in one form to another so that the CPU can understand the data. Fundamental input devices are the keyboard and mouse. Fundamental output devices are the video display and printer.

In healthcare informatics, inputs also include analog or digital signals from medical devices, digital signals from other computer systems, and analog signals from microphones. Digital signals are processed so that the input can be understood by the computer.

Analog signals first have to be transformed into digital signals by an *analog-to-digital converter* (ADC) (Figure 8.2). The ADC measures discrete intervals of voltage at discrete intervals of time. This means that for digitization of an analog signal that has a continuously varying voltage at a continuous epoch of time, samples are taken at specified times. If we sample every 4 milliseconds, that would be a sampling rate of 250 samples/s.[1] So, this means that if anything happens in the time frame of 4 to 10 milliseconds, this particular ADC would not be able to tell you much about it. There are not enough samples in this time frame. Similarly, the voltage is measured at discrete levels. If the measured levels are 5 mV apart, then a measurement of 200 mV would be 40 levels. If there were fluctuations in voltage that were as low as 3 mV, we could not see that with a voltage resolution of 5 mV. So, the ADC has *time resolution* and *voltage resolution*. These resolutions change depending on application.

Common inputs and outputs receive and transmit digital data from other systems. There are some agreed-on formats for movement of some data (e.g., Health Level Seven International [HL7], Digital Imaging and Communications in Medicine [DICOM]), but these standards have variations that complicate interfacing.

Hardware

Modern computers have multiple processors and are configured so they can perform multiple operations simultaneously. Regardless of the operating system used,

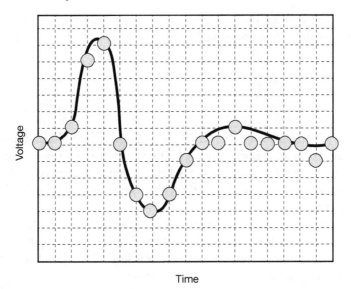

Time

Figure 8.2 An analog-to-digital converter (ADC) places essentially a piece of digital graph paper over the analog signal. The vertical lines are times of voltage sampling, and the horizontal lines represent the voltage levels resolved by the converter.

the ability to do multiple tasks is key to performance in healthcare. Among these applications are

- EHRs
- PACSs
- Specialty apps (e.g., for cardiology, gastroenterology)
- Productivity apps (word processing, spreadsheets, presentation graphics, email, remote conferencing)

Most of these rely on some degree of network access, although the specifics depend on the architecture. For example, the EHR app might be installed on the user computer and just read/write data through the network, or more commonly, the EHR application is running on a central server and only the user interface routines are running on the user computer.

Software

Application software resides at every level of the computer system. Applications will be local, meaning on the device, or remote, such as on a centralized server. If the principal computations are performed on central servers, the local client computer must have software responsible for making network connections, relaying information to and from the servers, and interacting with the user; software decodes keystrokes, mouse actions, and sometimes other inputs (e.g., audio) into a form to be handled by the server system. Local software is responsible for displaying the returned information on the screen and ensuring that the display is appropriate to the set resolution, dimensions, and orientation (e.g., portrait/landscape) of the display.

Firmware

Firmware is a form of software that is typically responsible for low-level functions of the computer, such as interaction of applications with device hardware. Firmware is not distinct from software but rather is a subset of it. Firmware typically resides on nonvolatile memory, meaning memory that is not cleared when the device is powered down.

BIOS is the *Basic Input-Output System*. This is firmware used to guide startup and has the instructions on how to load the operating system. Since computers have become more complex, what had begun as a very low-level system now has options for startup and configuration, some of which can be set by the user.

Memory

Computer memory is electronic and stored in different ways depending on the type of memory, discussed in the material that follows. This is in contrast to storage devices, such as optical and magnetic media. The terms *RAM* (random access memory) *ROM* (read-only memory), *EPROM* (erasable programmable read-only memory), and *CMOS* (complementary metal oxide semiconductor) *RAM* are often used to designate the type of memory and are detailed as follows.

When we think of memory, we usually are referring to RAM. But, this is just one sort. RAM is memory used for temporary storage for the purpose of computer processing. The data arrived there by being read from a storage device, by being loaded from more permanent nonvolatile memory, or by calculations previously performed by the computer. If power is suddenly lost, the data in RAM disappears unless there is some nonvolatile backup. This is because RAM stores data as states of individual circuits, which are composed in part of a transistor and capacitor.[2] The transistor acts as a switch to control charging of the capacitor. The capacitor can be charged or not, indicating whether this bit is a 1 or a 0.

Hence, RAM is usually *volatile*. When the power is turned off, circuits have no power, and the data are lost. *Nonvolatile* means that the memory continues to be stored without power. There is nonvolatile RAM (NVRAM), and a common form of this is flash memory, although there are cost and performance issues with this form.

ROM is nonvolatile memory, and the most typical use is for firmware. ROM might indeed be ROM only, but more commonly it means data can be written but with difficulty.

EPROM can be written and rewritten using special techniques, particularly ultraviolet light. *Electrically erasable programmable read-only memory* (EEPROM) is similar, but erasure is done electrically.

Flash memory was developed from EEPROM. Flash may be considered to be a more advanced version of early EEPROM, partly in how the memory is written, making it more efficient and less expensive than earlier versions of EEPROM.

Virtual memory is when the effective operating RAM of a computer is increased by assigning RAM addresses to solid-state or mechanical storage media. Writing and reading from this memory will be slower than that of RAM, but it can avoid shortages of memory that cause application failure, which afflicted earlier computers.

PROGRAMS AND PROGRAMMING

Programs are the instructions that direct the innumerable tasks of computers in healthcare systems. *Programming* is the writing of these instructions. Entire careers are built around the foundations of programming, so this chapter presents a brief overview and is not intended to bring the reader to programming proficiency. As with many information systems functions, it is important for informatics professionals to have an overview without needing to know the details. Informatics is not programming, although informatics depends on programming.

Overview of Computer Applications and Programs

The terms *application* and *program* are often confused and sometimes used interchangeably. There is even disagreement among computer scientists about the distinction. For our purposes, we consider *program* to refer to a set of instructions to accomplish a task for the computer. An *application* is a set of instructions, including programs that accomplish a task for a user. For example, a word-processing program is really an application because it not only processes words but also performs lower level tasks, such as print formatting for installed printers and screen formatting for dimensions and resolution of the display. Then, to take this hierarchy up one level, we have *application suites*, which are groups of applications with a common or entangled interface or that accomplish similar tasks. Microsoft Office is an application suite in that the elements do similar tasks but with differing data types and purposes, but they use many of the same program structures for handling data plus a consistent user interface look and feel. Our EHR is an application suite, bringing data from multiple applications into a single interface. In fact, some of the pages displayed in our EHR are merely display windows to other applications, such as for archived data from legacy electronic medical record (EMR) or cardiac echocardiogram displays.

Our enterprise information system has approximately 239 different *applications* running concurrently. Each application is multiple *programs* bundled together. An application can be the EHR, in which one program in that application can send direct messages, another can do orders, and another can deliver results. They function from a common interface. The application also usually depends on programs that are part of the operating system and not directly part of the EHR application.

Examples include some printer or other data-interface programs, which are not directly part of the EHR application.

Overview of Programming

Programming is writing the instructions that are then followed. These are traditionally written in a software language that is fairly easy to write and read by humans and then are translated into computer-readable instructions by a *compiler* program A wide variety of languages exists; these have different strengths and weaknesses. *Machine code* is the instructions actually used by the device, but this is not directly written by humans.

Among some of the common programming languages historically are BASIC, FORTRAN, COBOL, C, and derivatives of these. More modern programs are numerous, but just a few of the ones you may be familiar with are C++, Objective C, and Python.

Source code is a transcript of the instructions written in the programming language plus associated comments. Most languages allow for comments intended for the programmers so they can remember what specific sections of code are for and also so plans for future changes can be documented without having to keep a log outside the file. The computer ignores the comments.

A *compiler* is a program that translates a high-level language such as Python or C++ into a lower level language that is more ready for execution by the computer. We mentioned machine language, which is the actual instructions. The compiler might also translate to *assembly language*, which is one step higher than machine language. When a compiler has translated a program, it can no longer be easily read by a human.

An *interpreter* is a program that executes the instructions of a high-level language without it needing to have been previously compiled. Not all languages are amenable to one or more types of interpreting.

OBJECT-ORIENTED PROGRAMMING

As computer programs became more complex, their development became more time-consuming. In general, the time a programmer needs to write a line of code is the same if the code if the language is detailed and complex (e.g., C-langage code) or if the line is written at a higher level that in turn calls on more detailed code. Object-oriented programming is one way of ensuring that programs are more easily understood and created more efficiently. These code objects can in turn call on specific data or on lower-level functions that can be created once and used in many different objects and even different applications. Objects are defined by class libraries that describe what different object templates do.

An analogy we use is building a house. It is certainly possible to build a house from original materials (e.g., rocks, trees, clay, iron ore, etc.), with unique specifications, and do all of the building on ones own. A procedural programming approach would begin with a procedure "build a house" and this procedure in turn would describe methods for laying bricks, placing water pipes, running electric lines, installing light switches, and performing even minute tasks. To understand procedural programs at even a high-level, one must dig into a lot of details. A list of necessary house-building tasks and requirements would be extremely long.

An object-oriented program has more uniform ways of representing necessary data and procedures by specifying classes of objects and methods that an object uses to accomplish specific tasks. For example, one object may be of the class *contractor*. This class has common *attributes* such as price-list, start-time, specifications etc. It also contains *methods* (programs) required for the object to perform desired tasks. These methods and data differ between different objects in this class; *contractor-electrician-object* has different methods than *contractor-brick-layer-object*. When creating object-oriented programs, one can invoke an object through a message and rely on the object to perform the program tasks. A diagram of an object-oriented house-building program would be a high-level graph. Those seeking additional details can examine the data and methods of an object through a programming interface. But generally such an examination is not required.

It takes just as long to write a line in MUMPS as it does to write a line in an OOP language, and the latter gives a lot bigger bang for the buck. It's also easier to understand what's going on because one can stay at a high-level or dig in to whatever detail is required.

C++ is the best known foundational programming language to use an object-oriented approach and has been widely used. Most programming languages are able to do both object-oriented programming and direct command entry. For direct entry of commands, there is a specific vocabulary and syntax.

Terminology

The terminology of computer programming is extensive, and a glossary is included at the end of this book, but briefly, some of the more important terms we use in discussing programs are as follows:

- *Syntax* is the set of rules to which the language adheres. For example, a language might require a command sequence to begin with a command word such as PROCEDURE and end with END, whereas another might require SUB and END SUB. The first example resembles Pascal, and the second resembles BASIC.
- *Semantics* is the function of the commands, assuming the commands are syntactically legal.
- *Markup* is entries in a document, which can be a program or data document that give a nonprinting command. An example is HTML (Hypertext Markup Language), for which the header of the Web version of this section might be <h4>Terminology</h4>. This markup tells the browser to display the heading with the style defined as Heading Level 4.
- *Boolean* refers to logical operators commonly used in programming, with the determinant for each one being True or False; for example, "Misulis Age > 60" is either true or false, and there are no other possibilities.
- An *iteration* is a programming loop, described further in this chapter.

- A *subroutine* is a code set that is part of a larger program that accomplishes a specific task. Subroutines are often called from different parts of a program. For example, my program might have a subroutine to label each of my entries with the current date and time. There is no need to write the same subroutine repeatedly; the program calls the subroutine every time I make an entry, whether it is an order or a clinical note.

Pseudocode

Pseudocode is a term used for a hypothetical programming language for which there is not actually a compiler or interpreter. Pseudocode is typically easily readable, so that the purpose and the high-level logic of the code can be understood.

Pseudocode in this chapter is used as an instructional tool for those who are unfamiliar with the essentials of computer programming. Pseudocode is also sometimes used for the design of programs so the overall logical structure can be developed, which is later rewritten in a bona fide computer language.

Pseudocode does not have a defined vocabulary, syntax, and semantics because it is not a real language, but in general, the features of a program generally are similar to those of one of the genuine programming languages, such as BASIC, C++, or FORTRAN.

For our purposes, we will invent pseudocode that does not attempt to resemble most languages but can be used to illustrate the concepts. We might call our language *Anulap*, after the god of magic and knowledge in Micronesia.

START AND END OF THE PROGRAM

The compiler for our imaginary programming language needs to know when the program begins and when it ends. For Anulap, we use

```
Start of the program: START PROGRAM
End of the program: END PROGRAM
```

SUBROUTINES

Subroutines or subprograms will need to be delimited so the compiler and the programmer know the beginning and end of each. Because subroutines are called from different parts of the program, we need to put in the name of the subroutine, in this case called DisplayTime

```
Start of the subroutine: SUB DisplayTime
End of the subroutine: END SUB
```

Elsewhere in the program, the subroutine is called to display the time. For our language, we call the subroutine simply by entering RUNSUB and the name of the subroutine:

```
RUNSUB DisplayTime
```

and the time is appropriately displayed.

Sometimes, there are variables that need to be passed to the subroutine. In the example of DisplayTime, there might not be any variables that are passed, so the name would be DisplayTime( ), with empty parentheses. However, if we needed to display the language in a particular format, such as for British or Japanese users, we would pass a variable that indicated the particular format, such as DisplayTime(eng), where the *eng* indicated English format. Similarly, we might pass an integer variable to indicate time zone, as offset from Coordinated Universal Time (UTC).[3]

The following would be the command for displaying the date and time in Tbilisi, Republic of Georgia, in the Georgian language:

```
RUNSUB DisplayTime(kat,4)
```

where *kat* is the International Organization for Standardization (ISO) 639-3 code for Georgian language and Tbilisi is +4 time zones from UTC.

IF/THEN STATEMENTS
IF/THEN statements are among the first learned in programming. The logic is simple. If one condition is true, then do one thing; if not true, then do not do it.

```
IF (MisulisAge > 60) THEN PRINT 'Old man'
```

If the statement is true, then the phrase is printed; otherwise, nothing is printed.

IF/THEN statements typically include ELSE to indicate what do if the statement is false:

```
IF (MisulisAge > 60) THEN PRINT 'Old Man" ELSE PRINT
"Young man"
```

IF/THEN and ELSE statements are simple examples of conditional statements that are available in languages in a variety of forms.

FOR/NEXT STATEMENTS
FOR/NEXT statements are used for creation of iterative loops, which continue until a particular condition is met. If we wanted to make a simple table of squared numbers, the following code might be used:

```
FOR n = 1 TO 10
      PRINT n, n*n
NEXT
```

This produces a simple list:

```
1    1
2    4
3    9
4    etc . . .
```

If I wanted to only do the squares for every other n, then the code might be

```
FOR n = 1 TO 10 STEP 2
      PRINT n, n*n
NEXT
```

FOR/NEXT statements can be nested, so that multiple iterations of an instruction set are performed within each larger iteration. An example might be creating a multiplication table:

```
FOR n = 1 TO 10
   PRINT n,
   FOR m = 1 TO 10
      PRINT n*m,
   NEXT
   PRINT
NEXT
```

This program begins with n = 1 and prints that number, then goes through the subordinate loop, which prints n*m for each of the values. The comma after the print command means use a tab between printed values, not a new line. The last PRINT command outside the inner loop makes the display go to the next line.

WHILE Loop

Most programming languages have some form of WHILE loop construction. This differs from the FOR/NEXT loop, although it is in the same family of conditional instructions. The loop is defined by a Boolean condition, either true or false. The loop is executed until the condition is false. For example, WHILE (n > 0) would begin a loop that is executed until n is equal to 0 or is negative. The loop likely either alters the value of n or reads the value from some other location.

The WHILE loop must have some command that tells the compiler where the end of the loop is. A version of BASIC uses ENDWHILE, whereas Java uses curly brackets to delineate what is included in the loop iteration, such as WHILE (n>0) {n = n-1}. The parentheses indicate the evaluated condition; the curly brackets indicate the instructions to perform while the condition is true.

In our pseudocode Anulap, a program to divide numbers by themselves might be

```
n = 100
WHILE (n > 0)
      PRINT n/n,
      n = n - 1
END WHILE
```

This program starts with 100 and prints as n divided by itself, which will always be 1 until n is equal to 0, in which case 0/0 is not 1 but is undefined, or in the description of Apple's on-screen calculator, "Not a number." So, the WHILE loop exits when n reaches 0.

COMMENTS IN THE CODE

Code can become remarkably complex and, depending on the language, may be more or less readable by humans. We need reminders of what certain parts of the program are designed to accomplish, and we need to make notes to ourselves to alter a code. In BASIC, the command REM means this is a remark, and none of the characters on the same line as REM should be considered to be instructions.

```
REM This subroutine calculates square-roots.
```

Forms of BASIC such as Visual Basic (VB) use an apostrophe for the same purpose:

```
'This routine performs factorial.
```

In C, comments are delimited by slashes:

```
/ Rewrite the following commands as a subroutine to
use another time /
```

Exhaustive programming experience has taught us to make frequent comments.

Synopsis of Some Important Programming Languages

Not all programming languages can be covered here; there are excellent Wikipedia pages on almost all programming languages and even one that is a directory of programming languages.[4]

BASIC is actually an acronym derived from for Beginner's All-Purpose Symbolic Instruction Code. This was initially used mainly by end users of early personal computers to develop small custom programs, but with maturation of the language and development of different versions and extensive enhancements, descendants of BASIC have been powerful tools in the hands of professional programmers.

Visual Basic was developed by Microsoft on a BASIC foundation. VB is object oriented and can be assembled by dragging objects, which are sections of code. Although VB is no longer supported by Microsoft, it is still in use. A derivative, *Visual Basic for Applications* (VBA), is still implemented in the Windows and OSX versions of Office 2016. This is used by many, including data handlers, for automating tasks. An example is census report; the app queries the bed board database, crunches the numbers, and produces a PDF of numbers of occupied and empty beds for different services and different units of the hospitals and different hospitals in an affiliated system. This report is automatically sent to senior leadership every 12 hours. For example, if they are short on cardiac care unit or neuro intensive care unit beds, that is communicated to the on-call staff and transfer center.

FORTRAN originated from IBM in the 1950s and is still in some use today. The name is from Formula Translation. The original intent was to be a step higher than assembly language to facilitate larger and more complex programs, which are quite difficult to write in assembler. There are many versions of FORTRAN, and a new update is planned.

Python is an increasingly used high-level language. Advantages include readability by humans, which is better than that of many other languages, and efficiency, so fewer commands may be used than with some other languages. Python was developed by Guido van Rossum, who continues to be involved in its evolution. The name is from the Monty Python performing group.

The language *C* was developed in the early 1970s, and derivatives remain in extensive use. Typical functionality is available in C, but the structure differs somewhat from previous languages. Instructions are included in subroutines, and variables are passed to the subroutines. These are called *Functions* in C. C provided a readable language that could offer low-level functions and, importantly, could leverage the Function structure to allow for more ease of creating large and complex programs. The name C comes from its succession to the B programming language developed at Bell Laboratories.

C++ is an enhancement to C and includes object-oriented programming. It adds the functions of class (templates for creating objects) and inheritance (where an object created from another object or from a class inherits the features of that predecessor). These factors plus an extensive library of functions make C++ an efficient programming language. Inheritance can be illustrated by a brick-laying analogy where the objects in class *Brick* (such as *red-brick, yellow-brick,* etc.) inherit the features of the class: hard, heavy, angular. The objects *straight-brick-laying* and *corner-brick-laying* of class *Brick-laying* share the class features of difficult and exhausting manual labor using mortar.

Java is an object-oriented programming language developed by Sun Microsystems, which has a code that looks similar to C++ but the syntax differences make the code not interchangeable. The intent was to allow development of programs that run on different platforms, so that many different versions of an application would not be needed. Sun released Java in 1995, and it is still in widespread use today, with numerous updates. The name comes from coffee, this name having been chosen because the original working name for the project had already been trademarked by another company.

Microsoft Visual Studio is an *integrated development environment* (IDE) used to create programs for Windows devices. At least 36 programming languages are supported by Visual Studio. The development environment simplifies tasks such as user interface and communication.

Xcode is an IDE for most Apple devices, including tablets, computers, phones, watches, and Apple TV. There is support for multiple languages.

What the Healthcare Informatics Professional Needs to Know About Programming

We recommend that informatics professionals should be familiar with, but not necessarily proficient in, programming. Unless you are intending to write large programs, we recommend some familiarity with one of the IDEs. Both Xcode and Visual Studio have free versions for download. At the time of writing, Xcode was available only for MacOS, but Visual Studio had community versions for Windows and MacOS.

For fun and instruction, we recommend trying one of the free BASIC interpreters. These will not allow creation of useful custom programs but will be instructive of how programming works.

NETWORKS

Network, as an information systems term, can refer to an affiliated group of devices connected to share resources or can refer only to the connection infrastructure. Networks are at multiple levels, including internal and external to the healthcare facility.

Network Hardware

Computers connect to networks through *nodes*, which are communication points on the network. Nodes are of various types:

- A *hub* is a node with a number of connections; it is used to allow connection of multiple devices to the network.
- A *router* is a connection device between different networks. The networks are still distinct, and the router controls data transfer between the networks.
- A *bridge* is almost the flip side of a router. A bridge connects multiple networks so that they appear to act as a single network.

A *modem* is a device that translates signals into digital form, which can be understood by the network. The term *modem* comes from modulator-demodulator, owing to the design of modems to translate back and forth between analog and digital formats. Modems can work on a variety of signals, including modulated sound (e.g., telephone) and light (e.g., fiber-optic signals).

Two principal forms of networks are the *local area network* (LAN) and *wide area network* (WAN). A LAN is a network that is in a facility and does not rely on external connections for internal resource sharing. The WAN usually depends on third-party communication lines and equipment.

The healthcare system usually has multiple networks because each has different duties, and those duties have differing requirements.

An increasing number of devices used in healthcare communicate over wireless connections. For this, we have *wireless access points* (WAPs), which turn the network digital signal into a radio signal that our personal devices can decode. The WAP is connected to the router by a network cable.

A *wireless router* has the combined function of a router and a WAP, so there are wired connections on the box as well as radio transmission and receiving hardware.

Network Design

Most healthcare systems have multiple networks. In our facility, we have separate networks for the following tasks:

- Medical device (e.g., pumps, mobile charting and barcoding devices, nursing computers on wheels [COWs]) connection
- Provider devices (laptops, COWs, tablets, smartphones)
- Patient and visitor Internet access.

Bandwidth of these networks will depend on use. Providers who might be looking at cine on a picture archiving and communication system (PACS) or using other data-intensive apps require more bandwidth and are provided a special high-bandwidth network. Medical devices send widely varying amounts of data, but in one of our hospitals, we have over 3000 medical devices connected to the wireless network. Patient and visitor network access is usually with controlled bandwidth and sometimes limitations, such as no streaming videos or other large data movements.

Security and access control involving the networks are discussed in Chapter 18. Many networks are hidden from the casual user. Access to mission-critical networks should be tightly controlled.

KEY POINTS

- Knowledge of basic hardware and software design is essential for clinical informatics professionals.
- Computers perform calculations. Even when dealing with text and image data, they are performing calculations.
- Data are all represented ultimately in binary.
- There are multiple types of memory with differing strengths, weaknesses, and uses. ROM is mainly for firmware. RAM is used mainly for temporary operational storage. EPROM is used for computer firmware. EEPROM is used widely for flash memory in memory cards and programmable devices (car key fobs) and has replaced EPROM for BIOS systems because of the updating capability.
- Computer programming is usually performed in languages that are sufficiently readable for humans to write the code, yet of a structure and syntax that allows a compiler to turn the code into computer-executable instructions.

Design of the Core Healthcare Operating System

DOUGLAS J. DICKEY, KARL E. MISULIS, AND MARK E. FRISSE ■

OVERVIEW

We commonly use the term *electronic health record* (EHR) to indicate the extended manifestation of our clinical information systems. As these systems become more interoperable with other systems and extend into the cloud, an alternative term we use in this text is healthcare operating system (HOS), which takes the EHR up another level, at least conceptually.

SYSTEM GOALS

The HOS must meet the goals of the enterprise. All healthcare systems want to give excellent care at a low cost with the most efficient workflows and the best analytic and reporting systems. However, enterprise priorities have to be set.

The tasks of the healthcare system are

- Healthcare delivery
- Management and financial duties
- Sharing of information with patients, other facilities, and care teams

The tasks the system needs to accomplish are many, but among those are

- Storing and cataloging records
- Facilitating clinical workflows
- Producing and collecting bills
- Creating reports
- Complying with rules and regulations
- Providing interoperability with other systems

Most commercial EHRs exhibit economy of scale such that larger installations are proportionally less costly per user. This is mostly because there are basic core functionalities and resources needed by hospitals and clinics of every size. Scaling up these capacities produces more costs in training, user licenses, devices, and data space. But, in general, scaling up is proportionately lower cost than acquisition of the core system.

In this chapter, we discuss a generic architecture that would be employed to a greater or lesser extent in most healthcare systems where the information system has to service both the hospital and outpatient arenas. Some of the details would change depending on priority and scale.

SYSTEM ARCHITECTURE

System architecture is the high-level structure of the system. There are layers to this organization. On the top are conceptual models. Components of the conceptual layer include the care delivery system and the business system. Beneath these layers are sublayers as shown in Figure 9.1.

Components of the care delivery system include the patient, providers, clinical staff, the data systems that support them, and an extensive physical and coordinating infrastructure.

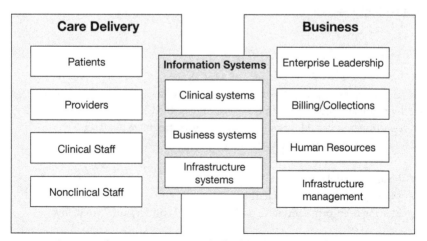

Figure 9.1 System architecture comprising the healthcare system. Information systems work with all elements to accomplish their tasks efficiently.

Components of the business layer include not only billing and collections, but also the entire business infrastructure, some of which includes scheduling, facilities management, material management, and human resources.

Data system architecture is a major component of our conception of system architecture, and this is the principal focus here. Some of the clinical systems included in the data system architecture are

- Acute EHRs
- Ambulatory EHRs
- Picture archiving and communication system (PACS)[1]
- Radiology information system (RIS)[2]
- Laboratory information system (LIS)
- Patient portal
- Population health system
- Device integration platform
- Specialty systems

Figure 9.2 shows these in a parallel organization for clinical and business healthcare components.

The components might all be from the same vendor, but that is uncommon. No one vendor has all requirements of a healthcare system adequately serviced by their products. Even though we tend to stick with a single vendor for ease of data flow and handling, we almost always have other vendor applications that will need interfacing.

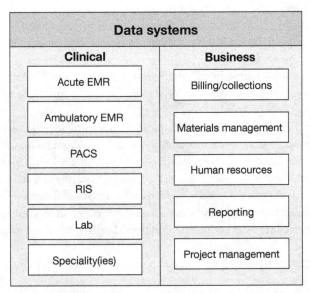

Figure 9.2 System architecture: Data systems include both clinical and business components. While we tend to think of these as separate, the clinical and business systems are increasingly intertwined.

Network

The EHRs depend on a local network so that the clinical devices can connect to the computers that hold the data and servers on which the user devices depend. Historically, wired devices have most commonly been used because they are considered to be lower maintenance and more secure. Neither of these assumptions is always true. Embedded wires need to be replaced, physical connections can be faulty, and there are security concerns with wired as well as wireless access.

Wireless networks are increasingly relied on for device connectivity. They can be secured so that it is difficult, although not impossible, for unauthorized access to the network to occur. Bandwidth used to be a significant problem, but presently it is not so much of a problem because of improved network capacities and better allocation of network resources. Network experts allocate sufficient bandwidth for medical devices while allowing public access, albeit on a subnetwork (subnet). However, wireless networks can be attacked and can fail. Damage to the access points, routers, cables connecting the network server(s) to the routers, or the servers themselves can cause network dysfunction. Older hospital buildings with thick, reinforced concrete walls can sometimes cause wireless signal penetration issues. Retained capabilities depend on the device strategy, discussed further in this chapter.

Network devices include routers, access points, and repeaters. These are often confused. In brief, a *router* is an interface between two or more networks, such as the network of your Internet service provider (ISP) and your home or work network. There may be more than one network in your organization so that you can determine the bandwidth for each. For example, you will likely create subnetworks with the largest bandwidth for clinical devices. Networks for the public and for personal use by staff would have a smaller proportion of your total available bandwidth. It is extremely important that you get the proportion correct so that all people and devices are satisfied. Bandwidth limitation can be a source of failure for an enterprise information system.

An *access point* is correctly called a wireless access point (WAP). This has a wired connection to the servers and has a radio for communications with wireless devices.

A *repeater* is a radio that communicates with your network wirelessly via an access point or router with wireless capabilities and then in turn communicates wirelessly with your devices. The repeater serves to extend a wireless signal without having to place new cable. This is like relay stations from the last century, where a series of radio or microwave towers received and retransmitted signals.[3] In hospitals, repeaters are used not only for in-house wireless network communications but also often for select cell services because penetration of cell signal into large facilities can be poor.

A virtual private network (VPN) occurs when the enterprise private network is allowed to be accessed from outside the enterprise, that is, through a public network. This arrangement is usually where there are secure connections (*tunnels*) which require a high level of security to prevent unauthorized access.

Connectivity

Internal connections are mainly accomplished through a network interface. Some equipment may be directly connected, but generally, network communication is favored for most applications. This allows for greater ease of connections and troubleshooting of connections. Some systems, especially specialty-specific applications, are directly interfaced without passing information through the network. For example, the PACS and the RIS are usually directly connected even if they are not products of the same vendor. Electroencephalography (EEG) machines usually pass data directly to the EEG database; as with radiology and cardiology images, interpretive and archival storage of raw raster-based clinical data are seldom a task for the EHR database. A single computerized tomographic (CT) study can be a much larger data file than all of the medical records of a long-term complex patient.

Security

Security has to be ensured from both internal and external threats, from intentional attack, unintentional error, and infrastructure failure. This is discussed in detail in Chapter 18.

Functions of an EHR System

To accomplish the tasks of the system, there are core functions that every HOS must be able to do. Among these are

- Data storage
- User interface
- Patient access services (PASs)
- Patient financial services (PFSs)
- External connections for
  o Population health
  o Research
  o Cloud functions
  o Interfacing with medical devices
  o Interfacing with other systems
- Access control

DATA STORAGE
Data storage is discussed in detail in Chapter 10, but briefly, data are received from multiple sources, including from patients, clinicians, support staff, laboratory, radiology, and business systems, to name just a few. Incoming data are classified into type, including string, integer, floating point, and Boolean. Categorical information,

such as whether a patient's status is inpatient, outpatient, observation, is generally stored as an integer, and each integer is associated with a specific status.

Data have rules, so that the data adhere to specific characteristics, such as limits. For example, if an integer field is used to indicate whether a patient is in one of five locations, with 0 being "unknown," a value of 6 or greater would not be allowed. Another example would be a medical record number (MRN); the system would not allow the same MRN to be given to two people.

Data are stored as elements and arrays, the design of which depends on type of database.

USER INTERFACE

The user interface is discussed in detail in Chapter 14. In brief, the interface simply displays information and receives input from the user. In the past, function was more important than design, but now that all systems have essentially similar and complete basic user functions, efficiency of use is of pivotal importance to developers as well as those healthcare organizations shopping for applications.

Among the many functions of the interface are creating and editing documents, placing orders, viewing results, and messaging with other providers and members of the care team.

PASS AND PFSS

Patient access services (PAS) include communications between patients and the enterprise and scheduling. They are generally done through the clinical interface but can be done through the business system; in either case, they require a close link between the two systems. *Patient financial services* (PFSs) include billings and collections.

EXTERNAL CONNECTIONS

External connections are many and include other clinical apps in affiliated clinics, hospitals, and other healthcare organizations, payer systems, payers for electronic submission of claims, and reporting entities for metrics.

Other connections are included with a health information exchange (HIE), especially as the backbone for a clinically integrated network (CIN). As the industry evolves to the HOS in the cloud, we expect important external connections to include

- Population health systems
- Patient portals
- Medical devices, both implanted and wearable
- Substitutable Medical Applications and Reusable Technologies (SMART) on Fast Healthcare Interoperability Resource (FHIR) applications
- Research registries and data repositories
- Affiliated enterprise connections

Access Control

The HOS has to allow appropriate access depending on position; a physician will have different privileges than an office medical assistant. Access is usually controlled by user IDs and passwords, but biometrics is sometimes used. Increasingly, single sign on (SSO) is used so that access is allowed by a single shell app, which then launches individual clinical apps on demand without having to sign in again. The most common would be the electronic medical record (EMR) and PACS. The SSO function also allows for context matching, such that the patient information being viewed on the EMR has the patient's radiology folder shown on the PACS. There are other, newer avenues of access control. Details are discussed in Chapter 15.

Core Design of an EHR System

Figure 9.3 shows a schematic design of the core of an EHR.
Essential elements of the EHR include the

- Data storage unit
- Servers
- User interface devices
- Peripheral and other system interfaces

Figure 9.4 shows a schematic design of the integration of the EHR into the HOS.

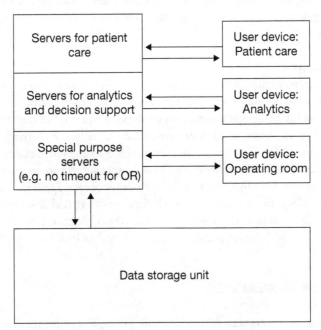

Figure 9.3 Core design. Design of the core system for a computer comprises a host of networked devices. When generating a diagram, it is difficult to determine how detailed to be, so this is a minimalist representation. OR, operating room.

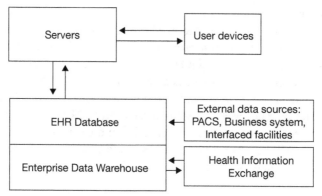

Figure 9.4 Integration with the HOS. The core systems integrate with other systems to form and enhance the healthcare operating system (all information systems used for all phases of healthcare, from hospitals to patient homes).

DATA STORAGE

The data storage unit is the physical storage for the data in the database. This is typically magnetic disk. Archive data may be kept on magnetic tape, but this is not used for day-to-day clinical work, termed *production*. Details of data representation and storage are discussed in Chapter 7.

Security is discussed in detail in Chapter 18, but is generally accomplished by both physical and technical means.

Data can be queried from within the EHR application, but often independent data analytics applications are used to query the database. All queries are documented for auditing.

USER INTERFACE

Chapter 14 discusses the user interface in detail, in brief, the user interface is created as part of the EHR programming and currently consists of a graphical user interface (GUI). Occasionally, the application runs on the user's device, but this is rare. More commonly, the user interface data are generated on servers, with the user device mainly the conduit for the input (keyboard and mouse) and output (display).

A virtual desktop, in our context,[4] is where remote servers are used to create an application environment that can have the appearance of local applications. The user device essentially is the communication platform to the virtual desktop so that no EHR apps or data reside on the user device. When the connection is terminated, data access is lost. Virtual desktops provide better security than local EHR applications.

How to Select Components

Selection of components is multifactorial, with principal factors including

- Function
- Interoperability
- Cost

Function is assumed. A selected component has to either have all of the required functions or be combined with another component that can complete the balance of the functions. An example might be interfacing with biomedical equipment. An interface bus might be able to join many disparate devices but might not be able to join some, in which case custom manual interfaces will have to be created; the interface engine cannot accomplish all interfacing, but it is of value in reducing the amount of custom work needed.

Interoperability is usually best accomplished when components are purchased from the same vendor or from a solution partner where there is prenegotiated and predefined interoperability. In this case, less work has to be done by the client to make the connection. Best-of-breed components have historically been desirable, but interoperability issues can produce a HOS that has the benefits of the best components eclipsed by the interoperability concerns.

Cost is always an issue and is negotiated in the initial contract. As discussed in Chapter 13, contracts have to specify exactly what is and is not included in the contract.

INTRODUCTION TO DATABASE

Data types are discussed in Chapter 3, and database structure is discussed in detail in Chapter 7.

The data are written into organized fields on the storage media. These data have to be indexed along with the logical organization so that the data can be efficiently located on demand. There are two commonly used database structures, again detailed in Chapter 7: relational and hierarchical.

A relational database has a series of data tables that are linked by keys that correlate data from one table to another. One table would be patient identification, another would be list of encounters, and so on. The hierarchical database is organized in a tree-like structure where nodes are connected by branches. There are relative advantages and disadvantages of these two models, discussed in Chapter 7.

Searching the database is accomplished by a variety of engines, including the EHR itself.

The database can reside at the healthcare facility or at a remote location. Increasing numbers of facilities are relying on remote hosting, where the computing power and storage media either are at a vendor-owned site or are under contract with a hosting service. Reasons for remote hosting include expense, because data centers are expensive to build and maintain and to expand. Also, security is an increasing issue, so leaving the security to a hosting service with robust state-of-the-art cybercrime defenses may be more secure. A hosting service, whether vendor owned or independent, is a larger target for intrusion, but the hosting services typically have far more security resources than an enterprise could afford.

Big Data

The term *big data* has a definition that is in evolution. Big data are more than just a large amount of data, especially because the handling capacity of databases has expanded in recent years. The term *big data* refers to large amounts of data that generally are beyond the capability of most analytic routines to process. Special data-handling processes are needed.

Big data are typically accumulated from multiple data sources, but a single source can be used. For example, Google Trends has the ability to correlate the search data for billions of searches. Google Public Data has access to many databases around the world. Most commercial data analytics packages would not be able to search, let alone analyze, these data.

The importance of big data is in learning to manage and maintain new associations, which can help advance medical care in quality and efficiency. There are many clinical questions that cannot be answered by a single-site randomized trial.

As clinicians, this is the utopia for which we all strive. We want to identify patients who are at high risk for disease and intervene before the event. This is a foundational element of population health (Chapter 26).

The learning healthcare system is another extension of big data analytics. Getting information to us at the right time helps us make better decisions and provide better patient outcomes.

HARDWARE

Storage Media

Database information is usually on magnetic media, often in the form of fixed disks, termed *hard disks*, as opposed to the historically important floppy disks. Archive data can be stored on removable disks or magnetic tape. Flash memory is used for some databases, although this is not in widespread use.[5] Backup is often done at regular intervals, sometimes nightly. Some enterprises have mirror data centers that comprise identical servers and data at two spatially separated installations; if one fails, the other can take over. However, this duplication is prohibitively expensive for many healthcare systems.

Server Strategy

Early computers had a central processing unit (CPU) and one or more terminals attached. The terminals had no computing power other than the ability to transmit information to the CPU and display the returned data.

Current HOSs use *client-server architecture*, where an array of servers runs the applications and the client devices connect to the servers for input and output. The servers reside in the data center. Each server has the ability to multitask so that it can support multiple clients. Yet, the experience to each user is that they are running their own instance; they cannot see the other users working on the same multitasking server.

Server Virtualization

Server virtualization gives increased flexibility to the processing capability of the servers. To understand virtualization, we must first understand the history of how processing used to work using traditional server architecture. Traditional server architecture uses an operating system on each server that is of a particular vendor, version, and configuration (e.g., Windows 7 running Internet Explorer [IE] 8). So, multiple users are on that server, running the EMRs and other apps. If that server fails, then the load is shifted to another server, and the experience of the user is unchanged, except for a brief interruption during the switch.

Figure 9.5 shows server virtualization, which is where the servers are running a program that creates virtual servers, so each user seems to have their own server. The servers are still multitasking, but unlike conventional client-server architecture, each instance need not be of the same configuration or even same operating system. So, if one user requires an instance of a specified version and configuration, then that can be linked to their user ID.

Updates to applications are common, and it might occur that the updated Web viewer for the PACS requires IE 10.[6] Or, perhaps a different version of the operating system is required for the voice recognition application. In that case, server virtualization can be useful.

The software that makes virtualization possible is called a *hypervisor,* a term derived from the word *supervisor,* which in computer-speak refers to the most privileged kernel mode of the operating system. Whereas the supervisor mode controls the basic functions of the processor operating system, the hypervisor coordinates the operating systems of the individual instances of virtualized servers.

Clinical User	PACS User	Business User
Virtual Machine Applications	Virtual Machine Applications	Virtual Machine Applications
Virtual Machine Operative system	Virtual Machine Operative system	Virtual Machine Operative system
Hypervisor		
Server Operating system		
Server hardware		

Figure 9.5 Server virtualization. Most enterprises use server virtualization; each server can support multiple virtual servers, which can have different code levels, different operating systems, and different active applications.

The purpose of virtualization is to make more efficient use of the servers. Advantages include flexibility of configuration, efficient use, and ease of updates and upgrades: New apps do not have to be installed on provider devices. Limitations of virtualization include poorer performance due to server sharing because instance configuration takes some resources.[7]

Client Strategy

Clients are the devices users employ to enter and view data. They can have minimal processing power or be robust computers themselves. Client strategy usually employs thick and thin clients.

Thick clients are standard desktop computers with our apps installed, which perform the tasks locally, and those apps could run even if the machine were not connected to the network. However, in the absence of network data, most of the clinical functions would be impossible.

Advantages of the thick client system are multiple. Performance is the principal reason for most thick client deployments. We have already discussed resource-hungry applications usually involving images or other large data files. Passing much information between the client and the server degrades performance significantly. Offline app function is usually limited on enterprise thick clients.

Thin clients are small computers with few resources. They are often so small that they sit almost invisibly behind or beneath the displays. Modern thin clients have just enough space for the connections. These connections include power, Internet connection, keyboard, mouse, and display. Thin clients are tasked with communicating securely with the servers. Commands are relayed to the centralized servers, and the display is generated locally. Processing of data takes place on the servers. Thin clients are inexpensive, and because they have minimal processing tasks, they do not have to be updated (software) or upgraded (hardware) often. Applications are only updated on the server side. Advantages include low price, small size, lower maintenance, and relative ease of securing from inappropriate use. Disadvantages include poor performance for resource-intensive applications, such as dealing with large arrays of data (e.g., EEGs or x-rays). For these, a thick client is usually needed.

A variation on the theme of thin client is sometimes called the *smart client*. This is a machine that tries to blend the thick and thin advantages. A shared library is stored and runs on the client, and that library looks to the network for data and instructions. The host server does not need to do all the operational tasks. Tools such as Adobe Flash and Java are used in some of these smart clients. These are faster than thin clients, especially when dealing with large chunks of data. The future of healthcare computing is expected to be increasingly using smart clients.

Zero clients are sometimes called *ultrathin clients*. These generally have no storage and no complete operating system, just the capacity to execute instructions to send information from user input and receive output to display for the user. The zero client has such elemental communicating abilities that the instruction set seldom requires updating and is relatively immune to attack.

Present and recommended client strategy can be as follows:

- *Thick client*: Radiology PACS, laboratory systems handling images; cardiology workstations reviewing catheter and echocardiographic visual data; office workstations for providers who need robust office capabilities
- *Thin client*: Nursing station devices; physician locations where only EHR basic input/output is needed
- *Zero client*: Clinical stations that do not demand more robust input/output and performance capacity
- *Smart client*: Likely will replace most provider and staff workstations, including thin and zero clients and some thick clients

Device Strategy

Device strategy is closely linked with client strategy, just discussed. In this discussion, we consider when each client type might be considered. Also, we consider some of the device options.

DESKTOP COMPUTER

The desktop is classically the thick client, with applications directly installed on the computer and the network used for data relay. Most processing is performed on the desktop. In reality, many desktops are used as thin clients; the EHR application is not installed on the desktop, but rather on centralized servers, and a gateway such as Citrix is used. Most of the local duties for the EHR are in reading and writing of data, so the local processing power is not optimally used.

Some apps are installed on the desktop and run locally, especially apps that depend on local processing power. Image-based apps are the most common in this category, such as radiology PACS, cardiology and gastroenterology imaging apps, and neurodiagnostic (EEG and electromyographic [EMG]) apps.

Apps for personal work use are commonly installed on a desktop designated for personal use (e.g., in an office). Common are office apps and enterprise communication apps, especially email and secure messaging apps. Alternatively, office apps can be run on the servers so that the worker can see the same desktop regardless of which user device is used.

Desktops can be installed in almost any area that has a surface, power, and an Internet connection. Desktops can also be placed on a cart that has an extended battery. These are often termed computers on wheels (COWs) or workstations on wheels (WOWs). The principal disadvantages of COWs are the need to be plugged in for recharging the batteries and the dependency on the wireless network. For most EHR tasks, this is not a critical factor. Desktops are used more commonly in inpatient settings.

LAPTOP

Laptops are predominantly used as mobile thin clients, with the use of a centralized group of servers that support virtual desktops. Laptops are only rarely used as thick clients because most devices with long battery life lack the processor power and resources to efficiently execute demanding applications, especially ones that depend on the wireless network for raw data. The wireless network is not best suited to movement of large amounts of data.

Laptops commonly have apps for personal use, such as email, secure messaging, office apps, and access apps, which aid the clinician in finding quick reference material. Laptops are used commonly in the outpatient arena. Because laptops are mobile, they must otherwise be secured to disallow unauthorized access.

THIN AND ULTRATHIN CLIENTS
Thin and ultrathin clients are commonly used for workstations used by multiple users. This would include nursing stations, pods, service areas such as the operating room, catheterization laboratory, gastrointestinal laboratory, and emergency department. Thin clients are seldom used for personal office desktop computers, although centralized access to productivity and communication apps can allow this to be done.

TABLETS
Tablets are commonly used for personal productivity purposes, and many EHR systems have apps for common tablet platforms. Portability and ease of use make these particularly efficient in hospital and office clinical practice, often obviating the need for devices installed in each room. There are limitations, however. Tablets commonly can do basic functions well but may have difficulty performing advanced functions, which might require a desktop or laptop. Tasks that tablets commonly can perform are document review, laboratory and radiology lookup, and single-order entry. Some allow for entry of field-based data.

The tablet version of EHR apps may have difficulty with more complex tasks, such as order sets, medicine reconciliation, and some decision support functions.

Security of tablets has to be carefully considered because many people share tablets with family members. Either this must not be allowed or the clinical apps must be configured such that unlocking of the tablet does not automatically unlock the clinical apps. Most organizations mitigate these issues using a medical device management (MDM) system. This allows them to quickly wipe any medical app if it is stolen so no patient information is at risk. The MDM system also enforces more stringent access controls to the personal device than would be required by the device manufacturer. Additionally, no medical information is stored on the device, but in a remote server. Some organizations decide to buy tablets for their clinicians, but most allow bring-your-own-device (BYOD) because of the MDM system.

The native EHR app usually used on a desktop or laptop can be used on most tablets. However, the client interface often has different abilities than the personal computer interface, making some tasks more difficult. It is usually, but not always, more efficient for the provider to use the EHR app designed for the tablet operating system than to use the tablet as a window to a virtual desktop.

Smartphones

Smartphones are pervasive in healthcare. An increasing number of healthcare systems allow use of enterprise phones for clinical and nonclinical purposes.

Viewing the desktop/laptop version of an EHR interface through a Citrix or similar farm is usually not optimal on a smartphone. The server farm may not support the resolution of the screen, and often the EHR app may not directly support the resolution of the phone. Some EHR vendors have smartphone apps with many functions, but often lacking some of the robust functions of the full desktop/laptop app. In Cerner's experience, 85% of clinicians choose to use their phone over a tablet when it comes to mobility. This is because of the convenience of having the phone with the clinician at all times. Most organizations have a BYOD policy with an MDM to manage the app. For those organizations concerned about infection issues, the phones can be placed in a plastic bag and can be used quite effectively.

Smartphones are likely to be used even more extensively in the future.

Device Ownership

Almost all healthcare systems provide devices for routine clinical use, usually as desktops but sometimes as laptops. Enterprise ownership makes control over updates and access easier than with personal devices. Most operating systems support the hardware and software infrastructure needed to secure the device.

Mobile devices such as laptops are convenient but easier to steal and harder to maintain because of their mobility. Our experience with enterprise-owned laptops has been that they have a much shorter work life than desktops because of the risk of physical and chemical damage. We have the general impression that users take better care of their personal device than an enterprise device, but we do not have proof of that.

There are advantages and disadvantages to enterprise versus user ownership of devices used for work (Table 9.1).

Mobile devices should be configured so that no Protected Health Information (PHI) or other confidential data are stored on the device, regardless of whether it is owned by the enterprise or users. We use virtual desktops for most clinical applications, so the user is only seeing a window to the application and not running the clinical application and storing data on the device. We use VPNs for some purposes, especially analytics and research access.

Hosting

Hosting refers to the computer system that supports the network of a client-server model. There is often confusion regarding definitions. A server is a computer that communicates with the client devices. The servers run the programs on which the clients depend. The host is a computer attached to a network and has an address on the network. The host may be a server or it might be an information resource, such as for PACS or laboratory information.

Table 9.1 DEVICE OWNERSHIP: ENTERPRISE VERSUS USER

Ownership	Advantages	Disadvantages
Enterprise	Easier to secure storage media. Easier to ensure access controls. Easier to ensure adequate performance.	May not be cared for as well as user-owned devices. May reduce productivity if devices are only available at the workplace. Costly to provide device(s) for users. Requires a support layer to maintain the devices.
User	Lower equipment cost. Productivity may increase with the mobile device, which the user takes home. Users can play a larger role in determining specifics of the device they use for work. Users often (but not always) prefer to have a single device.	Productivity may decrease if the users spend work time using personal applications on their device. The can be pushback from users because of their expense for work purposes. It is more difficult to secure data and ensure authorized access. Poor threat defense on personal devices may place the enterprise network at risk when connected. The user is more likely to install incompatible software on a personal device. User may claim enterprise responsibility for a personal device.

The servers often reside at the enterprise location, either in the same buildings or at least on campus. If there are multiple clinics or hospitals in a system, they usually use one data center to hold the servers, so at the outreach facilities, the computers are clients for most applications. This is *local hosting.*

Remote hosting is where the servers reside in a distant site, often hosted by a vendor or other third party. This arrangement depends on fast, dependable, and secure data movement between the remote hosts and the client devices at the clinical facility.

Local and remote hosting arrangements both have advantages and disadvantages. *Cost* is generally lower with remote hosting, which has the benefit of economy of scale. Setup and transition costs may make remote hosting more expensive in the short run, but we have found that remote hosting can be less expensive with contract times of at least 5–7 years.

Security might seem to be better with local hosting, but few healthcare systems have large security resources. Also, few healthcare systems have depth of knowledge of security threats and have difficulty keeping up with constantly evolving threats. Remote hosting services should have the scale of physical and technical security to protect from most threats.

Switching between local and remote hosting is expensive, so a possible change should be carefully considered. Local data centers are expensive and not only demand secure space for the servers but also require excellent power and Internet connectivity.

Domain Strategy

The servers are usually assigned to different groups termed *domains*. These are groups of servers that provide a network used for a specific purpose and group of users. For example, the domain in which we run our EHR and most active enterprise applications is the *Production* domain, termed *Prod*. We have other domains that are operationally separate. There are multiple others, but among these are *Build* and *Train*.

One way of thinking of domains is that they are separate *instances* of the system, for different purposes and living on different servers. New applications and upgrades are created in the Build domain. If this is a new application, then the Build domain is almost clean, just having the resources that emulate what is in Prod without the active application. The application is built in this Build domain. At the time of launch, the built application is copied to the Production domain and then turned on.

For an upgrade, the present Production domain application can be copied to the Build domain, the copy upgraded and tested, and then if all works well, the Prod application is upgraded with some assurance that the upgrade will work.

The Train domain is for training users for initial use or for training on upgraded functionality.

CONNECTIONS

Data is the lifeblood of healthcare information systems, so the connections are crucial. We consider some common methods of connecting systems.

Interfacing Versus Integrating

Interfacing is building a bridge between two or more systems to share data. The systems often have different inherent ways of dealing with data and may even be running on different operating systems.

Integration is making systems work as one, so that they share a common data structure and handle the information in a way that is fully compatible.

INTERFACING

Most premier EHR systems have integrated EHR, RIS, and PACS systems, but many enterprises have disparate systems for these tasks. In the case of different systems, interfacing is crucial. Diagnoses and other parameters of a radiology order have to be passed to the RIS and then PACS. Reports must be passed back to the EHR and be able to be directed to the inboxes of the ordering providers. These would be considered essential components of the EHR/RIS/PACS interface. In addition, the interface must be able to facilitate scheduling from within the EHR (requiring a push-through to the RIS), cancelations sent to the RIS must be able to remove tasks from the RIS list, and the PACS should be able to provide the capability of launching image viewing from links within the EHR. These functions are not available on all interfaced systems but should be.

There are hundreds of interfaces in our system. We accomplish these in two ways. First is a series of system-to-system, manually configured interfaces. This requires ensuring that the systems receive requests for information that they can understand, can deliver information that the other system can understand, and can transmit the appropriate data.

The second method of interfacing is using interface engines. This system is designed specifically to move data between disparate systems. We use two of these for many of our interfacing tasks. These are commercial systems with hardware and software components. While interface engines automate many interfacing tasks, they are not plug-and-play devices.

INTEGRATION

Integration is when systems are seamlessly able to share information, often giving the user experience of being a single system. In our healthcare systems, we have a mixture of interfaced and integrated systems for EHR and the LIS. The system with integrated EHR and LIS does not need further interfacing, although there are configurations governing how data are presented and handled in the EHR database.

In general, we try to select vendors such that as much of the system is integrated as possible, with interfacing used for other information movement needs. This does make best-of-breed selection for every application more difficult. Best of breed was a good approach to application selection when local niche data storage and retrieval were the focus. With the present and future demand for centralized data access, integrated apps become favored as long as they can do the job sufficiently.

Data Exchange

Data exchange between healthcare systems can be accomplished in a variety of ways. Among these are

- Point-to-point connection
- Direct messaging
- HIE

Point-to-point connections are similar to internal interfaces but with an external system. Cooperation between information systems staff of two enterprises can result in the ability to exchange data between them with certain rules and procedures. This is most commonly performed between a hospital and a community clinic.

Direct messaging is a protocol required for Meaningful Use. A document is created and sent in an encrypted format, which is then decrypted and available for display at the receiving facility. This is commonly used for transition-of-care (TOC) documents. These contain selected fields from the EHR, just some of which are identifiers, diagnoses, medications, and laboratory results.

A *continuity-of-care document* (CCD) is an XML[8]-based standard established by HL7 (Health Level Seven International). A document following the CCD format will have much of the information suitable for HIE. The CCD is a part of the CDA, Clinical Document Architecture. This HL7-established standard includes not only textual information but also tags and instructions. The CCD was developed with a view to the continuity-of-care record (CCR), an electronically transmittable document to help with care transitions.

The HL7 *Consolidated CDA* (C-CDA) is a combination of templates for implementation of the most common CDAs. This makes implementation of CDA easier but is not turnkey.

Health information exchanges have been established in many geographic areas with variable success. Many have failed. In theory, the HIE is supposed to facilitate care by bringing together data from a variety of systems. We belong to an HIE, and affiliates on the exchange can share clinical information with the exchange system providing not only the connection, but also the context to the connection; that is, data elements are associated with related data elements from the different systems. Some exchanges normalize the data so laboratory studies can be directly compared despite differences in laboratory methods and data configuration. This is discussed further in Chapter 25.

In the future, the HOS will allow EHRs from different vendors, patient portals, patient wearables, medical devices, data repositories, and other outside sources of data to connect seamlessly in a secured cloud via advanced interoperability. Many of these standards are being set today.

Faxing and Printers

Printing and faxing are still widely used in healthcare despite efforts to transition to paperless practice. Drivers of persistent printing and faxing include

- Anchoring in prior practice methods.
- Difficulty with interfacing EHRs.
- Slow and incomplete integration of EHRs.
- Difficulty with e-prescribing, either by unfamiliarity of process or lack of two-factor authentication for controlled substances.
- Some clinicians still prefer paper to electronic use for office visits, hospital rounding, laboratory check offs, and so on.

Faxing is the default method of transmission of information when interface status is unknown. It is easier to order a fax to be sent than to investigate the possibility of electronic transfer. Many fax machines continue to print paper versions of the documents, although others will store the documents digitally and then allow for screen viewing or incorporation into the EHR. The fax is reliable and a part of former workflows for decades, making it difficult to replace.

We need to move from printing and faxing to electronic data transfer, but this transition will continue to be slow. When there is no consensus on how data are sent, the lowest tech common method will be used; right now, that is faxing. We suspect the transition will only occur when there is technical consensus, when all EHRs can seamlessly transmit and incorporate the data, and when regulatory requirements include the need to have data in a format that is amenable to incorporation into the EHR.

We often consider the security of electronic transmissions, but we do not give sufficient attention to the security issues surrounding selected printing and faxing and paper records in general. Some examples of behaviors that place a clinic at high risk for HIPAA (Health Insurance Portability and Accountability Act) violation include leaving reports or laboratory results on a desk after hours, paper encounter scribble sheet with PHI visible in a clinic door bin, or faxes with PHI left in the fax machine after hours. Many clinics do not adhere to the requirement of securing paper records.

KEY POINTS

- Design of the HOS and the EHR must keep the aim in mind of excellence and efficiency of patient care.
- Device strategy depends on the practice and workflow of the user. Mobile devices are most often for bedside tasks. Desktop workstations are used more for prolonged epochs of EHR use and for resource-intensive applications.
- Client-server strategy with server virtualization results in optimal flexibility for users and for application environment requirements.
- Impediments to data access can jeopardize patient care.

Data Repositories

KARL E. MISULIS AND MARK E. FRISSE ■

OVERVIEW

Data types and modeling and an introduction to database technical theory are discussed in Chapter 7. In that chapter, we discuss data types and both relational and hierarchical databases. Here, we focus on data storage, retrieval, and database queries.

DATABASE CONSTRUCTION

The term *database*, in our context, means the entirety of the data storage and retrieval system. This includes the physical data storage and the database management system (DBMS). The DBMS determines the means of data storage and retrieval, the data type handling, the search capabilities of the system, and the rules that govern database function. In general, the physical database cannot be controlled by another DBMS.

Migration from one DBMS to another is possible but requires quite a bit of work. Reasons for changing DBMSs may be vendor issues, mergers, or acquisitions.

Relational and hierarchical databases both write data, but how the data are written and how they are searched differ. The first databases in routine use were little more than lists, but the next evolution was when connections between elements were created: the *navigational* database, where data elements point to other data elements with their relationships. IBM evolved this type to *hierarchical,* where the navigation connections are all *parent-child* or *one-to-many. Relational* database structure was subsequently developed, also at IBM, to efficiently deal with larger data sets, and this used the indexed multitabular arrangement we use today.

The grandfather of medical databases systems, Massachusetts General Hospital Utility Multi-Programming System, (MUMPS), used one form of the navigational structure. MUMPS provides efficient transactional[1] data storage and query. A descendent of this structure is still in use with some EHRs, including Epic.

The relational model of database structure was developed a few years after the generation of MUMPS. There are a number of differences between relational databases and MUMPS, including data type constraints, but the iconic element is the tabular organization. There is no tree to follow. Many EHRs use relational databases, including Cerner's EHRs.

The relative merits of the relational and hierarchical database systems can be debated, but effectively, the clinical user sees no significant difference in function or performance.

Database Rules

There is a series of rules that databases and the DBMS should adhere to. These serve to reduce the chance of database errors. Errors can develop especially when data from multiple users are being written to the database simultaneously, a common occurrence in healthcare.

Some of the rules are as follows:

- *Atomicity*: Each transaction is all or none, meaning that if writing part of the transaction fails, the database is left as it was before the change was attempted.
- *Consistency*: The database remains valid after changes are made, meaning that there are appropriate data types and constraints in place for the changes applied.
- *Isolation*: Transactions applied to the database simultaneously result in the same appearance as if they were applied sequentially.
- *Durability*: Transaction data recorded remain unchanged despite a number of events, such as a system crash or power loss.
- Only one user can write into a field at a time.
- No record can actually be deleted.
- All changes are logged.
- Data index keys must be unique and unchangeable.

The first four go by the acronym ACID.[2] Let us consider some details.

Atomicity uses the term *atom* from *atomos,* in Greek meaning indivisible. If the entire transaction cannot be written to the database, the database is left as it was before the attempted update.

Consistency refers to the expectation that all of the constraints on data types, string lengths, value limits, and other parameters of the entries adhere to the rules of the database. In short, this indicates that the database remains valid after the transaction. This is accomplished by the DBMS by not recording transactions that would violate database rules.

Isolation refers to the independence of transactions in updating the database. Specifically, this means that if two or more transactions occur simultaneously that were judged to be valid by the DBMS, then writing of one does not affect writing of the other. So, whether they are written simultaneously or sequentially, the database would look the same after the transactions.

Durability refers to the expectation that once the transactions are written, they are stable even in the event of power loss or system crash. Once power has been restored or system function is restored, the record of the transaction is still there. This is accomplished partly by physically writing the data to the media, but of course, later transactions can modify data on specific fields. This is also accomplished, and even more so in our opinion, by writing logs of changes to the database. These logs are kept and usually redundant.

One user at a time refers to a prohibition of more than one user writing to the same field at a time. This is covered in ACID, but deserves special attention because there are often thousands of concurrent users online with an EHR, with several users perhaps working on the record of a single patient.

Regarding *no record is deleted*, even entries in error are logged as individual transactions, so that the error can be audited. This is true even if there are errors in the database entry—not an error in the database itself, but an error in the data entered into the database. For example, if a patient is given two different medical record numbers due to confusion about date of birth or expression of name, the records are merged for clinical and business use, but the duplicate entry is not actually deleted.

All changes logged is a requirement for backup not only in case of damage to the database, but also in case of a system outage during the process of writing a transaction. Data-writing processes are designed to minimize partial entries, but the logs store records of all of the changes made.

In relational databases, *keys* must be unique and unchangeable. Otherwise, keys would point to the wrong records.

There are other rules, and these are mainly handled by the DBMS. Most databases are commercially acquired, either from the EHR vendor or from a third party.

DATA WAREHOUSES AND DATA MARTS

Data warehouses are *secondary databases*, meaning that they are not directly populated by data from the healthcare providers. The data include a subset of data in the *primary database*, which is the operational repository of data for patient care. Data from other sources are often incorporated as well. Therefore, the primary EHR database can be considered the transactional database, used for active healthcare transactions, and the secondary databases are derived from one or more primary databases and are used for analytics and sometimes data sharing. The data warehouse is not intended to be the complete record needed for delivery of healthcare.

Extract, Transform, and Load

A commonly used acronym for the processes of moving data into a data warehouse is ETL, for extract, transform, and load. *Extract* is where the data is obtained electronically from one or more data sources, usually EHRs, specialty clinical applications, and financial databases. Therefore, data populating the warehouse are very different from data in the primary EHR database, where data is stored in fields on a transactional basis. For extraction, the data are pulled according to specific criteria. Set criteria determine which data are to be uploaded because much of the information in the EHR does not need to be loaded into the data warehouse.

Transform is where the data are converted into a format for recording in the secondary database. Some of the transformations are related to different specifications of the warehouse. For example, the warehouse may be extracting data from two different EHRs, one from a hospital and one from a clinic or another affiliated hospital. In one EHR, gender might be coded by a number code, whereas in the other it might be coded by a letter. Additionally, duplicative data are often eliminated; for example, there may be a field for age as well as date of birth. Only the date of birth is needed, and age can be calculated. An important transformation is to reconcile differences in how data are expressed; certain laboratory values may be expressed with different units or may be performed with differing techniques, needing calculated transformations to make the data comparable between sources.

Load is where the data are uploaded to the secondary database. Part of the load task is also to ensure that the data conform to constraints of the warehouse. For example, data older than a certain date might not be loaded because the purpose of the warehouse may be to look at only recent data. Alternatively, there may be conflicting data in the pipeline from two data sources, such as identical medical record numbers but somewhat differing names; in this case, the patient may have different versions used for different purposes, business versus personal or married versus single versus divorced. Sometimes, these differences can be automatically reconciled during the load process, but at other times, this has to be sent to a queue to be handled manually.

Master Patient Index

The master patient index (MPI) is a database that can be part of an EHR or be a separate database with connections to one or more EHRs and other healthcare data systems. To accomplish this task, the MPI has a unique identifying number for each patient plus sufficient demographics such that matching patient identification can usually be ensured.

The MPI includes a variety of data elements but may typically include name(s), date of birth, gender, ethnicity, address, Social Security number, and modes of contact, including phone numbers and email addresses. Additional information can include diagnoses, recent encounters, or insurance information.

When the EHR searches for a patient to create an encounter, it queries the MPI so that there is a match between clinical and nonclinical systems and between data warehouses and health information exchanges.

With the term *enterprise* often used for the compilation of entities consolidated into a larger healthcare system, the term *enterprise master patient index* (EMPI) is increasingly used. Each EHR and specialty information system will have its own patient index, so the EMPI is a way to bridge these systems.

The MPI engine compares new registrations with those already stored, so that patients are matched. There are *deterministic* matches, with clear matching on the basis of name, date of birth, or other elements that, with agreement, make identity certain. There are also *probabilistic* matches, with a probability assigned to the parameters of comparative demographics. A specified probability may be judged to be sufficient to indicate matching. However, there will always be cases for which the computer cannot decide, and human judgment has to be used.

In routine medical practice, when searching for a patient's record, there will be cases where a patient is found to have two or more different records in the system. The user discovering the duplication should inform the health information management (HIM) department so the identity can be validated and the records merged. Much rarer is for the records of two patients to be merged into one; when recognized, it should be brought to the attention of HIM.

A national MPI has been discussed in the United States, but the present cultural and political climate make this unlikely to materialize.

Rationale for Secondary Data Storage

The primary database is not optimally configured for analytics. This is true especially for hierarchical databases but also is somewhat true for relational databases. Hierarchical databases with the parent/child structure make a query for patients of a certain characteristic somewhat difficult (e.g., searching for all patients between the ages of 50 and 60 years with diabetes but not congestive heart failure who have had an admission with diabetic ketoacidosis in the past year and who live within 25 miles of your hospital).

The secondary databases are populated with data that are likely to be used for analytics, and as such, many institutions have multiple data warehouses and data marts. One might be a general analytics warehouse with a subset of data on patients admitted to the hospital. Another might be a cancer registry.

Technical Aspects

Data warehouses and data marts are relational databases, stored on physical media, just like the primary EHR database. If the primary EHR database is hierarchical, the secondary database is still typically relational.

Data Warehouses

A subset of clinical and often financial data is populated into the data warehouse. Often, the warehouse has data from multiple sources, so there is information not contained in the primary EHR database. For example, the warehouse may include data from multiple clinical databases (e.g., if there is more than one EHR used by the enterprise), a financial database, and specialty databases, as would be used by cardiology, gastroenterology, and radiology (PACS and RIS).

William Inmon[1], a pioneer in data warehousing, defined the fundamental features of a data warehouse[2]:

- Subject oriented
- Integrated
- Nonvolatile
- Time variant

Subject oriented: The data warehouse is designed with the potential question(s) in mind. This is needed to select the appropriate data to extract from the primary database(s).

Integrated: Data from different sources need to be able to be considered together, and this sometimes requires transformation. For example, cholesterol levels and international normalized ratios are dependent on the equipment used to run the analyses, so different normal values may be applicable; a transformation may be needed so the numbers can be compared.

Nonvolatile: The data should not change and not disappear once they have entered the warehouse.

Time variant: Analytics often look at trends or performance, so keeping data for an extended time is usually warranted.

Data warehouses pull most data at times of lower overall system load so that the queries do not degrade clinical system performance. For example, one of our healthcare systems performs the daily queries at 2:00 AM.

Analytics are performed on the data warehouse using one of a number of software packages. We presently have multiple analytics packages with different purposes, only one of which is from the EHR vendor. In addition, we often extract queried data into an Excel spreadsheet. Analytics is discussed in depth in Chapter 16.

Data Marts

A data mart is similar to a data warehouse but with a restricted focus, typically on a single issue. For example, we use a data mart to follow the glucose values of patients admitted as inpatients or for observation to identify patients with incipient

---

1. https://en.wikipedia.org/wiki/Bill_Inmon

2. What is a Data Warehouse? W.H. Inmon, Prism, Volume 1, Number 1, 1995.

or poorly controlled diabetes. This task could not be performed with our data warehouse because not every point-of-care glucose is populated into the warehouse. Also, the warehouse only is populated once per 24 hours, whereas for the purpose of identifying some conditions, such as sepsis or poor glucose control, more frequent data queries are needed. While our point-of-care glucose is seamlessly integrated into our EHR laboratory data presently, this was not always the case; at an earlier time, the data mart integrated data from those sources independently.

Other common uses of data marts are for departmental metrics, specialty programs (e.g., cardiology), or trial analytics.

Data marts may be derived from data warehouses, but this does not have to be the case. Data marts can integrate information, including data not brought into an existing data warehouse.

Data Lake

A *data lake*[3] is a large data repository where usually vast amounts of data are stored for later query and analytics. Unlike warehouses and marts, the questions to be asked do not need to be considered on the front end. Data are dumped into the lake along with tags to facilitate query and are left there until a use is found.

The lack of defined purpose is a principal feature of a data lake. Also, a data lake often contains substantial unstructured data. This is less true for data warehouses and marts.

The data lake frequently does not perform the transformation or other organization of data that the warehouses and marts would perform. These tasks are performed during the later data study.

QUERY

A database query is performed for a variety of reasons. Some of them are

- Analytics
- Patient lists
- Patient search

Information on each patient is stored in multiple tables of a relational database, so to find the information we need, we have to be able to search beyond single tables. For example, if we want to pull a list of patients admitted within the past 24 hours who have glucose values of more than 300 mg/dL yet are not diagnosed with diabetes, we query for these three parameters:

- Admit time ≤ 24 hours
- Glucose > 300 mg/dL
- Diagnosis ≠ Diabetes

There are many diagnostic codes for diabetes, so when we specify "not diabetes," we have to use a search algorithm that specifically excludes records that contain any of these diagnostic codes.

Queries often are not completely automatic. For example, there will be patients who have known diabetes mellitus yet have not had diabetes added to their problem or diagnosis lists, so those patient names would be manually removed from the list after the fact.

Query Mechanisms

Queries are performed using applications that search the database using specified parameters. Historically, a command line interface was used, but presently, most queries are performed using scripting. Queries can use interfaces specific to the database vendor or from a third party. Queries of health information require advanced skills and experience, so most informatics professionals are unlikely to perform searches themselves, but it is instructive to see how they are written. When vendor applications are used, they essentially turn the menu commands into query script.

Structured Query Language

Structured Query Language (SQL) was developed in the 1970s at IBM for query of relational databases. SQL is in widespread use, and variations exist for specific systems. SQL has a fairly intuitive set of search commands.

To show an example of SQL, we have to create a sample database. Our database has three tables: *Patients, Diagnoses*, and *Genetics*.

The Patients table (Table 10.1) contains only three patients, and the ID number is the primary key for this table.

The Diagnoses table (Table 10.2) has primary and secondary diagnoses for these three patients. The first column is the index for this table and as such is the primary key for this table. The second column has the ID number for each patient, which points to the Patients table, and is the foreign key.

The Genetics table (Table 10.3) has the results of gene testing for each of the three patients. The first column is the index for this table, the primary key. The second column is the patient ID, which points to the Patients table, the foreign key.

Looking at the data, we can see that Patient Betty Beta is age 60, had diagnoses of stroke and breast cancer, and was negative on both gene tests. We get this by finding

Table 10.1 PATIENTS

IDNumber	LastName	FirstName	Age
1001	Alpha	Adam	50
1002	Beta	Betty	60
1003	Gamma	George	70

Table 10.2 Diagnoses

DxEntryNum	IDNumber	PrimaryDx	SecondaryDx
2001	1001	Lung cancer	Stroke
2002	1002	Stroke	Breast cancer
2003	1003	Pulmonary embolism	Melanoma

Table 10.3 Genetics

GeneticsEntryNum	IDNumber	GeneDelta	GeneEpsilon
3001	1001	Positive	Negative
3002	1002	Negative	Negative
3003	1003	Negative	Positive

the name in the Patients table, looking up the ID number, then going to the second columns of the Diagnoses and Genetics tables to find the additional data from the rows with the same ID number.

It we want a table of ages of the patients in the table, we might begin our SQL query like this:

```
SELECT Age FROM Patients;
```

This returns a list of ages of the patients from this table.

```
50
60
70
```

If we wanted a list of first and last names from this table,

```
SELECT FirstName, LastName FROM Patients;
      Adam Alpha
      Beta Beta
      George Gamma
```

If we wanted to display all of the columns in the table, we would use a wildcard:

```
SELECT * FROM Patients;
      1001 Alpha Adam 50
      1002 Beta Betty 60
      1003 Gamma George 70
```

So far, we have only been looking at data from a single table. The JOIN command will be used to combine outputs from different tables.

Now, we want to create a list of primary diagnoses side by side with Gene Delta results, regardless of the identity of the patients the data came from. The JOIN command can join lines between at least two different tables.

```
SELECT Diagnoses.PrimaryDx, Genetics.GeneDelta
FROM Diagnoses
INNER JOIN Genetics ON Diagnoses.IDNumber=Genetics.
IDNumber
```

Produces:

```
Lung cancer              Positive
Stroke                   Negative
Pulmonary embolism       Negative
```

Dissecting this a bit, the first line says we want to return the primary diagnosis (PrimaryDx) from table Diagnoses (Diagnoses.PrimaryDx) and the Gene Delta results (GeneDelta) from table Genetics (Genetics.GeneDelta).

The INNER JOIN statement means that we want to join data where the patient ID number from table Diagnoses (Diagnoses.IDNumber) is equal to the patient ID number in table Genetics (Genetics.IDNumber), meaning that they are from the same patient.

The JOIN command has several variations. INNER JOIN means to return records that have matching entries in both tables. In the case example, this means that the ID numbers were the same, indicating that the data are from the same patient.

LEFT OUTER JOIN returns all of the requested data from the first table and the associated data from the second table that is from the same patient. In our database example, because all patients are in all three tables, there will not be any null fields, but if we wanted to return the last name for all patients and primary diagnosis where one has been designated, we would use the following query:

```
SELECT Patients.LastName, Diagnoses.PrimaryDx
FROM Patients
LEFT OUTER JOIN Diagnoses ON Patients.
IDNumber=Diagnoses.IDNumber
```

This returns the last name for every patient and primary diagnoses for ones who have one entered. If a primary diagnosis field was empty or null, the name would be returned with a blank spot of NULL for the diagnosis.

RIGHT OUTER JOIN returns all of the records from the second table and associated data from the first table where there is a matching condition:

```
SELECT Diagnoses.PrimaryDx, Genetics.GeneDelta
FROM Diagnoses
RIGHT OUTER JOIN Genetics ON Diagnoses.
IDNumber=Genetics.IDNumber
```

Note that you would receive the same results if you switched your table references and used LEFT OUTER JOIN again.

FULL OUTER JOIN returns the data of both first and second tables, matching their data, leaving blank spaces if there are missing or null data.

```
SELECT Diagnoses.SecondaryDx, Genetics.GeneEpsilon
FROM Diagnoses
FULL OUTER JOIN Genetics ON Diagnoses.
IDNumber=Genetics.IDNumber
```

This table would be all of the data where there is matching IDNumber regardless of whether a secondary diagnosis or gene epsilon test resulted.

While we are using LEFT RIGHT and FULL for OUTER JOINs, the OUTER JOINs are often just called LEFT JOIN, RIGHT JOIN, and FULL JOIN.

The WHERE command is the last considered here. WHERE specifies conditions for the return of data. Using the data tables previously discussed, if we want to return a list of patients with a last name of Beta, we would do the following:

```
SELECT * FROM Patients
WHERE LastName='Beta'
```

Commands such as these and many others are used in combination to make complex queries.

The important aspect of this discussion is not to enable the reader to design and create database queries, but rather for the reader to have a basic understanding of how queries are done. In roles in analytics and data governance, it is important to understand the basics so that the strengths and weaknesses of the query functions are known.

HOSTING STRATEGY

Hosting refers to where the database and servers reside. Traditionally, healthcare facilities have had an on-site data center that contains the servers with their associated hardware—hubs, switches, routers, and myriad cables—along with emergency power supply (UPS—Uninterruptable Power Supply) and air conditioning. Even in cooler climates, the heat generated by the servers requires air conditioning. Overheating of electronics results in susceptibility to element failure.

If there is a single data center, then periodic backups are performed, usually daily, and the backup media are stored off site. Common locations include bank vaults or other physically secure locations.

Some larger healthcare systems have more than one data center. This has often evolved from a time when the system's first data center has been outgrown by the expansion of computer hardware requirements. A second data center offers some security in that a catastrophe in one data center does not affect the entire data systems, yet it does double the number of areas where disaster might strike.

Hosting Options

Hosting options include

- Local hosting
- Remote hosting
- Cloud services

This discussion concerns database hosting, not Web hosting, such as for an organization's website.

Local hosting is where the on-site enterprise data center has the servers and all associated hardware and software for the systems. This has traditionally been the most commonly used model. Advantages of local hosting include the lack of need for external data connection (see remote hosting, next), the ability to use on-site staff to replace servers or otherwise troubleshoot hardware problems, and the ability to actually see physical hardware security. Costs are great up front because of the need to purchase the hardware, but costs may be lower over time, although servers eventually do have to be replaced.

Remote hosting is where the physical servers and storage media are in a remote location, usually a contracted third party. This is sometimes the EHR vendor but does not need to be. Communications between the remote host and the enterprise are through the Internet or through dedicated fiber-optic connections. Remote hosting has a lower startup cost than local hosting, but there is an ongoing service charge, usually based on some measure of server load.

Cloud hosting differs from remote hosting in that there are no dedicated servers for the enterprise; rather, virtual servers are created with the applications needed. There is a limitation on the applications available in this type. Advantages include less concern about local physical security and the availability of additional tools that often come with cloud services. However, Internet security and ensured availability are concerns.

Often, healthcare systems use a combination of these options, with specifics for different purposes. Some applications are local hosted, some remote hosted, and some cloud hosted.

One of our affiliates uses remote hosting for acute and ambulatory EHRs, local hosting for most specialty applications, and cloud services for Web services, including patient portal, some analytics, and some decision support. To ensure security and availability, this healthcare system has two dedicated fiber-optic lines for communication between the remote hosts and the hospitals.

This affiliate relies on vendors for the security of the remote servers, and this is not a task some information systems executives are willing to give up. However, the resources for security in our large healthcare systems are a tiny fraction of the physical and technical security abilities and resources of the vendor.

DOWNTIME DATA REPOSITORIES

Downtime data repositories are the backbone of downtime procedures. The data are just one part of the issue. There are reasonable expectations that patient data will be available during downtimes. There are no specific requirements for how this is done, but there is an information source by the Office of the National Coordinator for Health Information Technology (ONC)[4] that healthcare systems use to assess readiness for downtime. We should be familiar with this information.

Mechanisms to mitigate downtime effects include

- Centralized redundancy
- Centralized downtime database
- Local downtime database
- Dedicated downtime apps
- Paper

Centralized redundancy means having a separate set of servers such that if the production servers are all disabled, there is a set of servers that can immediately be implemented. Sometimes, they are already on task but mirroring the production servers until the production server system fails. This is very expensive, essentially having a total duplication of your data center.

Somewhat less expensive is a remote hosting vendor having servers available to switch to our database in case of failure of our servers. In this case, the new servers do not already have our applications loaded, so it can take several hours for this material to load, and local downtime processes have to be used meanwhile.

A *centralized downtime database* has a duplicate of the present database that is queried by a program with limited functionality. Often, this is a database that does not have all of the data from the production files but rather records from recent transactions. For example, one downtime system provides 48-hour look back for some affiliated hospitals in our network. This is read only and includes notes, laboratory tests, radiology reports, cardiology reports, records of medication orders during the epoch, and a clinical snapshot, meaning orders and diagnoses active for each patient at the time the downtime system was activated.

The *local downtime database* is similar to the centralized downtime database, but this is local to the nursing unit. The provider has to go to that unit to see the records of the patient.

Downtime apps are of various types. They can be a subset of the native EHR with the same look and feel but with reduced functionality, or a document viewer, which is intuitive but not the same interface as the EHR. This is similar to CCD or PDF viewers, which frequently are executed from within EHRs. No user instruction is needed.

During downtime, *paper* may have to be used, especially for orders and for writing notes. After the downtime is over, the notes are scanned into the EHR, and the orders are entered after the fact.

If downtime is planned, we recommend that our providers print their patient lists and perhaps clinical snapshots of their patients shortly before the scheduled downtime. The clinical snapshot is a single-page document generated by the EHR and includes a variety of elements, often consisting of essential demographics, code status, diagnoses and problems, medications, 36 hours of laboratory reports, last vital signs, highest/lowest vital signs within the past 24 hours, and intakes and outputs.

Reasons for a downtime procedure needs are multiple; among the most common are

- Server failure
- Software crash
- Power failure
- Network failure
- Remote access communication failure
- Updates or new installations

Server failure could be in the server farm that is used for the EHR or in servers that control the network. Failure of a single server is unlikely to result in the need for downtime procedures because the load is transferred to functioning servers when one goes offline. The user may have to reconnect, but the other servers usually take the load. If there is sufficient data center damage so that all of the servers are offline, then redundancy is activated if available. Otherwise, the downtime database goes online on the network.

A *software crash* can occur especially after a recent update. More common is an error in execution rather than a total failure. But, if there is a software failure that makes it inoperable, then centralized downtime procedures are activated.

A *power failure* results in loss of function that depends on configuration. All hospitals have emergency backup power; however, there may be reboots caused by the switchover. Desktops may or may not have uninterruptible power supplies (UPSs). Routers and access points may be on a UPS. On-site data centers almost always have backup power to bridge the switch to emergency power.

Network failure can occur especially if there is a software or hardware failure affecting network control. Healthcare networks are quite complex and require sophisticated programs to control data flow, bandwidth assignment, and security. If this fails, local downtime procedures have to be used.

Remote access communication failure can occur if the connection between the facility and the remote hosting vendor is lost. This is less likely with dedicated fiber-optic connections and more likely with Internet access. Some fiber-optic connections can fail, however, so we have duplicate connections.

Updates may require downtime if all of the servers have to be taken offline for installation of the new packages. More commonly, servers are updated in a rolling fashion, so that the user either does not notice the change or only is kicked off and can immediately log in again.

Downtime procedures should be tested and performance assessed during scheduled downtimes to ensure that in the event of an unscheduled downtime the procedures are in place and the staff are adequately trained for the eventuality.

KEY POINTS

- Data are the lifeblood of the healthcare system.
- Database construction and function are foundational to the EHR.

- Data warehouses are used for tasks that include data analytics.
- Data marts are typically single-issue databases used for restricted queries.
- The MPI and the EMPI facilitate identification of patients, including those from different data sources.
- SQL is a commonly used database query language.
- Hosting of servers can be local or remote, with cloud hosting a form of remote hosting. Each has advantages and disadvantages.
- Downtime systems can have a variety of mechanisms, but most employ a select extract of the database.

Decision-Making

KARL E. MISULIS AND MARK E. FRISSE ∎

OVERVIEW

Decision-making consists of the logical application of information. Much of the discussion in this text concerns acquisition, storage, retrieval, and presentation of information. This chapter concerns the logical aspects of decision-making, including statistics and logic theory.

STATISTICS

Statistics is the analysis and interpretation of numerical data. Statistics is an extensive field, and the data handling we consider represents only a small fraction of the field. We first consider probability and then move to more advanced statistical analysis, covering some of the most important concepts for clinical informatics. This is not intended to be a comprehensive discussion of statistics but rather a description of some of the fundamental applications of statistics to healthcare.

Probability Theory

Probability theory is a method to describe and predict the outcome of events where there is a distribution of possible results. The specifics of probability calculation

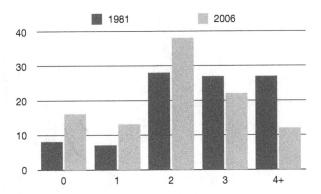

Discrete Distribution
Number of children per mother in Australia (%)

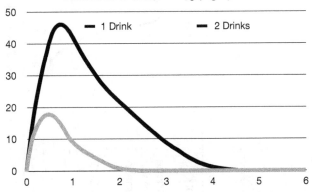

Continuous Distribution
Alcohol level after drinking (mg%)

Figure 11.1 Distributions. Top is a discrete distribution, which is real data on number of children per mother in Australia in two different years. This is a Poisson distribution. This is discrete because there can be no value of 1.2, for example. There is only one significant digit. Bottom is a continuous distribution, which is also an Australian study reporting blood alcohol levels after one or two drinks. This is continuous because there is a continuum of alcohol levels; so, for hour 1 we average the levels for a number of people, and each level has potentially infinite significant digits.

depend on the type of data and distribution. Figure 11.1 shows real examples of data in discrete and continuous distributions. Figure 11.2 shows a variety of distributions, idealized for illustrative purposes.

Discrete distribution is where the result is countable. In healthcare, discrete data include number of children a woman has had. A Poisson distribution is a discrete distribution. Age might seem to be discrete, but when we say someone is 37 years old, we are rounding; they are 37 years and some number of days, hours, minutes, seconds, and fractions thereof.

Continuous distribution is where the result can be any value or fraction thereof on a distribution. Most healthcare data are continuous (e.g., sodium level). The

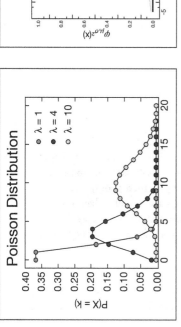
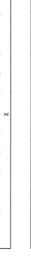
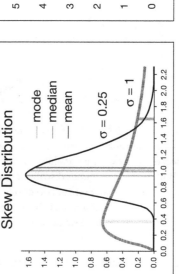
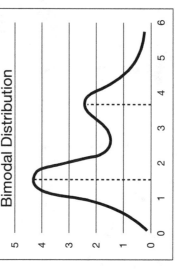

Figure 11.2 Distributions (for Poisson). Top left: Poisson distribution. A discrete distribution that could be represented by bars, but in this diagram, the indicator symbols are connected. Top right: Normal distributions: All of these are normal, with equal appearance of values and area on the two sides with a formulaic design. The difference between lines refers to differences in mean and variance. Bottom left: Skew deviation. The distribution deviated from normal by the mean not in the middle of the distribution. All of these are skew, but the level of skewness differs. Bottom right: Bimodal distribution. This has the appearance of two normal or two skew deviations summed, but it does not need to appear this way. This vector image was created with Matplotlib, CC BY 3.0, https://commons.wikimedia.org/w/index.php?curid=9447142. For skew, by Cmglee, own work, CC BY-SA 3.0, https://commons.wikimedia.org/w/index.php?curid=15147460.

bell-shaped normal distribution is a common continuous distribution, but often medical data are not normally distributed. They may have a skewed or even bimodal distribution. Some statistical tests depend on a normal distribution, but not all.

Continuous distributions are described by the *cumulative distribution function* (CDF). This is a function that describes the probability that a sample value will be greater or less than a specific value. The specifics of the formula depend on the distribution; a formula that characterizes a normal distribution is different from one for a skewed distribution.

Probability theory describes the behavior of events. Some of the questions that can be answered include the following:

- What is the chance of event A?
- Are event A and event B linked?
- If event A occurs, what is the likelihood of event B?
- If event A does not occur, what is the likelihood of event B?

The chance of event A is described by a number. A probability of 0 means that the event is certain to not occur. A probability of event A of 1 means that the event is certain to occur. Probabilities of greater than 1 or less than 0 cannot occur.

If one of two events has to occur, either event A or event B, the probability of event A plus the probability of event B sums to 1. An example is a coin toss, where the result would be heads or tails. We will ignore the theoretical possibility of a coin landing on edge.

If there are six possible events, A, B, C, D, E, and F, and one of them has to occur, then the sum of the probabilities of each has to be 1. An example would be dice, with each of the faces of the die having unique markings.

In the two examples, the probabilities are equal for the results. For the coin:

$$P_{heads} = P_{tails} = 0.5$$
$$P_{heads} + P_{tails} = 1.0$$

For the die:

$$P_{1dot} = P_{2dots} = \cdots = P_{6dots} = \frac{1}{6} = 0.1667$$

$$\sum_{i}^{P} = 1.0$$

which indicates that the probabilities P are summed over the six possible individual outcomes i for the roll of the die.

In healthcare, the probabilities of specific events are usually unequal. After administration of intravenous tissue plasminogen activator (tPA) for acute ischemic stroke, the probability of symptomatic intracranial hemorrhage is about 3% in many stroke centers. Healthcare becomes complicated when the probability is dependent not only on the biology of the condition but also on the timing of the measurement. Symptomatic intracranial hemorrhage is more likely several hours after administration of tPA but much less likely to be evident immediately after completion of the hour-long administration. The distribution of the probability of developing symptomatic intracranial hemorrhage as a function of time might look something like the lower image of Figure 11.1. The maximal probability is several hours after administration, with lower probability before and after. This distribution is a *skew distribution*.

In the stroke example, time from tPA administration to hemorrhage is a continuous variable. If the distribution is discrete (e.g., number of hemorrhages during each hour after the tPA), then there can also be a skew distribution, but in that case the *mode* (most common value) is different from the *median* (middle value) or the *mean* (average value).

Some laboratory values may have a distribution of biologically-normal results that appear to be in a statistically-normal distribution, but unfortunately, in healthcare, truly normal distributions are uncommon, with most only approximating normal distributions even for what we would consider to be laboratory values in the expected range of norms. In addition, the distribution of abnormal results is far from *normal*, in the distribution sense.

So, what is abnormal? To determine what is abnormal, we need to know what is the *variance* of the data. The variance is a measure of the variation in the values of a set of data. This is calculated by first calculating the mean, which is the expected value. Then, we take each value in the sample set, subtract the difference between the value and the mean, square that difference, and finally add all of the squares and divide by the number of samples. This is the *mean squared deviation*, or *variance*. The units of variance are the square of the units of measure, which is hard to conceptualize, so we then take the square root of the mean square deviations, and that is the standard deviation. The units of standard deviation are in the units of the original value, which is much easier to conceptualize.

About 68% of values will be within 1 standard deviation of the mean. About 95% of values will be within 2 standard deviations of the mean. About 99.7% of values are within 3 standard deviations of the mean. For most scientific purposes, abnormal is at least 2 standard deviations from the mean. This assumes that the deviation from the mean could be either greater or lesser than the mean. If abnormals are only in one direction (e.g., deviation on the high side is considered clinically abnormal but on the low side is not), then the percentages in the abnormal direction are the only ones counted. This is a one-tailed test and is treated differently from two-tailed tests.

Analysis of healthcare data is easy if there is a clear break point between normals and abnormals. An example would be the presence or absence of a gene. If the patient has the gene, the patient is either homozygous or heterozygous. Implications of the possibilities are clear. But, for white blood cell (WBC) count, there is overlap between normals and abnormals. If there is a large population of normals and a small population of abnormals, the distribution of WBCs for a typical hospital might look the solid line the lower right image of Figure 11.2. The solid line is the combination of values from healthy patients plus sick patients. The values from normal and sick patients overlap. There is no one value that clearly demarcates normal from abnormal. To deal with this difficulty, we have to interpret values in the context of other data. Does a patient with borderline WBC count have any other clinical or laboratory signs of infection? Clinical judgment will not easily be replaced by purely statistical analysis.

Sensitivity and Specificity

An event may be classified according to type, such as A or B, with additional classes depending on the number of possible outcomes. We consider the most common scenario, where a test is positive or negative. The test is performed on patients who at some point, either before or after the test, are determined to have a disease or not. So, a 2 × 2 table is created (Table 11.1). The table has more than 2 × 2 rows and columns because of labels and math cells, but the term 2 × 2 refers to the fact that in this table there are two possible disease states and two possible test results.

- True positives (TP) have the disease and a positive test.
- True negatives (TN) have no disease and a negative test.
- False positives (FP) have a positive test but no disease.
- False negatives (FN) have a negative test but do have the disease.

Sensitivity and *specificity* are measures of the performance of the test on identifying patients with or without the disease. Ideally, we would like the test to always be positive when the patient has the disease, a *sensitivity* of 100% or 1. Ideally, we would like the test to only be positive when the patient has the disease or, reworded, always be negative when the patient does not have the disease, a *specificity* of 100% or 1.

Sensitivity is the true-positive rate (TPR). Reworded, it is the rate at which patients with disease have a positive test.

$$Sensitivity = \frac{True\ Positives}{All\ patients\ with\ disease} = \frac{True\ Positives}{\left(True\ Positives + False\ Negatives\right)}$$

$$= \frac{TP}{(TP + FN)}$$

Table 11.1 TWO-BY-TWO TABLE

	Disease	No Disease	Sum of Rows
Positive test	True positive	False positive	TP + FP = All positives
Negative test	False negative	True negative	FN + TN = All negatives
Sum of columns	TP + FN = All with disease	FP + TN = All without disease	Total patients

Specificity is the true-negative rate (TNR). Reworded, it is the rate at which patients without disease have a negative test.

$$Specificity = \frac{True\,Negatives}{All\,patients\,without\,disease} = \frac{True\,Negatives}{\left(True\,Negatives + False\,Positives\right)}$$
$$= \frac{TN}{\left(TN + FP\right)}$$

The false-positive rate (FPR) is the rate at which patients without disease have a positive test.

$$FPR = \frac{False\,Positives}{All\,without\,disease} = \frac{False\,Positives}{\left(True\,Negatives + False\,Positives\right)} = \frac{FP}{\left(TN + FP\right)}$$

False-negative rate (FNR) is the rate at which patients with disease have a negative test.

$$FNR = \frac{False\,Negatives}{All\,with\,disease} = \frac{False\,Negatives}{\left(True\,Postives + False\,Negatives\right)} = \frac{FN}{\left(TP + FN\right)}$$

Sensitivities and specificities for most tests are both high but imperfect.

Predictive Values

Prediction of whether a patient has a disease depends not only on the sensitivity and specificity of the test but also on the relative proportion of patients with the disease.

What is the predictive value of a result? The positive predictive value (PPV) is the proportion of all who tested positive who have the disease.

$$PPV = \frac{True\,Positives}{All\,with\,positive\,test} = \frac{True\,Positives}{\left(True\,Positives + False\,Positives\right)} = \frac{TP}{\left(TP + FP\right)}$$

The negative predictive value (NPV) is the proportion of all who tested negative who do not have the disease.

$$NPV = \frac{True\,Negatives}{All\,with\,negative\,test} = \frac{True\,Negatives}{\left(True\,Negatives + False\,Negatives\right)}$$
$$= \frac{TN}{\left(TN + FN\right)}$$

Likelihood Ratios

The likelihood ratio is commonly used in evaluating the usefulness of a clinical test. There is a *positive likelihood ratio* (LR+) and *negative likelihood ratio* (LR-), although the likelihood ratio usually discussed is the *positive likelihood ratio*.

The LR+ is ratio of the probability of a patient with disease having a positive test (TPR) divided by the probability of a patient without disease having a positive test (FPR). This means the TPR divided by the FPR. Recall that the TPR is sensitivity. Also, the FPR is the complement of the TNR because false positives plus true negatives sum to all patients without disease. Therefore, the FPR is 1 minus specificity. *because Sens = % (+) that are test positive th 1- Sens = % False (+)*
spec = % true - that are test testing Then 1-spec = False (-)

$$LR+ = \frac{TPR}{FPR} = \frac{TPR}{(1-TNR)} = \frac{Sensitivity}{(1-Specificity)}$$

If the LR+ is greater than 1, then a positive test result is of clinical value in predicting the disease.

The LR- is the probability of a person with disease testing negative (FNR) divided by the probability of a person without disease testing negative (TNR). Because the FNR is the complement to the TPR (because they sum to all patients with disease), this means that LR- is equal to 1 minus sensitivity divided by specificity.

$$LR- = \frac{FNR}{TNR} = \frac{(1-TPR)}{TNR} = \frac{(1-Sensitivity)}{Specificity}$$

Odds and Odds Ratio

Odds are calculated from a probability and are a conceptual mechanism for describing the proportional likelihood of an event. For example, if patients with a specific gene have a 10% chance of developing a certain cancer, yet patients without the gene have only a 2% chance, then patients with the gene are said to have an odds ratio of 5.0 for developing the cancer. The odds ratio is used to describe both increased risk with certain risk factors and reduced risk with a treatment.

Some common uses of the odds ratios are as follows:

- Determine if a treatment is effective. Does it reduce the odds ratio?
- Determine if a potential risk factor affects disease prevalence. Does it increase the odds ratio?

In the examples that follow, the numbers are much smaller than would be used in clinical practice or research.

Table 11.2 TEST RESULTS FOR A DISEASE

	Disease (D+)	No Disease (D-)	Total Patients
Test positive (T+)	8 *a*	4 *c*	12
Test negative (T-)	2 *b*	6 *d*	8
Sum of columns	10	10	20

TEST EXAMPLE

A test is performed to determine whether it can identify patients who have a specific disease. Ten patients with a disease (D+) and 10 patients who do not have the disease (D-) are administered the test. Some patients test positive (T+), and some test negative (T-). The matrix and numbers look as in Table 11.2.

Of all patients with disease, 8/10 tested positive, for 80%. Of all patients with no disease, 4 of 10 tested positive, for 40%. To calculate odds, we compare the number of positives, not against all patients, but against the negatives. So, the odds of patients with disease testing positive is 8/2 or 4, designated 4:1. The odds of patients without disease testing positive is 4/6 or 0.667, designated 2:3.

To decide the overall odds ratio, we divide the first odds by the second odds, meaning the odds of positivity with disease over the odds of positivity without disease.

$$\text{Odds ratio (OR)} = \frac{8/2}{4/6} = 6$$

TREATMENT EXAMPLE

A new treatment for a very severe disease is being developed. For testing, 10 patients with the disease are given the new treatment, and 10 are given standard therapy. At some specified point in the future, clinical follow-up determines how many of the patients in each group are alive (Table 11.3).

Of patients who received the new treatment, 80% are alive, whereas only 40% of patients on standard therapy are alive. The odds of being alive for the new therapy

Table 11.3 RESPONSE TO TREATMENT

	Alive	Not Alive	Total Patients
New treatment	8	2	10
Standard treatment	4	6	10
Sum of columns	12	8	20

are 8/2 = 4 or 4:1. The odds of patients on standard therapy being alive are 4/6 = 0.667 or 2:3.

The odds ratio for being alive with the new therapy compared to standard therapy is

$$Odds\ ratio\ (OR) = \frac{8/2}{4/6} = 6$$

Relative Risk

Relative risk (RR) is a method of evaluating the performance of a test or response to treatments, but the calculations are performed on probabilities rather than odds.

For the previous treatment example, the RR is equal to the proportion of patients alive who received the new treatment divided by the proportion of patients alive who received standard treatment.

$$Relative\ risk\ (RR) = \frac{8/10}{4/10} = \frac{0.8}{0.4} = 2$$

Patients who received the new treatment were two times as likely to be alive as patients on standard therapy. If the RR of being alive was 1, then there would be no difference, and the new treatment would be no better. If the RR was less than 1, then the new treatment is worse than standard therapy, which unfortunately does happen in clinical trials.

Relative risk is often used to describe the risk of having an adverse outcome, so in the treatment example, the risk of death with new treatment is 0.2. The risk of being dead with standard therapy is 0.6. The RR of being dead with new therapy in comparison to standard therapy is 0.2 divided by 0.6 or 0.333.

Event Rates

Taking experimental evidence one step further, let us consider another 2 × 2 table (Table 11.4).

The Control group could be patients receiving standard therapy. The Experimental group is likely receiving a new treatment.

- CE = Patients in the Control group who had an Event.
- CN = Patients in the Control group who had No event.

Table 11.4 EVENT RATES

	Control	Experimental
Event	CE	XE
No event	CN	XN

- XE = Patients in the eXperimental group who had an Event.
- XN = Patients in the eXperimental group who had No event.

The *control event rate* (CER) is the number of control events divided by the number of controls regardless of events.

The *experimental event rate* (EER) is the number of experimental events divided by the number of experimental subjects regardless of whether they had an event. So,

$$CER = \frac{CE}{(CE+CN)} \quad \text{and} \quad EER = \frac{XE}{(XE+XN)}$$

Relative risk is the EER divided by the CER:

$$RR = \frac{EER}{CER}$$

Relative risk is sometimes called the *hazard ratio*.

Relative risk reduction (RRR) is the complement of RR: $RRR = 1 - RR$.
Absolute risk reduction (ARR) is the amount that risk was reduced:
$ARR = CER - EER$.
The *number needed to treat* (NNT) is the reciprocal of the ARR:

$$NNT = \frac{1}{ARR}.$$

The NNT is useful for assessment of the expected clinical benefit of a new treatment. For example, if the CER is 0.35 and the EER is 0.10, the ARR is 0.25, the reciprocal of which is the NNT to expect one patient to benefit, which is 4. This means that in clinical practice, 3 of 4 patients treated would not achieve benefit according to the metrics set. For many of our conditions, the NNT is much higher, often more than 10. Our patients often presume that every time treatment is administered a beneficial response is expected, but that is not the case.

BAYES THEOREM

The Bayes theorem represents a useful concept for determining conditional probabilities, that is, determining the probability of an event with knowledge that a separate condition is true.

$$P_{A|B} = \frac{P_{B|A} \times P_A}{P_B}$$

- $P_{A|B}$ is the probability that A is true given that B is true.
- $P_{B|A}$ is the probability that B is true given that A is true.

- P_A is the probability of condition A in the population.
- P_B is the probability of condition B in the population.

A clinical example would be a test for a specific disease. In our example, event A is having the disease; event B is having a positive test.

We want to know how much a positive test predicts having the disease. In general, with tests with high sensitivity and specificity, we would expect the positive test to indicate having the disease, but if the probability of the disease in the population is very low, then even a small FPR degrades the diagnostic utility of the test.

The following are hypothetical numbers for our disease and our test:

- Probability of disease: P_{D+} = 1% = 0.01.
- Probability of a positive test in the population: P_{T+} = 2% = 0.02.
- Sensitivity of the test is 99%, so the probability of a positive test in patients with disease is $P_{T+|D+}$ = 99% = 0.99.
- Specificity of the test is 98%, so the probability of a negative test in patients without disease is 0.98.

Let us change the abbreviations in the formula. D+ is with disease; D- is without. T+ is a positive test; T- is a negative test.

$$P_{D+|T+} = \frac{P_{T+|D+} \times P_{D+}}{P_{T+}}$$

The left side of the equation is what we want: the probability of having the disease given a positive test result.

On the right side of the equation, $P_{T+|D+}$ is the TPR or sensitivity, which is 0.99.

P_{D+} is the known incidence of the disease in the population, which is 1% or 0.01.

P_{T+} is a little more complicated. This is the probability of a positive test in the population. It is unlikely that a large study has been performed in a wide proportion of the population, but we can obtain this number from what we do know of the test. P_{T+} is the sum of patients with disease with a positive test and of patients without disease with a positive test, or the TPR plus the FPR.

$$P_{T+} = True\ Positive\ Rate + False\ Positive\ Rate$$

$$P_{T+} = \left(Probability\ of\ disease \times Sensitivity \right) \\ + \left(Probability\ of\ no\ disease \times \left(1 - Specficity\right)\right)$$

So,

$$P_{D+|T+} = \frac{P_{T+|D+} \times P_{D+}}{P_{T+}} = \frac{P_{T+|D+} \times P_{D+}}{\left(P_{D+} \times P_{T+|D+}\right) + \left(P_{D-} \times P_{T+|D-}\right)}$$

$$= \frac{(0.99 \times 0.01)}{(0.01 \times 0.99) + (0.99 \times 0.02)} = 0.33$$

So, this means that with an incidence in the population of 1%, a test with 99% sensitivity and 98% specificity grants only a 33% chance of a patient with a positive test having the disease. If we were considering a much rarer condition, the impact would be even greater.

DECISION TREES

Decision trees are aids to decision-making. They depending on *branch points*. Branch points are where more than one pathway exists because either a decision has to be made or there is more than one possible outcome. As we consider what happens, we consider both the chance outcomes and our decisions. This creates a series of hypothetical timelines starting from the present, and the branches become a decision tree.

Because nodes on the tree can be chance or decision, we usually use different symbols.

- Squares represent *decision nodes*.
- Circles represent *chance nodes*.
- Triangles represent *end nodes*, or *outcome nodes*.

Although unusual for a real tree, the decision tree usually starts from the left and progresses to the right. Nodes are only divergent; there are no convergent nodes.

The decision tree begins with the first decision to be made, for example, to give one treatment or another. The next node can be whether a patient has a response to the treatment. This diagram would look as in Figure 11.3.

An entire patient population enters the tree. This might be a group of patients with a specific disease. Some of the patients are treated with drug A, and some are treated with drug B. After treatment, the result may be outcome X or outcome Y.

For this example, drug A could be a new agent that may do better than standard therapy for a specific cancer. Drug B could be standard therapy. Outcome X could be survival for 1 year. Outcome Y would be not surviving 1 year. The decision tree can also take into account the probability of complications of treatment as well as consider the costs of specific decisions. For example, the new treatment might have a higher rate of side effects and likely has a higher cost.

Our example has only two possible treatment options and two possible outcome categories, but the model allows for more treatments and more possible outcomes. The outcomes do have to have criteria, meaning that the model does not allow for the outcome to be a continuous variable, such as tumor size; the

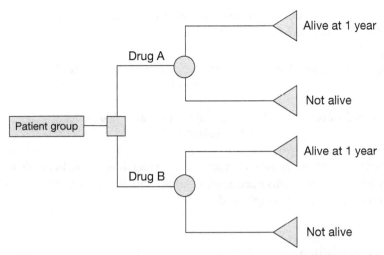

Figure 11.3 Decision tree. Simple decision tree where patients receive either one or another drug and are either alive or not alive at 1 year. Figure 11.4 is derived from this.

outcome must be in bins. Also, there should be some measurable value to the outcome. In the case of the cancer drug test, success would be equal to 1 patient-year. This allows us to calculate the probability and cost and risk of adverse effects of obtaining that 1 patient-year.

Many times, decision trees are not needed; the cost and risk of a treatment are far eclipsed by the potential benefit. But, occasionally, the decision is complicated, and not all decisions can be made by arithmetic calculation. Would you decide to have an expensive and painful treatment if it would prolong your life a few months? It would depend on your personal situation and assessment of the desirable quality of life. As physicians, we are surprised when patients make decisions that are different from what we would predict, in both directions.

Figure 11.4 shows an expanded decision tree based on the scenario just discussed. Patients in the group are selected for drug A or drug B. If this is a decision between approved treatments, then this is the decision of the patient. If this is a double-blind study, then the selection is made by the randomization process. Nevertheless, the square box is a decision point. Then, of the patients who receive either drug, some are alive at 1 year and some are not; this is indicated by the circle, indicating an event. The event has a certain probability, although this might not be known in the case of an experimental study.

Let us assume that we know the probabilities and place them on the decision tree. In addition, we have placed the value of each outcome: 1 life-year for surviving, and 0 life-years for not. This scenario considers years alive to be equivalent, but there could be significant differences, so we often adjust the value of life as quality-adjusted life-years (QALYs), which are discussed in the next section.

Drug A: Alive at 1 year: 40% × 1 LY = 0.4 LY
Drug A: Dead: 60% × 0 LY = 0.0 LY
Drug B: Alive at 1 year: 30% × 1 LY = 0.3 LY
Drug B: Dead: 70% × 0 LY = 0 LY

Armed with those data, we can calculate the expected value in life-years of using drug A or drug B, where we add the life-years of each.

Expected Value of Drug A = Value if alive at 1 year + Value if dead
$$- 0.4 + 0.0 = 0.4 \text{ LY}$$

Expected Value of Drug B = Value if alive at 1 year + Value if dead
$$= 0.3 + 0.0 = 0.3 \text{ LY}$$

This indicates that, on the average, a patient who takes drug A fares better than a patient who takes drug B. This calculation was simple but illustrative. The calculations can become much more complicated.

QUALITY-ADJUSTED LIFE-YEAR

The concept of the QALY makes the determination of outcome value much more interesting. In the previous example, we assumed 1 year of life had a value of 1 year. But, that might not always be the case.

Referring to the decision tree just discussed for Figure 11.4, perhaps drug A produces severe neuropathy, which results in pain and weakness. In this case, survival time might only be valued at 75% of a life-year if completely well. Therefore, that 0.4 LY becomes a lower LY: 75% × 0.4 LY = 0.3 QALY. If drug B does not

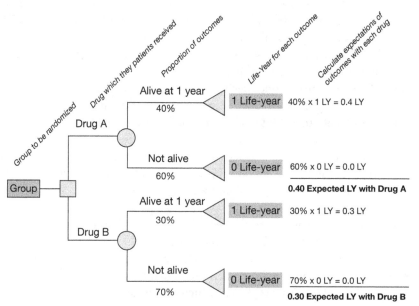

Figure 11.4 Decision tree.
Data and calculations added to Figure 11.3. This is discussed in detail in the text. LY, life-year.

produce the severe neuropathy or any other effect that detracts from quality of life, then the overall benefit of the two drug arms is equivalent at 0.3 QALY. The benefit of drug A over drug B is counterbalanced by loss of quality of life by adverse effects of drug A.

The numbers used on these trees are generated from a variety of sources. We do the experiment to determine the survival with the two drugs. We survey patients and ask them to estimate the adjustment in quality-of-life value. Some data have to be estimated, and there is often no solid data for some of the numbers plugged into decision tree analysis. This has to be remembered when considering the results of a decision tree. A precise number might not be accurate.

Figure 11.5 shows a more complex decision tree where quality of life enters into the calculations. Assume a similar study: Patients are randomized to drug A or drug B. The outcomes for each arm of the study are Cured, Alive but with residual disease, and Dead. Here, 1 life-year cured is equal to 1 QALY. But, perhaps living 1 year with residual cancer could be valued at half of a year without cancer, which is 0.5 QALY. At the end of the study, the proportions with each outcome with each treatment are calculated. All of the QALYs are added up for each arm of the study, and we can see that drug A is estimated to produce 0.5 QALY, whereas drug B produces 0.2 QALY.

We say *estimated* because turning deficits and residual cancer into a numeric estimate of quality years is far from perfect. In fact, it will differ markedly between patients.

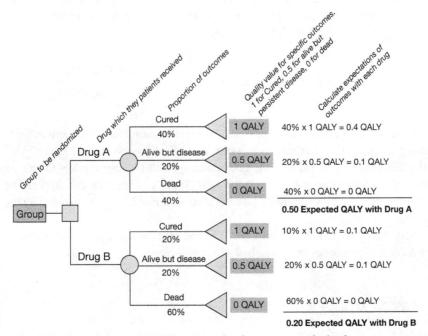

Figure 11.5 Decision tree: QALY. More complex decision tree, which takes into account a quality-of-life estimate. Discussed in depth in the text.

COST-EFFECTIVENESS RATIO

Cost effectiveness is the cost of a response. Medically, the purpose is to calculate the cost of a response to a treatment. If we consider a nonmedical example of us starting a company that makes bottles, and we purchase a bottle maker and supplies, the following formula clearly applies: There is a cost of the equipment (fixed cost) plus supplies (variable cost), and those together are the *cost of the intervention*, that is, creation of the business. The *benefit of the intervention* can be defined as value of sales:

$$Cost\text{-}Effectiveness\,Ratio = \frac{\left(Cost\ of\ intervention\right)}{\left(Benefit\ with\ intervention\right)}$$

From a business standpoint, this calculates whether we are making a profit. But, for medicine, the units and implications are quite different. In medicine, our intervention is a treatment for a disorder. There is a cost in currency to this intervention. The benefit is in improvement in survival, pain, or some other metric of value to the patient. So, the cost might be $10/point improvement in the pain scale.

In medicine, there is seldom a straight cost and benefit. There are different costs with different interventions. There are different benefits with different interventions.

For this example, we consider life expectancy with a certain stage of breast cancer with or without a new chemotherapy. The calculation is *incremental cost-effectiveness* because this indicates the cost associated with an increment in benefit and increment in cost. With standard therapy, there is a known cost of treatment and a survival probability. For these calculations, the costs of treatment are in total dollars per treatment, and the benefit is in QALYs.

$$Incremental\ Cost\text{-}Effectiveness\ Ratio = \frac{\left(Cost\ new - Cost\ old\right)}{\left(Benefit\ new - Benefit\ old\right)}$$

If the cost of the new treatment is $100 more than standard therapy and patients have 5 more QALYs, then the incremental cost-effectiveness ratio is $20/1 QALY, which is pretty good. Only $100 extra dollars would be absurdly low for a new antineoplastic treatment. If the cost is $100,000 per year for each QALY, then the implications of this incremental cost-effectiveness would have to be decided by the patient and society.

Sometimes, the benefits cannot be calculated with certainty, so a decision has to be made on the basis of estimated benefit.

MARKOV MODELS

The Markov model is named for the Russian mathematician Andrey Markov, who did his principal work during the waning days of Imperial Russia.

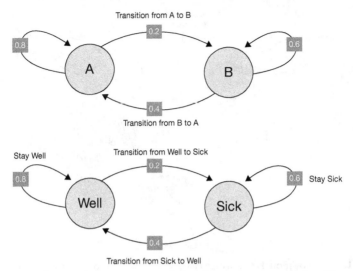

Figure 11.6 Markov process: patients can change from one state to another. The process assumes independence of the transitions.

Discussion of Markov models begins with a discussion of the *Markov process*. This describes the individual being in a state with a certain probability of transition to one or more alternative states. A series of these linked would be a *Markov chain*. All of these manifest the *Markov property*; that is, there is no memory. This means that each transitional event occurs without prejudice of what preceding events were.[1]

Figure 11.6 shows a diagrammatic representation of a simple Markov process. In the top diagram is a schematic of two states. One example might be membership at a golf club. Every year, 20% of the membership from club A goes to club B, and the remaining 80% stay with club A. Similarly, each year 40% of the membership of club B move to club A, with the remaining staying in club B. We could have added another node, those who quit each of the clubs. Similarly, the bottom of the figure is the same diagram but with a healthcare spin: Well and Sick.

Figure 11.7 indicates where we have added another state: Dead. People from either the Well or Sick states can go directly to Dead. The difference between these states is that there is no return from Dead.

The numbers on the arrows indicate the probability of making the transition to the target state. So, patients who are Well have a 70% chance of staying well, 20% chance of becoming Sick, and 10% chance of becoming Dead. Patients who are Dead have a 100% chance of staying Dead.

With these numbers, we can calculate what happens to a population of individuals in a time epoch. If there are 100 people in the Well category at time 0 and at each time interval there are the proportional transitions listed, then the results can be as in the table for each time interval (Table 11.5).

For each time interval, the number Well W_1 is equal to the number who were Well at the previous time W_0, minus the number who transitioned from Well to

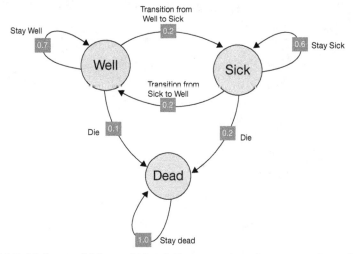

Figure 11.7 Markov model from which calculations made in the text were derived.

Sick (20% of W_0), plus the number who transitioned from Sick to Well (20% of S_0), minus the number who transitioned from Well to Dead (10% of W_0). Or:

$$W_1 = W_0 - (0.2 \times W_0) + (0.2 \times S_0) - (0.2 \times W_0)$$

Similarly,

$$S_1 = S_0 + (0.2 \times W_0) - (0.2 \times S_0) - (0.2 \times S_0)$$

and

$$D_1 = D_0 + (0.1 \times W_0) + (0.2 \times S_0)$$

or in tabular form as presented in Table 11.5.

We assume that whether the person was in the Sick category for three cycles or had just transitioned from Well to Sick had no effect on the probability of transition to Dead; that is part of the Markov property, yet that is not always true.

Table 11.5 MARKOV RESULTS

Time	Well	Sick	Dead
0	100	0	0
1	0 + (100*0.7) = 70	0 + (0.2*100) = 20	0 + (0.1*100) = 10
2	70 – (0.2*70) – (0.1*70) + (0.2*20) = 53	20 + (70*0.2) – (20*0.2) – (20*0.2) = 26	10 + (70*0.1) + (20*0.2) = 21
3	53 – (0.2*53) – (0.1*53) + (0.2*26) = 42.3	26 + (53*0.2) – (26*0.2) – (26*0.2) = 26.2	21 + (53*0.1) + (26*0.2) = 31.5

The calculations for Markov models are complex but not difficult. In practice, this modeling is used for prediction of clinical and economic outcomes in populations of patients. Although there are limitations in application of the models, they can be useful. In enterprise use, the models are quite complex, and manual calculation is impractical and unnecessary.

LOGIC

Logic could be discussed in Chapter 8 on computer programming but is included in a chapter on decision-making because we use logic in our decision-making processes. Also, we ultimately represent our knowledge base in protocols that have a logical organization.

Computational logic is best demonstrated by the use of logic diagrams. For these, there are some standard concepts and associated symbols. Here, we introduce the symbols with the concepts.[2]

For the following descriptions and examples, X and Y are operations with certain values or features (Table 11.6). For example, X may be all-things-red, and Y may be

Table 11.6 COMPUTATIONAL LOGIC

Symbol	Meaning
	AND: The expression X AND Y returns True if X and Y are both true. It returns False if either or both are false.
	OR: The Expression X OR Y returns True if either X or Y is true or both are true.
	XOR: Is exclusive or, where X XOR Y returns True if either X or Y is true but not both.
	NAND: Is Not AND, where X NAND Y returns True unless both X and Y are true. In other words, it returns True what would be False with an AND gate.
	NOR: Is Not OR, where X NOR Y returns True only if both X and Y are false.
	XNOR: Is exclusive Not OR, where X XNOR Y returns True if both X and Y are true or both X and Y are false. In other words, it is what would be false after an XOR gate.

all-things-circular. So, if we were to look for a large blue dot, we would find it in Y but not in X.

How might these logical concepts be used? In our hospitals we have a clinical decision support rule that looks at the medications used in patients with acute ischemic stroke. We want the engine to remind the provider to order an antithrombotic agent (blood thinner) for patients who are not on one, do not have an active bleeding problem, and have not had tPA (clot buster) within 24 hours. This algorithm uses a series of logical comparators to determine whether to alert the provider.

HEURISTICS

Decision-making depends not only on logic but also on our previous experience. We may use logic to say, "If a person has bleeding on the brain, do not order a blood thinner." However, research has taught us that patients who have brain bleeding because of venous thrombosis (blockage of the veins) benefit from blood thinners even though this can increase the amount of brain bleeding.

Heuristics in our context consist of problem-solving based on experience learned from previous similar situations, rather than foundational logic. An example of this type of heuristic would be if we were searching for our keys. We could begin by systematically walking through the entire house until we found them, but it would be more efficient if we tried to retrace our steps and used the complete search as a fallback plan. Alternatively, we would consider a list of places to look first on the basis of where we have left keys before or where they might be most likely put down, such as in the door lock, in the bathroom, in the kitchen near the refrigerator, or by the telephone.

There is another application of the term *heuristics*, and this pertains specifically to computer science, where the approach to a complex problem can be simplified, resulting in not necessarily the best answer, but a good answer. The *traveling salesman problem* (TSP) is illustrative: The goal is to calculate the shortest route to travel between multiple cities on a sales task. This is extremely difficult to compute, although it can be done. One approach is to take the shortest route to the closest city that has not been visited, then do the same again and again until all cities have been visited.

Where we use heuristics in medicine is to consider all available information and make decisions based on the compiled data that seem most relevant. A computer may know that most patients with a heart attack have chest pain, but the physician knows that some do not, so a heart attack is considered in a patient with jaw or left arm pain even without chest pain. If there are other clinical findings, such as specific abnormalities on electrocardiogram (ECG) or laboratory tests, the diagnosis of myocardial infarction will not be excluded on the basis of unexpected data. Heuristics in healthcare are best applied if they can be reduced to a degree of standardization. For example, ST segment elevation on ECG is more indicative of myocardial infarct than is a mildly elevated troponin. Therefore, a patient presenting to the emergency room with chest pain and ST elevation is evaluated for myocardial infarction.

KEY POINTS

- Statistics are fundamental to decision-making in clinical medicine. Rigorous metrics are superior to general impressions.
- Decision trees help with determining the best approach to a difficult decision, especially in conjunction with quality-of-life adjustments.
- Markov models, logic, and heuristics are important concepts for understanding how we do and should make decisions, but all have limitations.

Information Systems Strategy and Administration

JEFFREY G. FRIELING, KARL E. MISULIS,
AND MARK E. FRISSE ■

STRATEGIC PLANNING

Strategic planning is performed at many levels; those of principal concern here are those of the healthcare enterprise and the information systems (IS) division. Strategic planning extends beyond the enterprise, however, with the US Department of Health and Human Services (HHS) publishing detailed strategic goals approximately every 4 years.[1]

Commonalities of almost all strategic plans are the intent of

- Providing better patient care
- Making care more affordable
- Making care more accessible

Enterprise and HHS strategies depend on information systems to help them reach their objectives.[2] This is made both implicit and explicit in strategic plans, including that of the HHS. The enterprise expects information systems specifically to perform data management and to monitor and help optimize financial performance. Part of all strategic plans is individual accountability; for specific enterprise tasks, including IS, there are designated individuals who are accountable for performance.

Enterprise Strategic Plan

The World Health Organization definition of a *healthcare organization* includes a facility that has the "primary intent to promote, restore, or maintain health." There are further descriptors, but this is the essential phrase. This allows for a wide range of potential structures and functions. Enterprise strategic plans are designed to align with this definition.

Specific elements of the strategic plans differ but generally include many of the following goals[3]:

- Provide the best possible patient care
- Reduce inpatient mortality
- Reduce complications of healthcare delivery
- Increase patient satisfaction
- Improve financial performance to provide economic sustainability
- Reduce personnel turnover
- Integrate care delivery within the community
- Educate providers and staff regarding best practices
- Educate patients and the community concerning health awareness and healthy choices
- Improve timely access to healthcare for the community
- Achieve certifications and recognition for excellence in healthcare
- Enable research to promote advancement of healthcare in the community and beyond

The strategic plan is generated within the context of the *mission* and *vision* of the organization, with an eye to the specific needs of the community and the times.

Information Systems Strategic Plan

IS strategic plans and goals are principally focused on accomplishing a suite of support tasks for the enterprise. Among commonly held goals are the following:

- Support efficient healthcare delivery
- Provide knowledge resources to assist healthcare providers in decision-making
- Reduce medical errors through knowledge-based interventions
- Connect enterprise and community data sources to improve coordination of care
- Use advanced data analytics to identify issues needing intervention
- Leverage IS capabilities to identify sources of resource recovery
- Leverage IS capabilities to identify potential threats to clinical or financial performance

- Connect providers and staff to more closely coordinate healthcare
- Ensure security, privacy, and confidentiality of patient records

The IS strategic plan and goals should be reviewed periodically; we recommend yearly, and perhaps this is best done at the time that the budget for the next fiscal year is being assembled.

COMPONENTS OF IS STRATEGY AND RESPONSIBILITY

When we consider the components of our healthcare IS, clinicians first think of the electronic health record (EHR), picture archiving and communication system (PACS), and specialty systems; administrators commonly consider the revenue cycle system. Certainly, these are pillars of IS strategy, but there are many more IS functions required for efficient operation of healthcare systems. Some of these components are not under the direct leadership of IS, but they do require IS participation.

Room and zone access: Healthcare personnel have widely differing requirements for room and zone access. For example, IS security personnel need access to the data center but not the neuro intensive care unit, whereas access for healthcare providers would be the reverse.

Phones: Phones used by select providers and administrators are often configured so that if the provider quits the enterprise, access to email, secure messaging, and other enterprise applications is canceled, and the applications and permissions disappear.

Communication systems: Contacting individuals in specific circumstances can be complex, with multiple options. A different mode may be needed for different purposes, and this must be coordinated. For example, notification of a provider of a routine consultation can usually be performed by secure messaging; however, notification of a cardiac arrest would more likely require an overhead page plus a phone call.

Heating and air conditioning: These are functions that, while not controlled by IS, depend on IS to coordinate and notify personnel in case of failure. If an air conditioning unit fails in the data center, personnel need to be alerted prior to device failure. Heating and air conditioning are coordinated throughout the enterprise through the IS network.

Tube system: Tube systems are pervasive in healthcare buildings and are used for rapid movement of a variety of items, including papers, some medicines, and some laboratory specimens. The tube system is more complex than often appreciated. Sending and receiving have to be queued to avoid collisions and misrouting. If the tube receptacle is full at the receiving station, the system needs to know to alert the receiving station to clear the landing area or needs to redirect the container to a nearby station and then notify the recipient of the new location of the package.

Radiology equipment: Almost every radiological device is connected to the IS network, many through the radiology information system (RIS). Because of system downtime or network issues, we have occasionally had to station radiologists at computed tomographic (CT) and magnetic resonance imaging (MRI) scanners to read time-critical studies.

Provider and staff credentials and privileges: All personnel have credentials allowing differing functions. The chief medical informatics officer (CMIO) who practices medicine at the facility needs access to clinical applications not only as a provider but also for analytics to review provider and system performance. A provider who resigns as active staff of a hospital but maintains outpatient clinic practice in the same enterprise needs to have EHR privileges revised so that they can still work in the outpatient arena. A terminated employee must have his or her access to clinical, business, and physical access systems immediately revoked.

Upgrades: Upgrades to IS or non-IS functions require communication to those affected by the upgrade. Some upgrades are unlikely to be disruptive, whereas others will be known to affect workflow during and after the upgrade. Notification and coordination of staff during these transitions are essential.

Newborn tracking: The leg bands on newborns often have active radio-frequency identification (RFID) capabilities for tracking location. These systems can allow for automatic locking of doors and elevators in case of attempted theft of a child.

Security: Networked cameras allow for visualization of common interior and exterior space and every entrance to our facilities. In the increasingly common occurrence of a wanted fugitive in the facility, security services can avoid confrontation within the facility but rather follow the individual until the individual leaves the facility, at which point law enforcement personnel can be directed to the individual's precise location for apprehension.

Employee privileges: Employee access to fitness center or lounge or to obtaining a discount at the cafeteria is coordinated typically through magnetic card or RFID access, which in turn is dependent on IS resources and configuration.

INFORMATION SYSTEMS ADMINISTRATION

There are commonalities to running various healthcare system departments. Among the common concerns are budget, personnel, support infrastructure, and scheduling. This section focuses on specific considerations applicable to IS.

Leadership of IS consists of a hierarchy that differs somewhat between enterprises, but in general, there is an organizational tree with governance at the top and operational experts throughout.

Executive leadership is usually the *chief information officer* (CIO). This individual requires capabilities in business, medical, and technical spheres. The background of the individual may be as a provider with subsequent executive and technical training or as a nonclinical person who has worked in healthcare for an extended period. We generally favor someone with hands-on clinical experience, such as a physician, nurse, or allied health professional. The CIO is usually at a vice-presidential level.

The CIO works closely with CMIO and chief medical officer (CMO). The position of the CMIO differs between organizations, most reporting to the CIO or directly to the chief executive officer (CEO). The CMIO has a vice-presidential

appointment in many enterprises. The CMIO may be the CIO in some organizations. The CMIO should be board eligible or board certified in clinical informatics.
The CMIO is responsible for a variety of functions, some of which are:

- educating providers about enhancements and other changes in the system;
- coordinating implementation of best practices into the EHR;
- interfacing with data governance professionals at affiliated and referring organizations;
- advocating for the providers in decisions regarding clinical informatics;
- guiding clinical decision support efforts;
- ensuring that new projects meet needs of the stakeholders.
- working with medical staff to optimize EHR tools to reduce errors and improve patient care; and
- working with the CMO, business staff, and pharmacy staff to improve financial sustainability.

Directors of IS divisions depend on the size as well as the structure of the organization. There are usually directors for applications, hardware, security, interface, analytics, decision support, network, education, and informatics.

Organization: The subdivisions of the IS department must have a working relationship with leadership in other departments, including finance, patient access, utilization control, medical staff, nursing, pharmacy, and specialty services, especially including radiology, cardiology, and surgery. Some departments will have informatics-trained professionals separate from but working closely with the IS department.

Personnel selection: Information systems are constantly changing, so prospective employees must embrace change and be willing to spend a significant component of their effort either facilitating or supporting change. IS personnel must want to learn new skills. Change-averse applicants need not apply.

Trust: Information systems are so complex that it is impossible for any one individual to fully comprehend all systems. We trust that our security and privacy officers are aware of the current regulations and guidelines and are watching for threats. We trust that our interface engineers are ensuring that data transfer is valid. While we will always be observing our colleagues, we could get no other work done if we did not trust them. Micromanagers need not apply.

Budget: For most healthcare systems, IS is about 4% of enterprise budget but is more than 5% in about a quarter of systems. The budget is a combination of capital and operating expenses plus revenues. During the transition from paper to electronic records, IS budgets were particularly strained, and these projects have been a source of financial woes for many enterprises and a financial disaster for a few. *Capital budget* is for new projects, which are usually new equipment, applications, or both. *Operating budget* is for salaries; benefits; minor replaceable equipment (e.g., printers, phones); maintenance, including maintenance contracts; and other ongoing expenses, such as remote hosting or some consulting services.

Training: Included in the budget is training for staff and for users who are not in the IS department. Costs of training time and personnel for IS are reflected in the IS budget, but costs of reduced productivity and continuing medical education (CME) expenses for provider training time are not. Training for IS staff should include opportunities to enhance personal abilities, which benefits the enterprise by providing an employee with additional skills, and benefits the individual by virtue of new marketable skills. For example, a programmer may want to learn SQL (Structured Query Language) and the basics of analytics.

Consulting services: Consulting services are used because of required unique skills not present in the enterprise or because of lack of sufficient personnel. While these people are more expensive than full-time employees are, they are usually used for a limited project duration and are not retained.

Employee development: IS a continuously evolving field, so we recommend continuing to educate the staff. Allow employees to learn more so they can be used outside their initial focus arena and also have a potential path to career advancement. As part of a yearly review, career path, including ambitions and interests, should be evaluated.

KEY POINTS

- The IS strategic plan must be aligned with the enterprise strategic plan.
- Governance of IS requires coordinated work by experienced professionals.
- The IS departments are large and busy with many staff wearing multiple hats. IS is a team sport with closely defined roles of the teammates.

Large-Project Management

JEFFREY G. FRIELING, KARL E. MISULIS,
AND MARK E. FRISSE ■

OVERVIEW

Information systems (IS) actions are generally divided into projects, with some of the projects being ongoing maintenance of systems and applications. Our Gantt chart of projects is divided into major sections, with one maintenance and upgrade and another transitions and new installations.

Figure 13.1 shows the graphic section of a project list. There are maintenance tasks as well as new projects. Active times are indicated by the gray blocks. The x-axis is time. On the left are names of the projects.

In this chapter, we focus on large-project management, specifically the inception, creation, execution, and assessment of plans of the magnitude of an electronic health record (EHR) installation or conversion.

PROJECT PLAN

Most of the IS budget is dedicated to maintenance of present functionality, but there are always major projects that will demand careful and expert planning and implementation. The functional and financial survival of an enterprise may hinge on success of some large projects. While some project leadership has lost jobs when a project has not met expectations, few have enjoyed accolades when the projects are successful.

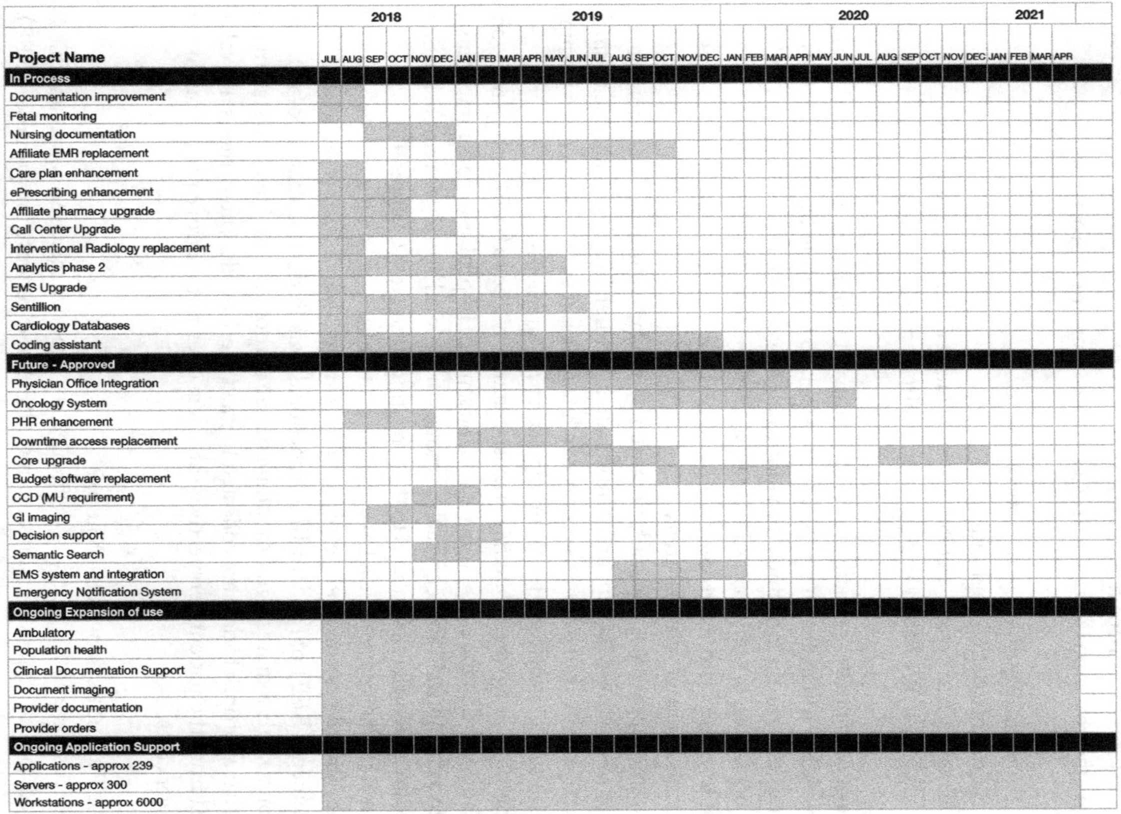

Figure 13.1 Project chart for one of our affiliates, with certain identifying information removed. Projects are divided into categories based on whether they are new, ongoing, or future.

Identify the Need

The need is often assumed in project planning, but this has to be clearly delineated prior to inception. We need to consider needs in the context of IS and enterprise abilities and strategy.

WHICH ISSUES TRIGGER THE NEED?
Among the common issues that trigger the need for a new project are

- Functionality missing from current state
- Sunset of existing application
- Transition in system architecture (e.g., merger of healthcare systems)
- Change in regulatory or reporting requirements

Missing functionality is usually from lack of capability of installed systems. Very few hospitals are still maintaining records on paper, so transition from one EHR to another usually means movement to a more mainstream application. However, at least 20% of outpatient clinics are still using paper, so these will eventually have to transition from paper to electronic records or cease to be participatory in the present administrative and financial arena.

Sunset of applications is usually because a particular application is not going to be upgraded or otherwise supported by the manufacturer. This is usually due to small market share but can be due to product architecture not being conducive to keeping up with accelerating functional and regulatory requirements.

Transition in system architecture is most commonly due to healthcare system consolidation, so that the entire system is on the same EHR platform. Sometimes, this is due to a change in IS strategy, such as moving from local hosting to remote hosting. There are practical implications to these hosting strategies (Chapter 9).

The *regulatory environment* has been frequently changing, with increasing burden on healthcare systems and personnel for analytics. Much of the request for enhancement (RFE) of modern EHR functionality is in documentation of metrics. Of course, this requires significant time on the part of the providers and staff to ensure that appropriate data are collected to meet these needs. Often, this is not value added from the patient perspective; the effort does not improve patient outcomes or lower costs.

WHAT PRECISELY ARE THE NEEDS?
The needs have to be precisely delineated for product selection to occur. This is needed for the request for information (RFI) and request for proposal (RFP). There have to be specifications that the system will have to meet.

Requirements can be separated into *must-have* and *like-to-have* elements. If we were to select a radiology information system (RIS) to interface with our EHR, essential requirements would be that orders and results are passed back and forth across the interface. An optional, but desirable, feature may be embedded decision support to ensure that the correct study is performed considering the clinical information. The time will come when the decision support tool bridging the EHR and

RIS will become high enough priority that this feature becomes essential. So, when discussing requirements for a potential IS installation project, we consider future possible enhancements and heightened expectations.

Appropriation of Resources

The two principal components of the resources are personnel and money. By the time that the project has begun, monetary resources have already been designated. The budget created for enterprise board approval usually has a bit of extra money allocated for inevitable overruns. Monetary requirements are often designated on a not-to-exceed basis.

The budget for the project is developed with the IS strategy and enterprise strategy in mind. This includes not only financial data, but also a timeline of the needed human resources.

Manpower is generally existing IS staff, but there will often have to be additional staff for the project, including partial- or full-effort personnel for select clinical and nonclinical tasks. For example, installation of an upgrade of a cardiology application can involve many cardiology clinical staff in addition to IS staff. Work on a financial application will require involvement of administrative staff in addition to IS staff.

Timing of financial and human needs is critical. Efficient use of staff demands that there be minimal unbusy time. Also, it is essential that there not be excessive demands of the staff; otherwise, there is the possibility of discontent and resultant personnel loss. In addition, an overextended workforce is more likely to miss target dates and fail to achieve success criteria.

Payments for vendor services and product (e.g., software) usually occur in stages, part at the beginning, part at certain intervals or on meeting certain milestones, and the remainder at the successful completion of the project.

Many projects are large enough and long enough that they can extend to more than one budget year. Depending on the financial condition of the enterprise, payment over multiple budget cycles is often more palatable to the enterprise and is often acceptable to the vendors, who are hoping to preserve a long-term relationship.

Options

If the project concerns the EHR or other core system, there are several options for meeting our needs. We may consider replacing the old system with a new system, upgrading the present system, or installing a separate system to cover gaps in the present core.

NEW SYSTEM
Installation of a new system could be a first install or replacement of a legacy system. We investigate the market of potential solutions. RFIs are sent to selected vendors whose candidate products seem to be of sufficient functionality that they meet the needs. RFPs are sent to vendors of candidate systems that seem to be able to meet

both functional and budget criteria. There is seldom a good rationale for installing a system that does not meet requirements unless the failed requirements are to be met using an alternative method.

MODIFY PRESENT SYSTEM
Modification of a present system is usually an upgrade. Upgrades are usually less costly and less risky than replacements or new installs, so they are preferred if they can meet the needs. We are offered upgrades to almost all of our applications. Most of these are not obligatory, but they can be, especially if there are regulatory requirements or there are dependencies that require an upgrade. For example, many healthcare enterprises have had to upgrade analytics systems to provide reporting for Meaningful Use and MACRA (Medicare Access and CHIP Reauthorization Act of 2015) or MIPS (Merit-based Incentive Payment System). Similarly, we had to update core code level order to support installation of a new financial system.

Potential upgrades are considered for benefits versus costs of each. If an upgrade does not have sufficient functionality to warrant installation, it is skipped. In most circumstances, upgrades do not have to be taken at the time they are offered. For example, we may skip upgrade v24 and v25, but we are able to upgrade to v26 when we see that it contains valuable added functionality.

Sometimes, a *bolt-on* can meet the need. This is a smaller application that is attached to the existing system for a specific purpose. A bolt-on differs from most apps in being dependent on the particular base app; it does not typically run as a freestanding application.

IMPLICATIONS OF OPTIONS
There are multiple implications for consideration. Among these are technical, financial, and strategic issues.

Technical
A principal consideration is technical integration with the rest of the healthcare IS. Ease of transmission of information and format of the transference is key. If the system does not share needed data, then it will be unable to meet the needs. Any two systems can almost certainly be interfaced, but the amount of work and the format of the interfaced data can be problematic.

Historically, best-of-breed applications and devices were desirable because data sharing between devices and other data sources was of secondary importance. However, with healthcare IS development, integration has become essential. This is often best accomplished by integrated applications. These are often from the same vendor or from aligned partner vendors.

Financial
Financial traditions would dictate that prior to any project, a pro forma be created. This is a financial document that sets out the estimated costs and return on the project, along with objectives, rationale, and a high-level discussion of the project. Part of this is a calculation of return on investment (ROI). Almost certainly, installing additional operating room suites would be expected to have

a positive ROI, but in healthcare, some projects are meritorious in the absence of being profitable.

Information systems are essential for functioning of the healthcare system, but they do not generate much direct income, so an ROI often cannot be calculated. Most of the financial impact is downstream, and much of it is essential. A modern healthcare system cannot function without state-of-the-art clinical, financial, and administrative information systems.

A method to deal with absence of a calculated positive ROI for IS projects is to do a cost-benefit analysis.[1]

$$Value = \frac{Benefits}{Costs}$$

The value formula is used, but with the numerator and denominator having different units and being more subjective (e.g., we saved X lives at a cost of Y dollars).

Cost accounting frequently includes equipment purchase for IS projects. User devices often do not change with a new project, but they have a fairly short life-time and must be upgraded or replaced regularly. New projects often demand new or expanded server space in addition to all of the support structures, from uninterruptible power supplies to air conditioning. For a new project, hardware is usually acquired substantially prior to need, so that the project is not waiting for physical delivery. Just-in-time approaches to materials management are often not practical for IS equipment.

Models of software acquisition include *ownership* versus *software-as-a-service* (SaaS). From a financial perspective, ownership generally has a larger front-loaded cost, whereas SaaS has costs spread over a much longer time, usually over multiple budget years. This can help with cash flow, although the long-term (7–10 years or more) costs are often higher with SaaS. This is not always the case because economies of scale for the vendor may be partly passed to the client. Also, updates to software should be somewhat easier in the SaaS model.

Budget creation must include some cushion for unexpected expenses. Separately from big-ticket unanticipated expenses, there are multiple incidental expenses that are difficult to include in the contract budget.

Enterprise and Information Systems Strategy
The strategic plans for the enterprise and for IS must be coherent, as discussed in Chapter 12. Some of the issues the IS strategic plans must consider include the following:

- Anticipated needs of the enterprise for new functionality
- Maintenance of existing systems
- Replacement of legacy systems, as needed
- Changes in business models, such as effects of acquisitions and divestitures

Among the decisions to be made for the IS and enterprise strategy are even whether to make changes. When a system is working, there is a risk of change, so while making almost any change has the promise of improvement, there is no certainty that this will be the case. There is risk.

Efforts to improve quality and reduce costs often involve making tasks automated. Among the elements that are being automated now are voice recognition rather than transcription for provider notes and report generation and dashboarding for provider performance.

While there will be one-offs, in general we recommend having most projects, especially of any size and risk, be on a list of future projects with an outlook of 2–5 years. Future projects should be stratified according to priority and estimated resource demands.

Stakeholders in enterprise and IS strategy are many, so the presumption is that no project will make everyone happy. So, when strategy is being considered and stakeholder impact is assessed, attention has to be given to how those adversely affected by a project will be handled.

For a hospital or a large clinic, a single centralized governance for strategic design is adequate. With more healthcare systems involving multiple hospitals and multiple clinics, both local and centralized governance structures with strong communication are recommended. Individual service lines and departments will need leadership to be involved in integrating what is desired and what is doable from their viewpoint into enterprise and IS strategy.

Contracts

Most informatics physicians will not be involved in contract negotiation and execution, but they should be. We recommend that the chief medical informatics officer (CMIO) and other clinical informatics professionals be involved in all levels.

In general, the vendors often have a foundational contract with specific conditions and clauses customized for the healthcare system. Then, the contracting method is a series of back-and-forth changes, some of which are more or less negotiable. For example, a common contractual concession is for a vendor to allow payment to be spread over more than one fiscal year. Yet, a vendor may have a hard stop if the healthcare system wants to replace an end-of-life system within a month. Most vendors will not have the resources to perform all the steps of an IS project in that time frame.

Vendor pricing is often based on users or licensed beds. These numbers are imperfect because users come and go, and not all users have equal utilization of the system. The count of licensed beds is almost an imaginary number. In our healthcare system, we have large tertiary facilities that almost always have occupancy greater than listed beds and small hospitals that are never at full occupancy.

A compromise is often for initial pricing and configuration to be based on some metric, such as user count, and then to have expansion based on net revenue. This builds in the expectation of growing business, a good guess for a large system, in these days of consolidation. It also provides the vendor with revenue growth with success of the client. Sometimes, an annual growth charge is contracted, regardless of load.

Expense is dependent on how much vendor support is needed for implementation. We have used vendor resources especially for system testing and integration testing. Greater vendor resource hours increase the costs, but this may be cheaper than adding temporary staff and training them for the intended tasks.

Software support is included in contracts. Upgrades are in the contract, although the precise expenses associated with those might not be nailed down. Services for upgrades are usually extra because it is hard to predict whether the enterprise will have the resources for the upgrade several years in the future.

Equipment support is typically included in the annual maintenance contract unless the system is remote hosted, in which case that is usually handled by a separate contract.

The total price will be a function of all of these elements and the payment terms. If we spread payment across more than one fiscal year, the vendor will often want a little more reimbursement.

Indemnification and liability are usually assigned to the enterprise. Vendors seldom assume much liability.

Warranties are common; these are legal assurances that certain conditions will be met, often in a specific time frame. This could be a guarantee of agreed-on functionality. There are usually specified remedies if the events or conditions are not met, such as termination of the contract without further obligation or financial penalty for not meeting requirements.

Legal review of the contracts is typical, with in-house counsel performing much of this function. With large projects or projects that step into a regulatory arena with which in-house counsel does not feel comfortable, external legal review may be needed.

During the stages of RFI and RFP, careful readers of these documents will identify multiple areas of uncertainty in the responses. The answers to these questions should be in the contract so that it is clear during contract execution what is and what is not included in the signed contract.

The term of the contract is specified and includes time of implementation and subsequent support.

Finalize the Project Plan

The project plan is brought to a final consensus, but it is understood that there will be changes along the path. The final plan is what is ultimately brought to the governing board for approval.

From the final plan, a contract is agreed on with the vendor(s); the plan includes the rationale, the project summary, the price and payment structure, anticipated contingency, the expected process changes, risks, and resources that will be needed, including for implementation, ongoing support, and upgrades. Senior leadership of the healthcare system and vendor(s) approve and sign the contract.

Board Approval

The contract is approved by the board or not. The contract is often more complicated than can be fully discussed and considered in a committee situation. Preparation meetings with individual board members are helpful so the essentials can be discussed and there are no surprises at the board meeting.

The plan is presented to the board, and the presenter often gives an executive summary. The presenter then is available for questions and tries to anticipate questions and concerns of the board and is ready to discuss alternative strategies.

IMPLEMENTATION

Plan Governance

Project governance begins with a project management team. The team leader is usually at the director or higher level, with the specific individual determined based on the arena, scope, and magnitude of the project.

Project management services may be obtained from consulting groups. These services are used especially when there is a lean leadership base or when the project depends on skills that are not readily available at the enterprise. For example, conversion from a legacy niche EHR to an enterprise EHR could benefit from the expertise of consulting project management personnel who have had experience making the same conversion at other healthcare systems.

Project management is responsible for supervision of the timeline, budget, and resources. If additional infrastructure or personnel is needed, the project management team informs enterprise leadership and is prepared to justify the changes and present alternatives.

Project governance includes assembly of teams for specific purposes, such as design decision, build, testing, and training. Leadership of these teams report to project management.

Timeline

A timeline is developed that considers the aggregate development and maintenance requirements of the IS department. A project timeline is just one of several timelines, which otherwise include the enterprise and overall IS timelines.

Visualization of the timeline is usually with a form resembling a Gantt chart. An IS project timeline is shown in Figure 13.2.

The x-axis is time, and the stages of the project are indicated by horizontal bars spanning the expected time for initiation to completion of each of the tasks. Vertical lines indicate specific events, timelines, or the time of day this image was captured.

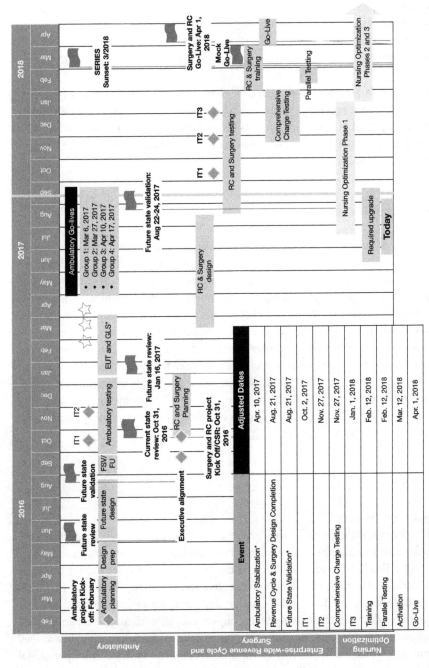

Figure 13.2 Project timeline for an affiliate. Some identifying information has been removed. The core of this project was replacement of a legacy ambulatory EMR and replacement of the surgery/anesthesia system.

Just some of the tasks illustrated on this project plan are

- Design phases
- Testing phases
- Required upgrade
- Optimization phases
- Go-live

The timeline is adjusted on the basis of changes in available resources (e.g., personnel leave), not meeting testing criteria, or other delays. Some wiggle room is commonly placed in a timeline, such as for extra testing. If delays are needed, then the estimated costs have to be calculated, and estimated adjustments to the timeline have to be determined.

Allocate Resources

Resources allocated include personnel and infrastructure. Personnel allocation is made on the basis of interest as well as need. Any large project will require dedicated staff who will complete the task, so interest on the part of the individual personnel will help with engagement. Among the common concerns of involved personnel is how tasking of previous duties will affect duties for the new project. There needs to be assurance that assigned tasks can be accomplished in a reasonable workday.

Infrastructure allocation includes space and equipment. The space is often physical, including data center space; meeting space for design, build, testing, and training; a command center; and domain space for build, testing, and training. Often, these resources are used for other purposes and projects, so availability cannot be assumed. If timelines need to be adjusted, the availability of these resources needs to be reevaluated.

The Project Begins

DESIGN DECISIONS

Design begins with review of the *current state*. This is so that all the design team members understand the tools and workflows currently involved in accomplishing the tasks. This is followed by design of the *future state*, what we expect the tools and workflows to look like operationally after launch. Then, there are often hundreds and sometimes thousands of design decisions. These decisions are made by cooperative discussion involving technical, vendor, clinical, and operational staff. The vendor considers the decisions on the basis of available functionality as well as model experience in other installations of the same system. The operational staff considers what they will need to accomplish their jobs, and the technical staff considers these decisions in view of the enterprise systems. Topics and decisions are usually recorded on a spreadsheet, from which builders can configure the new system to meet the anticipated future state.

BUILD

Build is directed by the vendor, but involvement of enterprise staff is recommended because they need to be aware of how the build is done to help with later troubleshooting. During build, there is some custom code, but most is often accomplished by setting the value of variables in the design matrix.

TESTING

System testing runs procedures or scripts to determine if the individual systems perform as they should. This is usually done in a domain that is a partial replication of the domain in which the production application will run.

Integration testing evaluates whether tasks that rely on interdependencies work as designed, for example, a test to ensure that an order for a charge placed by a provider in the EHR is transmitted to the business system in a format that can be turned into a charge to the payer. There are multiple links in this process chain, any of which might fail during integration testing. The testing domain is not a perfect representation of the production domain, so not all scripts are expected to pass, but we will have an idea, ahead of comprehensive testing, of which are more or less likely to fail.

During development of the system, there should be defined go-no-go criteria for entering and exiting testing. Pass-fail criteria need to be outlined, although during testing, many test scripts will not pass completely because of the difference between the build domain and the production domain.

The process of working on build, testing, assessment, and further work on build is just one of multiple iterative cycles that help to perfect the build. Assessments during the build include not only quality of the build, but also assessment of adherence of the process to the timeline and budget.

Changes to the Plan

TIMELINE

Changes to the timeline are common but should be minimized. Common reasons for timeline delay include

- Insufficient staff or resources to accomplish tasks within the anticipated timeline
- Failure of adequate testing performance
- Insufficient functionality
- Delay in infrastructure availability needed for project completion

We have encountered timeline delays due to all of these during our many projects. *Insufficient staff* can occur because of loss of key personnel. New projects are stressful to staff and demanding of their time during not only normal business hours but also often after hours. This can cause burnout and occasionally departure of some personnel. Finances may make hiring of additional personnel or expertise impossible, thereby delaying development, testing, and launch.

Testing failure is not expected to be 0% for reasons already discussed, but if testing completion is not satisfactory, the project should not proceed to the next step until the deficits have been fixed. Integration testing generally has a greater risk of failure than system testing.

Insufficient functionality should be unlikely with due diligence during the product evaluation and vendor negotiation phases prior to contract signatures. However, insufficient functionality may result in having to develop functional or technical workarounds for missing functionality or rarely having to dispense with the product altogether. There are usually penalties in the contract for a product not meeting the promised specifications. Although rare, this has resulted in legal action against vendors.

Delay in infrastructure availability is usually in the realm of domain backbone, where upgraded servers, increased server space, or core system code upgrade needs to be performed prior to copy into production and subsequent launch.

Rarely, a timeline must be accelerated, for example, if the legacy system fails or becomes increasingly unreliable.

Guides to minimizing timeline expansion include the following:

- Provide reasonable times for tasks.
- Add a small amount of wiggle room in the timeline.
- Involve participants and stakeholders in creation of the timeline.
- Encourage individuals to voice potential threats to the timeline as soon as suspected.

Involvement of participants and stakeholders serves to communicate the planned timeline with people who might otherwise be critical of any constraints or changes. Also, it gives those individuals project equity, so that expectations on adhering to the guideline extend at least partly to them.

Potential threats to the timeline or budget must be discussed with leadership as soon as recognized or suspected. Psychology might urge participants not to discuss these until they become certain, but adjustment to the timeline is easiest if done as early as possible. But, do be aware of Parkinson's law[2]: Time for work expands to fill the budgeted time.

RESOURCE/BUDGET
Budget changes are almost always overruns. There is seldom an unexpected budget surplus. Common causes of budget overruns include

- Upgrade to a component needed
- Timeline extension due to any difficulty
- Additional personnel needed
- Additional equipment needed
- System not meeting need or expectations

Timeline extension increases expense by requiring longer duration of vendor resources and having to provide for internal staff being dedicated longer to the project and away from other duties.

Participants should be encouraged to discuss potential budget overruns with leadership as soon as recognized or suspected, so that plans may be made to mitigate some of the expense and to make the administrative arrangements for the additional funding.

Training

Training is not required for all projects. Upgrade for a group of servers or a version upgrade that does not change the interface or functionality means staff needs minimal training, only perhaps a bit for support staff.

For the majority of projects requiring user training, this is accomplished in multiple ways. If this is an upgrade with added features, announcements and a slide or two can suffice. If it is a new application, then training should ideally begin with an introduction to the application even during the first phases of the project. Then, when launch is approaching, a combination of web-based, classroom, and individual training is accomplished. At the time of launch, at-the-elbow instruction is often needed. Most healthcare systems employ individuals who have training as a major or exclusive component of their jobs.

Each area often has superusers—individuals who use the system for the same tasks but have received more in-depth training than most users and not only can efficiently use the system for intended purposes but also guide others in their service area. Post-launch *optimization* is recommended for many launches and is anticipated and planning begun for this prior to launch. This is complex and requires analysis of individual and collective application use. Observers, analytics, and queries of users should determine areas of inefficiency, duplicative clicks, nonintuitive workflows, and other impediments to optimal use of the system.

Training and education for users is often included in the initial budget, but there is often need for additional resources to help with launch and optimization, with some of these resources not in the budget. This may include a subject matter expert from the vendor for a particular problematic area.

Launch and Go-Live

Launch is often called *Go-live*. Strictly speaking, launch and go-live do have slightly different meanings. *Go-live* is activation of the project product, whether new install, upgrade, or bolt-on. Activating a new application is *launch* because this is the first time the system is working within this healthcare enterprise.

Time for go-live is announced far in advance, and if appropriate and possible, user workloads are reduced for a few days and sometimes for weeks after launch.

Depending on the needs of the users, there is support centrally and often at the elbow. Trainers should remember to teach only the basics, the essentials, at this time. Showing a new user three ways to look for documents will be confusing to the user and reduce user effectiveness and satisfaction.

Prelaunch Preparation

Prelaunch preparation usually requires tasking staff with both on-site and centralized support. This includes at-the-elbow support for most user-facing apps. These personnel not only need to know the system well, but also need to be knowledgeable about model experience—the best way to accomplish tasks—and effective mechanisms of communicating with their assigned users.

Contingency plans must be in place in case the new system or upgrade does not work. The new system might fail to initiate or may be found to not function adequately after launch, with a need to be turned off while fix is under way.

Downtime procedures should be tested and staff trained in downtime workflows. This is not only for an anticipated downtime during launch, but also if there is failure of the new system at some time after launch.

If the new system does fail, in some instances reversion to the previous system is possible, but often the change is irrevocable.

Command Center

A command center is organized that serves to coordinate efforts, often at multiple sites. The command center will receive information on use of the system during the go-live period and also receives the issue reports. Issues are triaged according to severity and category and directed to the appropriate individuals. The command center is usually staffed 24/7, but for some installs 24-hour staffing is not needed (e.g. for an ambulatory install).

Method of Launch: Big Bang, Phased, Rolling

Launch approach depends on the application and the expected adoption characteristics of the users. Common approaches include the following:

- **Big bang**:
  - The new system is launched throughout the affected areas of the enterprise simultaneously.
  - This is the easiest to do, but risk is highest if there is difficulty using the new system.
- **Phased**:
  - Launch is performed in individual or multiple areas in stages.
  - This is less risky to perform because the effects of changes are in a smaller arena, but both new and old workflows and systems have to coexist for a while.
- **Rolling**:
  - The update is rolled out to one group of servers at a time, in a rolling fashion. Users often have to log off and then log in to the updated servers, but system downtime is not needed.

    o This method can be done only for select launches, such as an update that does not change interfaces or global functionality.

THE LAUNCH

Copy from Build to Production: The launch is often associated with a period of downtime at which time the software is copied from the build domain to the production (Prod) domain. The duration of downtime is variable. It might be an hour or so for a small application, or 8 hours for a complete EHR installation. Longer downtimes are seldom needed.

    Activation: Users begin to use the system in the production domain. Whether the activation is phased or big bang, the transition is sudden for the individual users. Depending on the magnitude of the workflow change, at-the-elbow support and superusers can help ensure that staff and providers are able to continue their healthcare duties.

    Issues: Users report problems to their local IS staff. Many of the problems are related to unfamiliarity with the application, and immediate instruction is all that is required. Other issues are problems with the system. Among some of the common types of issues are the following:

- System freeze or crash
- Nonfunctioning links
- Nonworking interfaces
- Failure of data movement

A *system freeze or crash* is especially likely if there are insufficient technical resources, such as excessive server load. Also, breaks in interfaces can cause apps to crash. With a client-server architecture, crashes are usually to single or small groups of users, but sometimes the instability is so pervasive that transition to downtime procedures may be needed. Seldom does the legacy application have to be reactivated, and this is often not possible. Our modern fault-tolerant systems are so termed because they can function even if there some errors, but this results in the potential for loss of some function for users.

    Difficulty with links and interfaces is common. The Build domain is different from Prod, and the expected interfaces often have to be adjusted. This may result in one or more sets of functions not performing as needed, even though other functions are preserved; this usually does not necessitate downtime procedures.

Postlaunch Training

Optimization begins with postlaunch training. When users have developed some familiarity with the system, they will identify difficulties that impede their workflow. At-the-elbow training is most beneficial for this. Some of the difficulties can be resolved with training. Some require filing of issues with the command center or help desk so that configuration fixes can be made. If the requested function is not doable with present system capabilities, then a request for enhancement is made.

Key to postlaunch training efficacy is willingness to learn on the part of the user. The user must be willing to change processes and workflows rather than trying to adapt the new system to the old workflows.

During postlaunch training, some problematic workflows may be identified that need to be changed with the new system. Well-intentioned informatics staff should not enable unsafe or noncompliant workflows. Potential examples of these could be medical assistants logging in as a provider, documentation without performance of the claimed task, or turning off of essential notifications. Failures in our systems can arise from being too accommodating.

Most users are willing to obtain basic instruction, but many are not avid participants in retraining and optimization. If they can get their work done, they do not want to spend uncompensated time in more training. We recommend giving little suggestions at the elbow and also at select meetings. One or two suggestions at each department meeting may accomplish something.

OPTIMIZATION

Optimization is not always needed but is recommended for any project that significantly alters workflow or presents a different user experience. Users often have a tendency to use the new tools to do the same tasks they did with the old tools; some do not embrace a new recommended workflow. Also, many users, when faced with a task for which they do not understand model experience, develop workarounds or otherwise-suboptimal workflows.

Optimization begins with evaluation of the system performance and user experience. While analytic metrics can obtain some of this information, such as number of clicks per order, direct observation is invaluable. In fact, when informatics staff are not in the midst of another busy project, observation of individuals who exhibit or express difficulty with the system should be performed.

POST-PROJECT ASSESSMENT

Assessment is ongoing from the moment of launch until the project has achieved its goals and needs. Early in the process, the focus is on technical issues, ensuring that the issues are fixed. The second phase of assessment is of the user experience. What is the provider efficiency and satisfaction with the system? What can be done to improve these? This is usually a combination of additional training, workflow redesign, and configuration changes where appropriate.

A key phase of post-project evaluation is to determine whether needs and objectives were met. This consists of not only assessment of functionality but also evaluation of the timeline changes, budget implications, and pain points. Lessons learned are delivered to senior leadership and the vendor(s).

Did the Project Meet the Needs?

Post-launch needs assessment considers present functionality in the context of legacy functionality and functionality outlined in the initial plan. The scope of the project will usually have been changed, but the overall target functionality of the program has to be met.

If the needs have not totally been met, then the remedy depends on the type of deficiency. Some deficiencies can be remedied by changes in workflow. Others may need consideration of other solutions, but it is hoped at not too high an additional cost. Still others may need a workaround until a better solution is forthcoming from maturation of the enterprise system.

What Is the Difference Between Contract and Reality?

For most projects, the contract is periodically reviewed during and even after build and launch because there may be fuzzy memories of what is stated in the contract. A careful comparison of contract to reality is performed after go-live to see if the future state imagined at the time of the contract differs from the new state.

The final budget plus any additional remedies for project insufficiencies are compared to the proposed budget and significant cost overruns analyzed so that similar events are not repeated in future projects. Some cost overrun is expected. While it is theoretically possible for a project to be under budget, being under budget on an IS project may mean that shortcuts were taken or tasks were not performed, and those could jeopardize ultimate success. Note that some projects, particularly business systems and decision support tools, may not reveal deficiencies for some months after go-live. Reports of successful go-lives followed by lost jobs several months later are unfortunately not rare.

Total cost of ownership (TCO) includes not only the actual project expenses, but also loss of productivity during and after transition, maintenance fees, subsequent patches and upgrades, incidental expenses, and resource commitments. TCO will always be greater than contract price.

Is the Implementation Process Complete? Is There More to Do?

Assessment reveals if there are still incomplete portions to the project. While much of this is troubleshooting and optimization, part of the implementation for many projects is identification of what needs to be done next. For example, successful implementation of a new EHR functionality in one site of a healthcare system will then turn to implementation in other sites of the enterprise. Similarly, successful connection with a health information exchange with bidirectional data flow will then lead to integration of affiliated entities in the practice area for the purposes of individual patient care. When these connections are complete, population health functionality will be added to capitalize on efforts to improve quality and cost of care.

We are never finished with technology. Our technology will continue to evolve.

How Well Did the Project Meet Stakeholder Expectations?

Part of how well the project met stakeholder expectations is basic functionality, but part is psychology. Psychologist John Fisher described an N-shaped curve for adoption of change.[3] There is anticipation at the beginning and happiness as change happens, but then there is reassessment of the new state and comparison with what was lost from the old state. From the low point of this "valley of despair," we should then anticipate that we will embrace the new normal, but there will be a few who will either complain and not work to embrace the new system or might quit altogether.

As leaders, we should educate our colleagues on the phases of transition and adoption. Yet, we need to also ensure that we address concerns and fix what can be fixed. Even if not every concern can be fixed to the user's satisfaction, every concern can be understood and internalized. We usually take requests and fixes that cannot be done with present technology to the vendor for subsequent enhancement.

At the end of the project, there may be individuals who refuse to adapt to the new systems, and a few who are vocally or operationally obstructionist. As leaders in the enterprise, we must be willing to let disruptive people work elsewhere. Otherwise, they could be not only ineffective teammates, but also toxic to the culture and operations of our enterprise. We want what is best for us and for them.

KEY POINTS

- Key elements to project planning include
  - Identify needs
  - Assess options for meeting needs
  - Submit RFIs and RFPs as needed
  - Plan the project with wiggle room in time and resources
  - Train users well before, during, and after go-live
  - Test and test again
  - Close the loop with those reporting issues
  - Have a positive attitude
- Some of the problems that risk increasing costs include
  - Loss of personnel
  - Increase in the timeline
  - Need for additional interfaces
  - Need for additional hardware (e.g., servers, access points)
  - Need for updates for build of new application
- Some of the problems that increase the risk to launch include
  - Prod domain is not the same as Build domain
  - Anchoring of the staff inhibits adoption
  - A different system breaks
- Some of the problems that reduce the chance of meeting performance and financial expectations include
  - Optimization not done or done too soon or too late

- o Functions not as expected
- o Financials not as expected
- Mitigation strategies can include
  - o Engaging users at every stage of the project
  - o Informing users of the anticipated steps to successful adoption
  - o Project management consultants may have knowledge of potential potholes from previous similar projects
  - o Being willing to "pull the chain": stop progress until a specific problem is addressed
  - o Adhering to entry and exit criteria for specific stages, especially testing

Clinician Interface and Experience

PAUL WEAVER, DOUGLAS J. DICKEY, KARL E. MISULIS, AND MARK E. FRISSE ∎

DESIGN STRATEGY

Expectations of the user interface (UI) begin with expectations of the electronic health record (EHR) itself. The Health IT Dashboard states that, of providers with an EHR that meets Meaningful Use criteria and have used it for at least 2 years, 85% believe that the system has made their practice more efficient, 92% have seen clinical benefits, and 72% have realized financial benefits.[1] Yet, study has found that for one cadre of neurologists, EHR use in their practice was one of the principal irritants affecting career satisfaction.[2] Human nature is to attribute troubles to a common identifiable cause, and for many, the mandatory use of EHRs is seen as an unnecessary expense that impedes efficiency and adversely affects patient engagement. The EHR may be blamed for required reporting, additional required documentation, and other tasks that are not due to the implementation of the EHR per se. All of this places the EHR at a disadvantage. Only a few providers will look forward to the technology; the vast majority just want to do healthcare.

Compounding frustrations with the EHR is the propensity of providers to use more than one EHR. In our travels as educators and consultants, we have met providers who use as many as six different EHRs. These have markedly different looks and feel, to the point that casual inspection of the UIs might not make it apparent that the programs were written for the same purpose. The Agency for Healthcare Research and Quality (AHRQ) has asked for research in usability to address these concerns.[3] With study and further development, perhaps the time will come when moving from one EHR to another will be comparable to moving from one brand of automobile to another—the purpose is the same, so the general UI should be similar.

Change from one EHR to another is common, and this adds to the angst of the provider and significantly affects provider perceptions. Transformation from a locally grown EHR to a highly respected commercial program at major academic medical system resulted in declines in some key perceptions, including satisfaction, productivity, and patient care, yet the conversion was to a system with far advanced functionality.[4]

Form Versus Function

Early versions of EHRs had a focus on function, and now that the basic tasks are part of core EHR capabilities, more attention is given to the UI and user experience (UX). Major EHR vendors have entire teams tasked with improving the interface. These efforts are laudable and essential, but they must be cognizant of the anchoring of providers: We cannot make too many changes too fast. In an era of increasing shortages of physicians and nurses, we cannot slow them down. We must make them as efficient as possible. The Health IT Dashboard data show us that when a provider has used a specific EHR for at least 2 years, the provider's perception of efficiency is much improved.

Expectations of the UI depend to a certain extent on the individual user, but there are some obvious general commonalities that users want:

- Intuitive layout
- Efficient workflow for basic tasks (e.g., documentation review, results review, documentation creation, orders, placing charges)
- Flexibility to accommodate different workflows depending on roles, specialties, and personal preferences
- Tools to make tasks easier and more efficient
- Fast response to data entry and commands
- Consideration of new form factors, including tablet and mobile devices, allowing end users to take their work on the go, retaining the same expected behavior

The long view of UI expectations is that the EHR will evolve into a virtual medical assistant, reducing times of tasks and mediating decision support efforts. Among the tasks we expect to be standard are

- Disease prevention and disease management decision support tools
- Best practice guidelines embedded into the system
- Assistance with pharmaceutical stewardship, such as antibiotics, opiates, and other drug classes

When users are making specific complaints that can be turned into recommendations, some of these include

- Too many clicks
- Inefficient placement of fields and click spots
- Hard-to-find data
- Too much data
- Too many alerts
- Poor quality or incomplete documentation
- Possibility of errors specific to the EHR: wrong chart, wrong encounter
- Loss of context and personal information about the individual patient: loss of the patient story

While complaining about the EHR, we should remind ourselves of the problem of the UX of the paper world[5]:

- Illegible handwriting
- Lost dictations
- Lost charts
- Only one person can use the chart at a time
- No ability to audit inappropriate changes to the chart
- Paper placed in the wrong chart
- The need to physically secure charts to adhere to privacy and security requirements
- Too long to refill multiple medications at once
- Orders that may be lost in the chain of transference: provider to clerk to pharmacy to nurse
- Great difficulty to share, transmit, and search paper records.

We focus in this chapter on the UX, how the EHR vendors are working with users and experts to improve this experience. Among the enlisted personnel are not only software and hardware engineers, but also psychologists, physiologists, cognitive neuroscientists, data scientists, stakeholders, and users.

USER EXPERIENCE

Definition

The term *user experience* (UX) has been used broadly over the past decade, with experts in the field slowly morphing their job title in this time period from *UI/UX designer* to the now more commonly used term *UX designer*. The operational definition is more nuanced, as there are designers with varied, specialized skill sets, including, but not limited to, interaction design, Web design, instructional design, visual (graphic) design, industrial design, and even game design.

The best UX can only be obtained by listening directly to the intended audience and using their feedback to objectively improve the design. This is a difficult task and requires a very specific skill set, utilizing not only a wide variety of techniques but also a great deal of empathy. Human factors researchers not only hear from clients, but also listen to them.

Human factors researchers have to obtain the information from the end user in a careful, scientific, and methodical manner. This is a combination of compiling direct feedback from users, as well as indirect observation. Only by taking this approach can we understand the issues that users are facing and work to improve the system.

User experience is the nexus between the human and the machine, a combination of design and human factors research that works to close the gap in making human-computer interaction more meaningful and pleasurable and not just usable.

Humans

Each human has unique perceptions that, while similar, are yet quite different from that of other individuals. We unconsciously ascribe an aesthetic value to our experiences. Therefore, we can resent being forced to interact with a device that is unpleasant to use. It would be optimal if our software addressed the aesthetic as well as functional needs of the user, especially because 25%–50% of our clinical workday is spent interacting with the computer.[6]

Computers

Details of computer architecture with particular reference to healthcare are discussed in Chapters 8 and 9. Here, we consider the computer from its role as a tool, a black box with the output to display and speakers and input mainly from the keyboard and mouse but increasingly voice and ultimately sight. The user's experience is determined by his or her working relationship with the software, with a well-designed and user-centered approach to the solution leading to a more pleasant experience.

Software Development

Software development involves composition of thousands to millions of lines of code. The days of a small group of programmers have passed. The user never sees that code because it has been compiled into human-unintelligible instructions before execution. Programming is discussed in Chapter 8; here, we discuss the issues that guide our design.

The programming core begins with addressing the functions of the system, including data acquisition and storage; data retrieval and display; data manipulation; option selection (such as patient, location, and medication dose); and placing orders. Recent efforts have tried to improve the UI to reduce user fatigue and frustration and improve the UX, thereby improving user satisfaction. This makes obvious sense from the viewpoint of the healthcare provider. But, it also makes sense from the viewpoint of the software developer; improved UX improves user assessments of the product and the company.

In order to develop an understanding of how we got to the point where clinicians do not like EHRs, we have to understand how they were originally developed. Let us consider two potential development scenarios, the first with a historical foundation and the second being more progressive.

SCENARIO 1: CONVENTIONAL SOFTWARE DEVELOPMENT

Our development team has been tasked with creating a new piece of software. We have met with the client, taken diligent notes, and formulated a list of functional requirements that have been prioritized and signed off. Our project management team has worked with the engineering leads to create a development plan. It is going to take 6 months to create the application. Confidence is high. The work begins.

As it turns out, the project was tougher than anticipated and ran late despite us demanding long hours from the team. The release goes out to the public, and they hate it. The customer feedback is damning, our app store rating is in the tank, and the team is demoralized. The code has to be edited and portions rewritten to accommodate the complaints logged in the reviews in the app store.

This story is not uncommon; the "hit-and-hope" strategy is still alive and being used to this day by many software development teams.

SCENARIO 2: USER-CENTERED DESIGN

Our team has met with the client, taken diligent notes, formulated a list of functional requirements, prioritized the work, and is ready to get started on build. However, rather than immediately engaging with the engineering team, we lean on our UX team to examine these tasks:

- *Research*—Our human factors team engages with the end users of the solution to understand how the users work—how they need the software to work minute by minute. This helps to refine the list of requirements into tangible goals.
- *Design*—Our design team, utilizing modern prototyping software, is able to convert the research into usable prototypes that are initially functional, clickable boxes that represent the solution (*wireframes*), progressing to highly developed versions of the solution, all without a single line of executable code having been written by the development team.
- *More Research*—The human factors team tests the prototypes with the end users to see if the team has successfully translated the wants and needs of the customers into an experience that meets their expectations. Measuring the intuition, cognition, and behavior and even observing the emotional response of the user, the research team is able to deliver a report that allows the design team either to go back to the drawing board and think of different ways to approach the experience and improve it further or to give the development team a high degree of confidence that the system can proceed as designed.

While there was more up-front research and design time, the development team was excited by the vision, bolstered by the validation of the interactive prototypes, which not only improved morale, but also enabled the team to produce better time estimates and deliver a much higher quality product to market.

Designing with careful consideration of the UX elevates the quality of the solution, but it has to be remembered that this is still a team effort of research, design, and software development. Next are some of the techniques that can be utilized by human factors teams to help understand the end user better.

User Research

User research is both science and art. There are two main measurements for good user research:

- *Attitudinal Versus Behavioral*: This is the distinction between what people say versus what they do. If we pay attention only to one, we are likely going to skew the research data.
  - A *survey* is an example of attitudinal research; this is a common research method and allows the investigators to ask direct questions of the user and grade their experience on a scale defined by the researcher.
  - *Clickstream analysis* is an example of behavioral research; investigators use analytics built in to the solution to look at the route that a user takes through the solution to see what the user's intuition was telling them.
- *Qualitative Versus Quantitative*: Qualitative user research involves the researcher working directly with an end user and observing the user's actions, while quantitative research involves indirect observation that can be performed remotely.
  - *Qualitative research* is typically best achieved with smaller groups. Extremely useful research data can be gained from as few as 8–10 users. A common example would be a small group of users attending and participating in a laboratory study, where they use the software, allowing the researcher to observe their actions.
  - *Quantitative research* can allow the research team to test at scale, examining usability metrics of hundreds or thousands of users. These techniques are usable for all software development projects, with healthcare applications benefitting from direct quantitative data.

Products are tested in multiple phases of development so that the end product more closely meets needs and expectations:

- *Product Ideation*: Early in the development process, we start with a list of known, functional requirements. The research team engages internal and external subject matter experts to help with element prioritization.
- *Early Development*: Workable prototypes allow users to validate ideas and implementation early in the process.

- *Live Products*: If a product is performing poorly, is due for an overhaul, or needs to be tested for regulatory purposes, it is practical to subject it to rigorous tests to help focus efforts to improve and evolve the product.

Cerner User Research Activities

At Cerner, the user research team uses a wide range of techniques to improve our solutions. These techniques highlight many of the requirements mentioned for better user research and can be used in a variety of settings and stages in the development and improvement process. Similar processes are used by other vendors.

Task Analysis: This is performed by the human factors team providing a scripted scenario that the user performs from either a personal operational workstation or a usability laboratory. This allows us to analyze how the user interacts with the system and works his or her way through the solution. This research allows us to monitor the behavior of the end user with the solution and measures intuitiveness, effectiveness, efficiency, time, and overall satisfaction.

Usability Testing: There are two types of usability testing: *formative* and *summative*. With formative testing, human factors researchers work directly with our end users, who are interviewed episodically during development, determining what is and is not working with the early design of the software.

Once the software solution is complete, *summative testing* is performed on the final production model ahead of it going to market. Summative testing is done with a smaller group of end users and measures their performance both objectively and subjectively. Objective assessments may include time taken, number of errors that occurred, steps taken to complete the task, and metrics at successful completion of the task. Subjective assessments may include whether the user was satisfied with the experience and how intuitive the user felt the solution was. The output of a successful summative test is that it validates the work to that point, ensuring that the decisions and changes made have had a positive effect on the UX.

Information Architecture Mapping: This process is a detailed discussion regarding features and functionality within the solution and how they relate to each other. Information architecture mapping can be aided by both *tree tests* (Figure 14.1) and *card sorts* (Figure 14.2).

Tree Test: One can imagine productivity software needing drop-down menus, such as File, which may then have New, Open, Close, Save, and so on as options underneath the File header. In a tree test, the relationships are displayed to the end user as headers, and the user is then asked to locate a function, it is hoped with the result that the user finds that function underneath the expected parent in the hierarchy.

Card Sorting: This is similar to tree sorting, but with the reverse effort. Historically, a user would be given a stack of cards, each listing a key word, function, feature, or task. The user would then sort these into a visual architecture. This task is now performed electronically, but the *card sort* name persists. This test creates prototype architecture, allowing the development team to see where people expect the features to be listed and accessed from within the software.

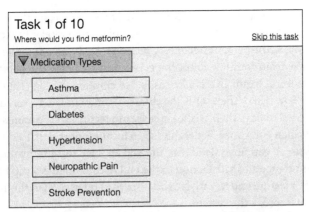

Figure 14.1 Tree test. In the tree test, following from the card sort example, we ask the user via questions where they would expect to find each medication. In this study, they simply click on the header in the tree where they would expect to see it. This is a very simple example, but the trees can go very deep, requiring the user to click on the first option, then choose from a secondary or even tertiary list of options.

Surveys: Surveys are used at almost every stage of the development cycle and can be administered online, via dedicated websites such as SurveyMonkey or by phone or email. Surveys allow the research team to build a statistical database of user preferences, feelings, and opinions that can be applied to early prototyping work or existing solutions or even help to identify a seed idea.

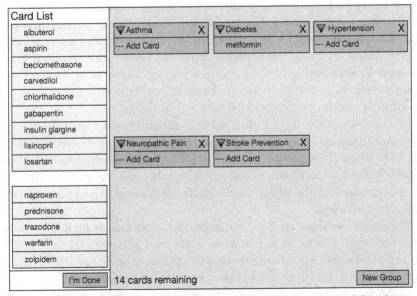

Figure 14.2 Card sort test. In this example, the user is asked to drag the "cards" on the left into the five sections to group them by type. (They also have the opportunity to create a new section if they feel the available ones are insufficient/inappropriate.) Once the test is complete, the researchers can compare and contrast the groupings to find the most appropriate location for each of the medications and then validate it using the tree test study.

Personas: These are fictional characters created by the UX team that embody the traits of important end users. Personas are assembled from research, accomplished in a variety of ways. The persona becomes a beacon for subsequent design decisions, encouraging the team to think about the *person* first and how the person will feel about the decision at hand. This is a key aspect of emotional design thinking.

Stakeholder Interviews: The user is the principal target of UX research, but other stakeholders need to have their wishes, needs, and technical constraints registered. This would include enterprise leaders and even local support staff.

Gap Analysis: A gap analysis allows the stakeholder to rank features by their perceived importance and satisfaction to the end user. If there is a gap between the importance of a feature and its satisfaction from the end user, then this indicates an opportunity to improve the system.

Discussion Groups: The user research team brings together project stakeholders and users in organized, structured, and productive conversations to help focus on the needs and perceptions of the end user. Among the discussion points are prioritization of features and methods to address specific issues.

Competitive Analysis: Researchers look at competitors' products and break the feature sets down into measurable, objective elements that allow stakeholders to see where their solution stands in the marketplace. This can help to identify missing or substandard features.

Ideation Workshops: Structured workshops involving the UX and research teams can address problems, seed ideas, or other issues for which a remedy is not immediately evident. Ideation workshops bring diverse subject matter expertise into a room and can generate a unique working dynamic.

Journey Mapping: A journey map tells the story of a fictional persona or real person working their way through the software solution. This is not only a map of clicks and entries, but also the need for the solution and expected emotional responses over an extended period. In addition to routine workflows, perturbations are considered. For example, what happens when an emergency occurs? Role-playing through these scenarios helps to promote creation of a better UX and tells an inspiring story that can aid design thinking and inspire the team.

On-Site Observation: On-site observation is essential to determination of solution function and experience in an actual working environment. The research team can learn about unanticipated interruptions, unexpected workflows, and operational bottlenecks. This allows the research team to become more familiar with the user's interaction with the software and is invaluable in design of the solution for the working environment.

User Interviews: These are one-on-one conversations, usually performed when on-site observation is under way. The researcher can assess attitudes, frustrations, and expressed recommendations regarding what needs to be changed. The data can apply specifically to the specialty and arena of the health professional.

Analytics: Data science and the effective, proactive use of analytics is becoming the norm in every software industry. We can use data to create compelling data visualizations and easily display actionable metrics, of both the system and the users. UX analytics results that were actionable include identifying providers making more than 20 clicks to place an antibiotic order. This was improved by building favorites and more complex order sentences. Another was identification of users who were doing ambulatory charting beyond midnight, prompting discussions to help avoid burnout and improve work-life balance.

Heuristics Analysis: This is a high-level analysis that takes an established set of best practice design principles, or heuristics, and benchmarks a given solution against them. This is a first pass that can be applied to software that is in development. This allows the team to pinpoint major issues in design that would almost guarantee a bad UX.

Content Strategy: Lastly, UX efforts can help to generate a consistent standard in content generation through the enterprise, from written content and formatting of documents, to the consistent use of specific words on buttons across the applications. Creating these standards allows the organization to align goals, procedures, and best practices and not create different sets of rules for different elements of the enterprise.

By utilizing these tools and techniques we have discussed, UX and human factors teams are working to improve the quality of solutions. Every EHR vendor is a business and has a focus on improving market share and profits, but at the end of the day, we are all on the same team.

KEY POINTS

- User experience is dependent on the design and function of the UI.
- Design is an iterative process with direct and indirect feedback from users.
- Stakeholders should be involved in all stages of the interface design process.
- There is a science to user interface design, with multimodal assessments of usability.

15

Access and Access Controls

KARL E. MISULIS AND MARK E. FRISSE ■

OVERVIEW OF ACCESS, AUTHORIZATION, PRIVILEGES, AND PERMISSIONS

Definitions

Authorization is the process of identifying the individual and determining what the individual can do. You are authorized to access your electronic health record (EHR) system.

Access controls are the method of enforcing authorization through mechanisms and policies. Access controls generally require single-factor authentication (password or fingerprint) to access the EHR, but require dual-factor authentication (e.g. routine access plus securely messaged code) to e-prescribe opiates.

Privileges and *permissions* are sometimes used interchangeably, but they are different terms. *Privileges* are what a particular user or user group is able to do. *Permissions* are what is allowed to be done to a particular file or function in a system.

We are authorized to use the hospital EHRs. We go through access controls to use the EHRs. We have privileges associated with being a credentialed provider of our specialties. We have permission to read and create documents and place orders, but we do not have permission to directly edit the data tables.

Access Control

Access controls depend on position because privileges and permissions depend on position. Here, we discuss some of the mechanisms of controlling access.

USER ID AND PASSWORD

Historically, access to clinical and nonclinical programs has been by user ID and password; the credentials are directly entered into the application interface. Most healthcare systems have requirements for changing passwords periodically.

The risk of this workflow is that with a multiplicity of user IDs and passwords that an individual has to remember and the encouragement not to use the same credentials for multiple sites, the user is likely to store his or her credentials in an easily discoverable place or use credentials that can easily be guessed.

An argument for not using the same credentials for many applications is in the availability from nefarious third parties of user ID/password combinations that have been captured by keyloggers or other mechanisms. Because many people reuse credentials, thieves will try these credentials on a multitude of sites to see if there are any hits. This is automated, so even if the yield is 1 in 1000, access will be gained occasionally.

Modern access systems generally have requirements for user ID and password selection which are relatively secure, but they have no way of preventing users from using the same credentials for multiple purposes.

SINGLE SIGN ON

Single sign on (SSO) has largely replaced individual sign on to applications. The user logs in to the SSO application, which presents a menu of applications in list or icon form. Clicking the menu item activates the app and passes login credentials. Hence, the user does not need to remember each user id/password combination, making it less likely that they will write them down in an easily discoverable location. Also, advanced SSO access, such as with two-factor authentication (2FA), is easier to implement. The configuration information is usually stored using a Lightweight Directory Access Protocol (LDAP), which is an open application protocol for distributed directory services, like an address book holding user ID/password sets as well as other configuration information such as roles.

SMART CARD

Smart cards are most familiar to us as the chips in modern credit cards. These cards contain digital information that is used to give some degree of assurance that the card is authentic. While security is not guaranteed, smart cards are more secure than legacy cards with magnetic stripes.

Most smart cards have contacts that make a physical connection with the reader equipment. Some are contactless and essentially a passive radio-frequency identification (RFID) chip (discussed further in this chapter).

Smart cards have two principal uses in healthcare. One is for access to computer systems, and the other is for transport of records. Smart cards can have sufficient storage capacity for essential portable information.

RADIO-FREQUENCY IDENTIFICATION

Radio-frequency identification is a mechanism to give identification through proximity. In healthcare access control, RFID is often employed by being part of the badges of healthcare workers. *Passive RFID* is most common: The power source for the badge electronics is obtained from induction from the reader, and there is no battery on the card. Very close proximity to the reader is essential for the chip to obtain the power needed. This is commonly used for the tap-in function for devices equipped with the readers.

In *active RFID*, there is a small battery on the card, which gives the card a shorter lifetime but does allow for much greater range. Range is less important for access control than for materials management (e.g., the location of the infusion pumps). An active RFID tag can be read by a detector at a much greater distance than for a passive RFID tag. We know of at least one enterprise that uses active RFID for their desktop workstations. When the employee walks away the workstation locks without the employee having to tap-out.

Credentials Management

User identification (user ID) is the defined variable used for access control by our systems. We may select a user ID that is easy to remember and often part of our name. User ID usually does not change over time but can be changed if needed. Some individuals will have multiple user IDs for different roles. For example, a chief medical informatics officer (CMIO) will have not only a user ID for clinical practice but also perhaps several different ones for testing the system with the positions of nurse, midlevel provider, clerk, or database administrator.

The password is the key used by the user presenting the associated user ID. This combination is usually sufficient to unlock most granted privileges on the system.

Some general password guidelines include the following:

- A password is changed at intervals, and when changed should not be to a previously used password.
- Passwords should not be the same between purposes (e.g., EHR vs. Microsoft vs. Apple accounts) and should not be the same for each access if the user has multiple user IDs.
- Passwords should not be shared or written down where they can be seen.
- Passwords should not contain any significant portion of the user ID.
- Passwords should be significantly complex that they cannot be guessed. Most systems have specific requirements (e.g., at least 8 characters, at least one from each of number, letter, special character, etc.).

Alternative methods of access include

- RFID badge or token
- Passcode sent to a pager or phone

- Fingerprint
- Face recognition

Access is often location specific. For example, access for some purposes may not be able to be made from off campus, such as core maintenance, which may require the user to be on site. Also, some healthcare systems restrict access to networks from outside the country or from select countries, similar to streaming services restricting access.

Two-Factor Authentication

For two-factor authentication, the typical user ID/password combination is supplemented by another method. Most commonly, this is something that only the authorized user would be expected to have. For example, many large corporations and some US federal agencies require a passcode sent to a phone or pager assigned to the user. Other examples would be swiping or tapping a badge assigned to the user. A newer technology is display of a QR (Quick Response) code, which is then scanned by the user's phone, which has been paired with the system.

Two-factor authorization is required for electronic prescription of controlled substances by the Drug Enforcement Agency. They define 2FA as previously mentioned, with use of two of the following:

- Something we *know* (e.g., password for the user ID)
- Something we *have* (e.g., a token)
- Something we *are* (e.g., biometric)

In the future, 2FA will likely be used increasingly for routine EHR use.

Context Management and Clinical Context Object Workgroup

Context management in healthcare refers to the ability of a user to open multiple clinical applications and see the records pertaining to the same patient. A common scenario is reviewing the EHR of a specific patient and being able to launch the picture archiving and communication system (PACS) and immediately viewing those study images. While not all healthcare applications have this capability, most do, and this is because of a standard protocol developed by Health Level Seven International's Clinical Context Object Workgroup (CCOW).

Context management is usually functioning in an SSO system, so that login is not required by the user for each application. If the basic access control is not SSO, then the context management process may pass user authentication from the first app to the affiliated app; for example, the PACS may presume authorized access from the EHR without asking for another authentication.

Profile Management

Profile management has two components: individual and group profiles.

Individual Profiles: Privileges are designated to each user according to a profile. This profile should extend to the user regardless of how they access the system. For example, a user might access the EHR from the two-screen desktop thick client or from the user's laptop. A profile should give the user a fairly consistent appearance and functionality between the different devices, yet allow for device-specific capabilities. In the example just given, the two-screen desktop could not be emulated on the laptop, but the remainder of the application display and access should be consistent.

Group Profiles: Individual groups will a have consistent look and feel and functionalities that are most appropriate to the workflow of the members of the group. For example, the profile for a hospitalist would be different from that of a clinic physician. However, a specific user might have different roles, so the profile is often able to be changed without having to have a separate login. For example, providers in our facilities have different profiles depending on whether they are in clinic, in hospital service, in obstetrics, or in the emergency department/urgent care.

CLIENT AND DEVICE STRATEGY

Specifics of thin and thick clients are discussed in Chapter 9. Here, we discuss some practical considerations of client and device strategy.

Enterprise-Supplied Devices

Enterprise desktop devices depend on use. For nursing units, thin clients are usually used. Thick clients are used when more robust local computing capability is needed, such as provider and administrator desktops or in procedural areas where interfacing with equipment is needed. Thick clients are usually needed for PACS, neurodiagnostics, and cardiology diagnostics, among others.

Phone apps for EHRs are increasingly being deployed, and all of our hospitals have this functionality even though they use different brands of EHR. These are convenient, though the look and feel of the application are far different from the computer user interface. This difference plus limitations in functionality have limited provider adoption. Access controls on phones and tablets offer particular challenges. Some SSO solutions will not work well on mobile devices, although this functionality can be retained by using a remote desktop virtualization application.

Laptops are often supplied by healthcare systems, although we generally do not recommend this. Limitations of security, battery life, update control, and physical safety place these devices at risk. We recommend that users who want to use a portable device have their personal device configured for hospital and clinic purposes unless the personal device is going to be a replacement for point-of-care devices.

LOGIN RESTRICTIONS

Most facilities restrict a user to one device login at a time. This is not universally true, but the risk of multiple logins is the potential for users sharing their credentials with their staff or the potential of an active session being unsecured. For example, a provider may ask a medical assistant to login as the provider to place preoperative orders. Or, a clinic patient may see data on the device that is already logged into by the provider, who has not entered the room. Unfortunately, these examples are not just theoretical.

TIME OUT

Time out of a login generally has two components. First is a time-out to lock screen. This is often set to 5 or 10 minutes of inactivity. This is generally a local device function, although configuration is pushed down from information systems (IS).

System time out refers to the time before the application terminates, often 30–45 minutes of no user activity. This is long enough for most clinical uses, but might not be for some slow-moving scenarios.

System time out cannot be allowed for apps under certain circumstances where there is critical background operation. For example, one of our affiliates disables time out of the PACS in the operating room so that a crucial image does not disappear in the middle of a case. Similarly, they have their anesthesia system configured so there is no screen saver and no time out. Because this is a server-level configuration for the implementation, they have separate dedicated servers for these purposes.

VIRTUAL DESKTOP

A *virtual desktop* has been discussed several times and refers to the applications not running on the user device but on servers with the user device as a communication platform. On a Windows, OSX, iOS, or other platform device running the client software, the desktop looks like a Windows desktop. Advantages are multiple but in this context provide the possibility of the active desktop following the user from device to device. For example, we use the EHR on our tablets and view the results while in a patient room. We then go to a desktop workstation to do orders and a note, and the virtual desktop is precisely where we left off on the tablets, but reformatted for the display parameters of the workstation.

This functionality can be efficiently used in conjunction with RFID, allowing for tap-in/tap-out to the desktop presence.

Personal Device

Personal devices are commonly used, particularly laptops and tablets for EHRs, and phones sometimes for EHRs but more commonly for secure messaging.

Clinical applications can be vendor apps or virtual desktops. Virtual desktops often do not scale well on small-screen devices, so specific platform apps are preferable, if available.

SECURITY CONCERNS

We allow providers to install and configure the virtual desktop client software on their devices, but IS staff perform the installation and configuration for many. There are some unusual configuration issues that can be encountered that are beyond the scope of expertise of many users.

We do not allow people to install and configure some enterprise apps themselves on their own devices; we require IS to do this and also install the ability to remotely wipe our enterprise apps from the user device. There can be some expected push-back from this approach, but it is fairly standard among nonhealthcare as well as healthcare enterprises.

FUTURE DIRECTIONS OF ACCESS

Evolution of healthcare systems and the constantly changing regulatory landscape continuously alter all facets of health information technology, including access. While it is impossible to precisely predict the future, the following are some of our expectations for the coming years.

Two-Factor Authentication: 2FA should become standard due to the increasing effort and sophistication of intrusion methods. User ID/password is not sufficient security for healthcare systems. Of the 2FA methods previously discussed, biometrics may be the easiest to avoid circumvention.

e-Prescribing: e-Prescribing will undoubtedly become more prevalent, and we predict that it will ultimately be required. The lack of security and high overhead associated with paper prescriptions should sunset that method. Similarly, with EHR assess on phones and other devices, telephone verbal prescriptions should sunset, especially with controlled substances.

Multiple Logins: These are disabled at most of our facilities and should be disabled in almost all healthcare systems. Where efficiency would be degraded, such as in a clinic setting, virtual desktop infrastructure can regain workflow efficiency.

Patient access: Patients initially had access to portals that were read only, but now the information is bidirectional, and most portals are able to facilitate appointments and communication with physicians. We foresee that patients will be able to access records from more than one enterprise on a single portal and, ultimately, have a centralized portal process where all medical enterprises can feed into a single access. Also, we expect functionality to improve so that patients can more easily add to and edit their records, complete forms prior to visits, authorize access to new providers, send records to other individuals and enterprises, and complete financial transactions associated with their visits.

KEY POINTS

- Access controls are key to ensuring authorized access to health IS.
- Access controls must balance security and efficiency.
- Virtual desktop infrastructure is increasingly common in healthcare IS.
- Mobile device use for health IS is increasingly used, and we must deal with security and access control but not impede efficiency.

16

Analytics

MARK E. FRISSE AND KARL E. MISULIS ■

OVERVIEW OF ANALYTICS

Analytics have two broad clinical goals:

- One is overall improvement of a group of patients. For example, do patients in our hospital have a higher or lower surgical site infection rate than expected?
- The second is for care of a specific patient. For example, is Mr. X showing early signs of sepsis? Or, does Mr. Y have findings suggesting a high risk for coronary artery bypass grafting?

The first goal is in the arena of institutional quality control. The second has two components: the analytics for Mr. X is in the arena of *clinical decision support,* while the analytics for Mr. Y is in the arena of *predictive analytics.*

Financial analytics has the purpose of monitoring costs and billing. *Cost accounting* ensures that the system is meeting expectations for utilization of materials and personnel. *Revenue accounting* seeks to ensure that bills are submitted and paid. This includes ensuring charge capture. These data are essential for financial viability of the system and for negotiating with payers for fees and bundled payments.

Payers and governmental agencies perform analytics as well as request reports from healthcare systems so they can ensure that they are getting their expected amount and quality of service and that costs are adequately controlled.

Healthcare analytics is pivotal to all informatics professionals, from providers to payers to regulators. We must respond to the results of collective and individual analytics on collective and individual levels.

But this is not easy. People and enterprises must increasingly respond to financial incentives involving more complex data sets and incorporating multiple care events. The expectation is that these approaches will improve care and lower costs. Of necessity, these approaches all require more complex and expensive analytic systems usually integrated with clinical data warehouses. But even if insights are gleaned, they are meaningless unless providers and patients can act on the results in substantive ways. Knowing health status or degree of risk does not necessarily mean that one can easily improve health status or mitigate risk. On the bright side, reporting requirements or initiatives may lead to positive behavioral change, but on the darker side, reporting without appropriate incentive structure can also lead to behaviors that are counterproductive to quality improvement aims.

Examples of the *bright side of analytics*:

- Widespread reporting of common quality metrics
- Reduction in the rate of ventilator-associated pneumonia after reporting was required.
- Reduction in the rate of catheter-associated urinary tract infections (CAUTIs) after reporting was required.
- Better means of assessing risk for sepsis, depression, and other medical conditions.
- Better means of assessing necessary care after hospitalization.
- Improved public health reporting.

But anecdotes on the "dark side" of analytics abound:

- Surgeons and other clinicians who care for complex patients may change their referral patterns or cease performing needed procedures altogether if outcomes are not appropriately adjusted for severity of underlying illness.
- Meaningful Use payment analytic requirements have triggered several facilities to report metrics that were not supported by their capabilities and led to severe penalties
- Complex and expensive analytic requirements may lead institutions to drop out of advanced Accountable Care Organization initiatives.

The potential—indeed the necessity—for advanced analytics is great. Although the focus of analytics may be on the organization, one must remember that the same data are being employed by payers and government agencies as well. While watching one's own organization, remember that others are watching you!

Clinical informatics professionals must work to ensure that efforts meet several criteria:

- Include the complete and accurate data set necessary to do the analysis
- Utilize competent analytics systems and professionals to implement the program

- Use realistic educational programs and workflow integration that will ensure that results from an analytics effort can lead to meaningful behavioral change

There are many good analytics efforts that can serve as models. These include efforts to:

- Reduce care variance
- Reduce hospital length-of-stay
- Reduce hospital readmissions
- Reduce care gaps
- Reduce medication errors
- Monitor costs and resource utilization
- Monitor billing and other administrative activities
- Identify individuals at high risk for complications and other adverse events

Our discussion is of necessity brief. Readers are encouraged to study this topic in greater detail. Analytics and data science books and other resources are abundant .[1] Other chapters in this book also touch on topics related to analytics.[2]

ANALYTICS METHODS

Data analytics begins with knowing what data we have and where it is. Every enterprise has multiple data sources, and most queries retrieve information that has more than one original source.

A recent vignette is illustrative. At one of our larger hospitals, administration asked the business systems analysts for information on who was ordering large amounts of certain high-cost antibiotics. They retrieved a list that included patients' accounts that had been billed for the specific antibiotics plus the IDs of the admitting and discharging providers. The initial results were misleading because the antibiotic data were associated with the admitting physician and hence attributed prescribing patterns to primary care physicians when often these drugs were ordered by infectious disease or other consulting specialists. This only came to the attention of institutional leadership months later. To clarify this point, the institution's CMIO (not involved in the original study) quickly performed a query through the institution's EHR and extracted accurate and actionable data within a few hours. The central lesson was that the CMIO and others who understood the clinical context and data sources were not involved in the initial reporting initiative.

Analytics and Reporting

The cornerstone of analytics has historically been reporting. While this is what many people think of when we talk of analytics, reporting is only a subset of what is done and what will increasingly be essential roles for these technologies. Reports can be generated automatically or manually. Many EHR and business systems have an array of preset reports that query for the relevant data, aggregate the data, and perform needed calculations. Reports are most commonly presented as a PDF or spreadsheet.

The series of steps invoked in preparing a report includes

- Decide on a question that can lead to actions
- Decide what data are needed to answer that question
- Design the query to extract the data from the data source(s)
- Run the query
- Aggregate the data
- Perform needed calculations
- Present the data
- Determine if the report answered the question

This is the beginning of an iterative cycle, which is seldom perfected on the first attempt.

Defining the question is key. A valid question is not, "Why do we spend so much on antibiotics?" That question is not actionable in its present form. A better first question might be "What antibiotics do we prescribe the most?" and perhaps team that with a second question: "What antibiotics do we spend the most money on?" Before proceeding one must be certain that the questions raised can be answered unambiguously.

Deciding what data are needed includes determining where the data are. Generally, larger organizations incorporate necessary data from multiple sources into a separate data warehouse. Clinical informatics professionals should play a key role in the acquisition, design, management, and governance of these data warehouses.

Previously in this chapter we gave a true story of a failed analytics effort because the analyst was looking in the wrong database. Historically, claims-based analysis could be very helpful for the utilization management side of business analytics. However, claims do not have granular clinical data to answer many clinical questions. Also, existing claims data may not contain all necessary information; low-cost generic drugs, for example, are not always included in health plan pharmacy claims databases.

Presentation of the data is performed in countless ways. Spreadsheet programs remain the mainstay for early exploratory analysis. Often they are sufficient either to answer a question or to identify additional steps necessary to realize valid results. Only after these issues have been identified can one employ general-purpose statistical software packages and more advanced data visualization techniques.

Data sets are often too small or incomplete to provide statistical insight. In these circumstances, simple exploratory data visualization may be the may provide insight into flawed study assumptions. An example from one of our affiliated skilled nursing facilities concerned an analysis of whether occupancy levels correlated with frequency of medication administration errors. A simple data plot made obvious that variations in occupancy were too small to yield statistical significance and, when discussing these simple results, investigators realized that the study did not account for lower staffing rates in the rare times that occupancy was lower.

Hence, an iterative approach to report generation and evaluation is needed. And, analytics professionals need to remain connected to providers who will have a current clinical context the analysts often do not have.

Organizations are tasked with generating a host of reports mandated by government regulations, others that are mandated by professional societies, and still others that are performed for local quality improvement processes. Governance of the reporting process is complex but should include participation by the department(s) involved in the issues under study as well as informatics and administrative leadership.

Just some of the reports generated include rates of certain complications of hospital stay (e.g., catheter-based urinary tract infection, central line–associated bloodstream infection, postsurgical infection), length of hospital stay, and readmission rates.

There are numerous analytics packages that can accomplish reports. None of them can perform all needed analytics and reporting. We suggest care and caution in selecting packages.

- Select reporting packages that will work with your information system.
- Ensure reporting packages meet the claimed reporting needs.
- Avoid extensive use of niche reporting packages, as much as possible. Many of these do not offer value-added capability over other capabilities already in our systems.
- Avoid duplication of reporting and analytics.
- Spend time looking at the report to ensure the report is accurate, the data seemingly valid, and actionable conclusions evident.

There are a number of challenges with reporting and analytics.

- *Data sources*: Many reports need data from different data sources. To facilitate a commonly used report, aggregation of these data into a data warehouse or data mart is often helpful.
- *Unstructured data*: Many clinical data are unstructured, such as that from provider and nursing notes. There are many efforts to address this, including natural language processing (NLP), but this remains a problem in developing clinically actionable analytics.
- *Missing data*: Some analytics will want data that are not available. For example, a patient may have had a follow-up visit at another hospital for a complication of a surgery at our hospital. Unless we are informed of this event, we will not be aware of the complication or readmission.

When studying reports, one must have realistic expectations. There are some general truths to financial analytics:

- Not every service will be revenue positive.
- Information systems are typically not revenue positive.
- Line items in budgets not clearly associated with any specific outcome are easy targets for inappropriate cuts.

If an administrator is looking at the revenue balance for clinical services, the conclusions will commonly be made that cardiology is revenue positive and the obstetrics service is often revenue negative, especially in public hospitals with poor payer mixes. Primary care may also be revenue negative but primary care provider referrals are essential to the financial performance of an overall care network.

These same concerns also plague the CIO. Information technologies are essential for healthcare organizations but the measuring the value of different components is elusive. Traditionally, information technologies comprise less than 5% of a hospitals budget, but this misleading figure does not incorporate the true value in terms of patient care and the true cost not just of the technology but the planning, maintenance, and overall contribution to organizational productivity. Small savings on technology may lead to enormous costs if systems decrease clinician and staff productivity or do not help an organization reach its aspirations.

Organizational budgets generally do not show the interdependencies among technology, processes, people, and attainment of corporate goals. Without a full appreciation of these dependencies, for example, a chief financial officer (CFO) might postpone to the next fiscal year an interface engine upgrade that, unbeknownst to the CFO, will delay installation of an essential new revenue cycle system that depends on the interface engine upgrade. Critical thinking about these matters is essential. The Information Technology budget is really an organizational budget.

Analytics and reporting are tools which must be used but can be misued through mistake or intent.

Statistics

Basic statistics of data analysis is introduced in Chapter 11. Healthcare analytics uses advanced statistical methods, particularly examining statistical differences between populations and identification of developing trends.

We summarize several common tests here. The test used depends on a number of factors. Some of these include type of data, number of samples, distribution of the data, whether the data are paired.

Common types of data are continuous, discrete, or Boolean. Continuous data could be the level of a chemical: An infinite number of results exists because a measurement could have infinite significant digits. Discrete data are counting data, such as the number of children or number of metastases. There are no fractional values. Boolean data are one of two states: true or false. Examples can be with or without disease, did or did not have a specified treatment.

The *Student t test* is used mainly for comparing two groups of continuous data. The data typically have a normal distribution (symmetric bell-shaped curve). Are the groups sampled from the same or different populations? Do patients with disease X have higher levels of chemical Y than the normal population?

The *Fisher exact test* is used for data in a 2×2 table. An example is data for patients with or without a trait (such as having a certain gene mutation or taking a specified medication) who did or did not get a disease.

A *Chi-squared test* is also used for tabular discrete data, but more than two columns or rows can be used (e.g., disease cure, or not, with four different treatment groups).

The *Analysis of Variance* (ANOVA) is for comparing more than two groups of continuous data that have an expected normal distribution, such as comparing the seizure frequencies of patients with four different seizure types who were on one of three different anticonvulsants.

The *Pearson correlation coefficient* is for determining whether two variables have a linear correlation. While that does not diagnose causation, it is scientifically helpful. For example, a recent analysis at a prominent medical school examined the correlation between students' performance on basic science classes versus clinical rotations. The correlation was positive but was remarkably weak.

The particular statistical tests to be used depend on what is being measured. Often the greatest failures are a result of a sloppy application of the right statistical method or, worse, the thoughtful application of a method that is not appropriate to the problem at hand. Consultation with expert statisticians and data scientists is often essential.

Data Mining

Data mining is application of one or many different methods to search for patterns in data. Sometimes, the term is used for delving deeply into analytic data sets, but this is not the intent of the term. Rather, data mining incorporates a range of techniques. Machine learning techniques are at one end of a range of data mining techniques. For some, data mining can be thought of an essential step in transforming data into information and into knowledge. When applied to a vast database, these approaches may identify patterns and relationships (e.g., between medications and complications) missed by initial conventional analyses. This cyclical process of providing evidence-based care and, through data mining, using new findings to improve care is a fundamental component of learning healthcare system (Chapter 6).

Knowledge discovery in databases (KDD) is one form of this process. It of necessity begins with a database of sufficient size to infer new findings on subsets of interest (e.g., patients with diabetes in the population of patients admitted to a hospital system). With this subset, outliers and clearly erroneous values are removed, the problem of missing data is addressed and assurances are made that all data are standardized (e.g., blood glucose levels are converted to LOINC standards.) Only then can analytic methods be applied. For example, for a diabetic population, an algorithm can correlate the effect of baseline Hemoglobin A1C and in-hospital glucose levels with mortality, surgical infection rate, length of stay, readmission rate, whether or not a standardized glucose control protocol was used. Subsequently, the results are evaluated for apparent validity, clinical implications, and operational utility.

The findings are then applied to practice. For example, use of a standard glucose control protocol designed for perioperative surgical care may have to be refined to adjust for underlying severity of illness. Conversely, the analysis may show that that inadequate near-term in-house glucose control might correlate more with surgical infection rate than long-time control metrics such as hemoglobin A1C.

A potential pitfall of data mining and the KDD process is so extensive an analysis of a large data set that relationships are identified that are specific to this data set alone and are not replicated in a similar data set or may be the result of overfitting or other methodologic errors. Expertise and validation are essential.

Predictive Analytics

Predictive analytics identify patterns in historical data and use these results to predict future events.

Health plans may look at historical data for millions of customers over multiple years and discover a patterns predicting risk of vascular events, other complications or even death. (Health plans are indeed examining these topics.) With these analyses, one can stratify patient risk and personalize interventions. One hope is that by sharing these data with patients and clinicians, medical interventions and lifestyle adjustments may be more effective.

Genomics is a major player in the field of predictive analytics. On the basis of genomics, we can often determine if a particular patient is likely to get breast cancer (BRCA1 and BRCA2) or if another patient might not respond to clopidogrel (CYP2C19 variants). Many other associations will be identified by similar methods.

Machine learning and other techniques are very powerful but, by virtue of the way the neural network computations are performed, may not be able to identify specific causative factors. The inability to explain findings is one reason why clinicians sometimes think of analytics—and especially machine learning—as a "black box" meriting suspicion. Others argue effectively that much of the evidence-base developed through advanced regression analyses is already the product of a "black box." Given the growth of these approaches, clinical informatics professionals must master this field.

The power to peer into behavior, genetics, imaging, and clinical care reveals both the promise and threats of these practices. New findings have already helped tailor better therapies in oncology and other fields. One the other hand, knowing the future also can lead to discrimination. As more genetic tests appear, the risk of neoplasia can be more accurately determined and this risk in turn could in theory allow employers to discriminate against these individuals when hiring. Particularly in the United States and other countries without universal health care coverage, future predictions of Alzheimer's disease and many other illness may have great social and actuarial consequences. In these areas, policy and legislation are often forced to play "catch up" with advancing technology. Although the Genetic Information Nondiscrimination Act of 2008 prohibits hiring and employment discrimination on the basis of genetics, these same findings may and do impact life, disability, and long-term care insurance. With respect to health care coverage, the impact of these findings will depend more on politics and perception than on science.

ORGANIZATION AND GOVERNANCE OF ANALYTICS

Increasingly, data sources will be centralized either though common physical storage or widespread data exchange. At the same time, many different groups seek these data for clinical care, epidemiology, research, or simple commercial profit. The result can be data access and use by many different organizations that use the data for different purposes and have different perspectives on ethics, security, and privacy. Given the virtual and distributed nature of data, the traditional idea of "data ownership" no longer makes sense. Rather, one should think of data in terms of three different rights—the right to collect, the right to aggregate and analyze, and the right to disclose data for specific purposes. As is the case in music or other intellectual property issues, the central question is not the location of a "master copy" but instead one of balancing individual preferences with societal expectations regarding data use. Governance principles, therefore, must be applied across the spectrum of data use. The governance of data is a complex balancing act between centralized and decentralized approaches and among the various needs and cultures of those in search of data.

Data security (to prevent unauthorized modification or disclosure) is not the same as data governance, but remains a primary responsibility of any organization in possession of a database.

Particularly with respect to hospitals and other health care delivery organizations, we recommend a multilayer approach to the organization and governance of both data and analytics:

- Enterprise analytics leadership should have representation of clinical leadership, operations and finance leadership, informatics leadership, information systems leadership, quality leaders, and analytics leaders. Among the C-suite representatives will often be the CMIO, chief information officer, chief medical officer, chief quality officer, chief nursing officer, CFO, and often chief executive officer. Analytics staff participation is essential so that the questions and requests are understood and estimates can be made of time and resources needed for the requested tasks.
- Service line and departmental analytics should be maintained so that focused reporting and metrics can be easily validated and deficiencies promptly investigated and corrected.
- Operational analytic leadership should be coordinated so that focused and enterprise tasks can be assigned to specific individuals with expectations on completion time. Also, this layer is best in a position to determine if metrics are duplicative.
- Processes for data security and governance are essential and are arguably the most important aspect of institutions relying on personal data.

Ultimately, health care must be built on a foundation of trust. Such trust cannot be achieved if an organization insufficiently considers data rights and cannot consistently ensure effective data governance practices.

KEY POINTS

- Data science is arguably one of the most important and emergent aspects of clinical informatics.
- Effective data science and analytics requires a continuous process of learning and collaborating with diverse experts.
- Effective analytics will help improve healthcare delivery outcomes and control healthcare costs.
- Effective analytics requires new expertise and state-of-the-art statistical judgement, methods, and visualization techniques.
- The governance of data and analytics is critical and requires coordination across many areas of an enterprise.

17

Decision Support

CHRISTOPH U. LEHMANN, KARL E. MISULIS,
AND MARK E. FRISSE ■

MAKING CLINICAL DECISIONS

Clinical decision-making methodology depends on the complexity of the patient's case, the certainty of a diagnosis, available treatment and diagnostic resources, reliability of information resources, training of the clinician, and psychological makeup of the clinician. In general, two major forms of decision-making exist: *algorithmic* and *syndromic*. While algorithmic reasoning is used predominantly, there are advantages of the syndromic approach.

Decision Theory

Algorithmic decision-making consists of reasoning using a systematic approach. For example, a patient presenting to the emergency department (ED) with fever and confusion has a large number of differential diagnoses (e.g., pneumonia, enterovirus, flu, substance abuse, meningitis, neoplasm, head injury, epilepsy, to name a few). Our algorithmic reasoning may describe this as encephalopathy and then develop a more granular differential diagnosis depending on additional data. Statistically, in the ED, encephalopathy with fever is most commonly due to a concurrent illness in a patient, who is elderly or otherwise debilitated from coexistent disease. The fever raises concern for an infection. We know that an infection causing encephalopathy could be from a primary central nervous system (CNS) infection, such as meningitis or encephalitis, or more commonly from systemic effects of a non-neurologic infection, such as a urinary tract infection or pneumonia in a patient with advanced age or baseline cognitive abnormality. The presence of stiff neck or other findings suggesting meningitis would lead us down that path. The presence of focal seizures would suggest encephalitis. Absence of either of these findings would not rule these diagnoses out but would make non-neurologic concurrent infection more likely. We perform computed tomography (CT) to look for the unlikely possibility of subarachnoid hemorrhage, and if bleeding or no other structural lesion is seen, then lumbar puncture (LP) is performed to look for infection in the cerebrospinal fluid (CSF). We gather more data, and we add those data to our algorithm. With each datum considered, the differential diagnoses change, making some subsequent investigations more useful than others. Evaluation and testing continue until the cost of the most useful next test is larger than the benefit from altering the likelihood of a treatable diagnosis.

Syndromic decision-making consists of recognizing a constellation of findings that suggest a syndrome, a clinical profile with specific implications. Experienced clinicians can recognize patterns of symptoms and findings that lead them immediately to recognize a pattern previously seen in another patient. These syndromes/patterns are not perfectly sensitive and specific, but they are helpful. Returning to our patient with fever and confusion, we discover neck stiffness. Jumping to the conclusion of meningitis will be correct some or most of the time. Other times, the patient may have a concurrent illness with fever plus the red herring of chronic cervical spine disease causing the stiff neck. Or, the patient might have a subarachnoid hemorrhage with an almost identical presentation.

Academic clinicians will generally prefer an algorithmic approach, mainly because they are responsible for training new clinicians, who cannot rely on patterns from personal experience. But, syndromic reasoning results in the correct answer often and allows for rapid diagnosis, which may be needed for rapid treatment.

Consider the example of a patient who is brought to the ED with acute onset of right hemiparesis and aphasia. This is almost certainly a stroke, most likely ischemic (lack of blood flow) but possibly hemorrhagic (a bleed). Because this patient requires immediate intervention, the provider does not have the time to perform a 45-minute neurologic assessment. A rapid, 5- to 7-minute neurologic assessment must arrive at a provisional diagnosis. If the CT shows no blood and there are no other confounding issues, the patient receives intravenous tissue plasminogen activator (tPA [clot buster]) before the physician has performed a complete history and physical.

The principal drawback of syndromic/pattern recognition decision-making is an inherent bias: anchoring at the first diagnosis considered. Contradictory information may not be given the appropriate weight or considered at all. Once a diagnosis is entered into a patient's chart, there is inertia at reconsidering or challenging the diagnosis unless the contradictory information is overwhelming.

Most illnesses seen and treated in community medicine are common and can be diagnosed straightforwardly. Because the physician recognizes a pattern, the diagnosis is evident early in the encounter. For most clinicians, syndromic diagnosis allows them to select a treatment plan faster. If this approach is not successful, then most clinicians step back and move to algorithmic reasoning.

If algorithmic reasoning does not arrive at a definitive diagnosis, there are multiple options. Among them are researching literature, consulting a colleague, treating for what is most likely, and waiting.

None of these is wrong, depending on the clinical scenario. Often, a clinician judges that a clinical presentation is confusing, unable to establish a single certain diagnosis, but considers the likelihood of serious illness as low. The low risk allows the clinician to try a potential treatment or follow the patient clinically while allowing time to add additional information. Clinicians have a tendency to perform tests, partly so the patient perceives that the clinician is doing something. However, medical tests should not generally be performed if the tests are not expected have actionable results. So, tests must either narrow the differential diagnosis for treatable illnesses or rule out serious illness.

Treatment trials can be helpful, especially if a likely diagnosis is expected to respond to a treatment, the risks of not treating another diagnosis are low, and the response to the treatment (or lack thereof) helps to narrow the differential diagnosis list. For example, a patient with a mixed tremor appearance, with some elements of essential tremor and some of parkinsonism, might be tried on levodopa/carbidopa (Sinemet), which usually helps tremor from parkinsonism—the risk is low and the likelihood of response is high.

Clinicians-in-training are taught to consider other diagnoses, even if a specific diagnosis seems evident and obvious. They are also trained to look for disorders that would be ruled out by certain findings. In addition, they are taught that uncommon presentations of common disorders are more common than common presentations of uncommon disorders. They are taught to develop pattern recognition. They are taught to not ignore the little internal voice that says, "We have missed the diagnosis" or "This patient is going to crash." This is not superstition; this is parallel processors recognizing a pattern that raises alarm with the consciousness.

Medical decision-making is made considerably more difficult because often the etiology of a complaint is multifactorial. Comorbid conditions and multiple causes have to be considered.

Medical decision-making is made more difficult because we have to live with uncertainty. We have to live with the fact that we will not always be correct and the fear of making the wrong decision can also lead to cognitive bias. The medical student who attempts to practice his or her career without mistakes is destined for disappointment.

The best methods to make the best decisions we can in the absence of decision support are the following:

- Avoid anchoring.
- Always derive a list of differential diagnoses.
- Consider alternative diagnoses.
- Document carefully history, examination findings, provisional diagnoses and differential diagnoses, plan, and thought process.

These elements not only can improve clinical decision-making and save lives, but also can help keep us out of court or help to defend our actions in court when we are wrong.

FIVE RIGHTS AND TEN COMMANDMENTS OF CLINICAL DECISION SUPPORT

While clinical decision support (CDS) can be invaluable to providers, there have been many reports of provider fatigue from useless, nonactionable, interruptive, or incorrect alerts. A recent experience by one of the authors (C.U.L.) highlights how unhelpful and poorly configured alerts can be: When documenting a progress note on a 2-day-old infant in the newborn intensive care unit, the author was interrupted in his work by an alert suggesting to "initiate smoking cessation on this patient." Providers are constantly alerted, and frequently these alerts can interrupt complex provider tasks, sparking frustration in providers, which may, in turn, lead to reduced information recall.[1]

Rounding on a complex patient can be compared to juggling. A juggler adds one ball at a time and can drop them entirely if interrupted. A clinician adds one fact at a time to the mental gymnastics that are clinical decision-making and if interrupted by a decision support alert, may lose the entire train of thought which our patient's care depends on.

However, if done well, CDS can reduce medical errors,[2,3] improve patient nutrition,[4,5] prevent orders on the wrong patient,[6] and reduce costs.[7-9]

The Centers for Medicare and Medicaid Services (CMS) developed the five rights of CDS,[10] which suggest that decision support systems (DSSs) should deliver the following:

- the right information (evidence-based guidance, response to clinical need, and pertaining to the specific patient);
- to the right people (provider, nurse, pharmacists, entire care team—including the patient);
- through the right channels (e.g., electronic health record [EHR], mobile device, patient portal, secure messaging);
- in the right intervention formats (e.g., order sets, flowsheets, dashboards, patient lists);
- at the right points in workflow (for decision-making or action).

Bates et al. further defined the 10 commandments for CDS.[11] The reader is encouraged to read the cited source publication, which is freely available at PubMed Central. The commandments include the need for information systems that have the following characteristics:

- Are speedy
- Anticipate user needs and deliver information in real time

- Fit into the users' workflow
- Have high levels of usability
- Recognize the psychology of users and tailor information so that is most likely to be heeded
- Avoid interrupting users and redirect them instead
- Use simple interventions
- Ask for information from users only when absolutely needed
- Be self-monitoring and correcting
- Include up-to-date knowledge

We want to add one important rule for CDS governance. When a group of individuals asks to generate an alert for other providers, any chief medical informatics officer (CMIO) should eye the request critically and involve the affected group of clinicians. Often, these requests turn out to be intended to reduce the workload of the requester, frequently at a significant expense to the affected providers.

While we understand how CDS systems should be designed, the reality is that providers still operate with less-than-complete information. This quality issue needs to be remedied.

The intent of using CDS systems is to improve the care delivery by reducing errors, achieving more timely and accurate care, and ultimately improving outcomes.[12] We will only achieve these goals if users accept the recommendations that CDS systems provide, which will only occur if they are perceived as helpful and acceptable to the provider's workflow.

DECISION SUPPORT SYSTEMS

Decision support systems can be divided into active or passive systems. Passive DSSs present relevant information but do not offer recommendations specific for a case (e.g., a link within the EHR to a medical reference source). Active DSSs use information known about the patient to offer information that is specific to the patient and clinical scenario.

Historically, decision support has been passive, but active decision support is prevalent in modern EHRs, and informatics researchers are working on enhancing active decision support to improve the effectiveness of the DSSs.

Active and Passive Systems

There are a multitude of passive DSSs. Passive decision support, by definition, does not give advice specific to a particular case. Among them are the following:

- Standard textbooks
- Online knowledge base (e.g., UpToDate)
- Facility-specific antibiograms
- Information on regional disease incidence

- PubMed and other medical information retrieval services

Passive decision support resources accessible from within the EHR (usually via links) include UpToDate, facility-specific antibiograms, and informational documents, such as medication reference information, guidelines, and protocols.

Active DSSs target a specific clinical scenario and are usually more complex. They generally use rule-based inference to guide recommendations. Examples of some of these can include

- Knowledge embedded in order sets
- Gap-in-therapy analysis
- Appropriateness of therapy tools
- Medication allergy or duplicative therapy tools
- Documentation reminders

The most prevalent example of active decision support is embedded knowledge in order sets. When admitting a patient in sickle cell crisis, the physician may decide to use an admission order set for patients with sickle cell disease. The order set has been built with predefined orders for hydration and pain management that are based on clinical evidence.

One of the principal roles of the CMIO and informatics support staff is to ensure that order sets are evidence based, up to date, and aligned with current guidelines. Outdated order sets that no longer conform to current guidelines and knowledge bases facilitate the practice of poor medicine. Similarly, *standing orders* (triggered by certain conditions, such as a patient becoming febrile) and *protocols* (provider initiated) must be maintained to be congruent with best practices. Only appropriate orders and options can be included in the order sets. Some orders will only be executed when obligatory fields are completed, which can be used as a form of decision support.

Order sets often have some textual information that is usually limited and designed to remind the clinician of certain tasks, such as to ensure that renal function is checked when nephrotoxic antibiotics are prescribed or to select the appropriate antibiotics for a specific indication.

We use *gap analysis* to prevent oversights or errors of omission. For example, antithrombotic therapy is supposed to be held for 24 hours for most patients who receive tPA for acute ischemic stroke. After 24 hours, an alert reminds the clinicians to order antithrombotic therapy and provides a short list of the most commonly used agents. Other examples of gap analysis include identification of patients who should be considered for screening colonoscopy or vaccination. Gap analysis is only as effective and useful as the underlying clinical data used to create the prediction. Incomplete data, such as vaccinations that have not been documented in the EHR, will result in false alerts.

Examples of *appropriateness of therapy* decision support include alerts to providers when duplicative therapy is ordered (e.g., the provider orders more than one statin). Another example is an alert to the nurse when retrieving warfarin for a patient whose international normalized ratio (INR) is high, in which case warfarin may be contraindicated. Of note, alerts are only useful if the patient data are correct and the underlying knowledge source is accurate and complete. For example, generally the concurrent use of clopidogrel and heparin is contraindicated but may be recommended in patients who had a cardiac stent. The implementation of a commercial drug-drug interaction knowledge base at a regional hospital that did not include the stent exception resulted in patients only receiving monotherapy because providers followed the CDS alert's recommendation, leading to potential patient harm.

Medication allergy alerts are generally prompted to the ordering provider prior to signature. As with most alerts, decision support alerts can usually be overridden. Providers must have the option to use their clinical knowledge as there are times when a medication has to be given regardless of an allergy. Allergy data are notoriously inaccurate, complicating the implementation of alerts. Side effects previously experienced with specific medications are often listed as allergies, creating false alerts. Patient preference not to receive a specific medication is frequently listed in the allergy section of the EHR, even though the patient has had no personal exposure to the medication. The CDS is only as good as the underlying data structure, quality of the data, and the logic of the CDS intervention.

Documentation reminders may prompt providers to enter required information, such as smoking status, referring provider, or vital signs. Embedded or bolt-on applications can assist with *International Classification of Diseases, Tenth Revision* (*ICD-10*) coding or *Current Procedural Terminology* (*CPT*) coding by suggesting appropriate specific codes or indicating whether the documentation fulfilled requirements for a particular level of service.

Decision support engines may be embedded within the EHR or bolted on. The latter sometimes is accessed via application program interfaces (APIs) or Web services. The level of integration within the EHR affects utility, and the method of presentation affects use of the notifications.

Decision support is frequently interruptive: The alert stops the provider from completing a task. This can be frustrating for the busy user. Less interruptive alerts have less of a negative effect on providers and reduce alert fatigue. Unfortunately, little work is being done in today's vendor EHRs to reduce interruptive alerts and build tools that prevent the provider from choosing the wrong choice in the first place. If a provider wants to order a contraindicated medication, the medication should be grayed in the menu of available medication to indicate that it should not be used.

Knowledge-Driven Decision Support

Knowledge-driven DSSs use complex logic and knowledge that may be gained from existing clinical systems to aid the decision-making for clinicians. For example, a risk model for acute kidney injury may be developed using EHR data. These models may use many variables, such as medications, blood pressure, hemoglobin, age of the patient, gender, and so on. The risk model can be implemented in complex event-managing machines that monitor all new data for these variables and recalculate the risk for the patients on an ongoing basis. These systems consider a multitude of diverse variables, and the risk models can be refined and reimplemented as new data are gained over time. These systems with complex models can see patterns that busy clinicians may not recognize. As genetic data increasingly are integrated into EHRs, the knowledge of how certain mutations can affect disease risk or response to a certain medication will require increasingly complex knowledge-driven DSSs; providers will not be able to manage the volume of knowledge on their own.

Another example of a knowledge-driven DSS is a sepsis-detection engine, which is implemented in a variety of hospitals in the Vanderbilt Health Affiliate Network. This system evaluates a number of parameters of all patients in the hospital and alerts the medical team if the engine suspects sepsis or SIRS (systemic inflammatory response syndrome, related to sepsis and septic shock). The system requires human analysis to confirm the suspicion. Another example of a knowledge-driven system is an antibiotic decision support engine that compares ordered therapy against the patient's microbiology results and suggests more effective therapy to the infection control staff, who then review the data and engage treating physicians.

Reasoning and Logic

Core to many of the decision systems is reasoning. There are fundamental methods of reasoning that can then be supported by more complex rules and procedures to create a reasoning capacity that emulates some of the features of human reasoning: artificial intelligence (AI).

In *deductive reasoning*, statements that are believed to be valid are used to derive a conclusion. An example is the following series of statements:

- All basketballs are spherical. (statement)
- My ball is a basketball. (statement)
- Therefore, my ball is spherical. (conclusion)

Unless there is an error in the statements, the conclusion is true.

Deductive reasoning presents a rule and then applies the rule.

Inductive reasoning uses a statement as probabilistic evidence for a conclusion:

- Most balls are spherical. (This statement can be interpreted that more than 50% of balls are spherical.)
- My ball is most likely a sphere. (conclusion)

Given that the majority of balls are spheres, the conclusion is correct, but it is not certain because a minority of balls are not spheres, such as footballs. The conclusion only provides a probability based on the relative prevalence of types of balls.

In medicine, this type of reasoning is used frequently. Imagine that a certain test is positive in 30% of all patients, and that, of those having a positive finding, 20% of cases turn out to have disease A and 80% have disease B. Knowing these facts, then one can conclude from the prior belief of the likelihood of either disease how much this test will alter the likelihood of each diagnosis. This methodology is discussed in detail in Chapter 11. This understanding is combined with the utility of diagnosing and treating the disease—is it treatable or not?—which gives the provider guidance on whether to recommend the test.

Inductive reasoning uses data to create a rule based on probabilities. As a result, for the individual patient, the rule may predict the wrong result. However, for a cohort of patients, more decisions will be correct. Inductive reasoning is frequently used in diagnostic decision-making, but also may be used in treatment. For example, while treatment A may be generally more effective, in patients with certain mutations, treatment B may provide better outcomes.

Abductive reasoning uses a set of statements or observations and makes a logical inference to determine the most likely explanation. This is the most commonly used logical method in medicine.

- Patients with acute bacterial infections develop fever.
- My patient has a fever.
- Therefore, my patient may have a bacterial infection.

The conclusion is not certain but is more likely than a diagnosis that is not associated with fever. There are certainly other potential causes for fever, but combined with the probability of similar patterns that were ultimately diagnosed as sepsis, this reasoning may be helpful.

The results of logical predictions, and specifically abductive reasoning, can be tested. An experienced clinician working in a hospital setting only with inpatients, might believe that most patients with fever have a bacterial infection, but our ongoing analytic view of our predictive accuracy of inpatients and outpatients shows that more patients with fever have fever with a viral cause than a bacterial cause. We also find that the relative proportion of bacterial versus viral infections in febrile patients depends on other factors, such as peripheral blood white blood cell (WBC) count. Adding these together, we come to the new rule: *Most patients with fever and elevated blood WBC count have a bacterial infection.* We are now correct most of the time. The healthcare system has learned. This example is not as trivial as it seems but is an illustration of how data used in a rule-based manner can add to operational knowledge.

The terms *forward chaining* and *backward chaining* are often used in discussing logical processes. In forward chaining, an engine starts with available data and rules and searches for more data until a conclusion is reached. A simple example would be the following series of rules:

- If a patient has large plate-like scales, then the patient has Godzilla disease.
- If a patient has Godzilla disease and has a fever, then the patient should be treated.

The question could be, Does my patient need to be treated for Godzilla disease? The following facts are known:

- The patient has large plate-like scales.
- The patient has a fever.

Forward chaining begins with the data and applies the rules.

- The patient has the scales, so the patient has Godzilla disease.
- The patient has Godzilla disease and a fever; therefore, the patient needs to be treated.

Backward chaining uses the outcome as the premise. In this case, Does the patient need to be treated?

- Does the patient need to be treated? If the patient needs treatment, then the patient must have Godzilla disease and a fever.
- Does the patient have a fever? Yes.
- Does the patient have the scales typical for Godzilla disease? Yes
- The patient meets all the criteria, so the initial statement is true: The patient needs to be treated.

MYCIN, an early artificial intelligence system that identified bacteria causing severe infections and recommended antibiotics, used backward chaining in its logic. In contrast, most other expert systems in healthcare use forward chaining.

Expert Systems

Expert systems in healthcare are an application of AI to attempt to emulate the decision-making of clinicians. Expert systems use rule-based logic and an extensive knowledge base. An inference engine is the part of the system that applies the rules to the knowledge base to create new knowledge.

Two of the best known expert systems in healthcare are INTERNIST-1 and MYCIN. INTERNIST-1 was developed by Dr. Jack Myers and colleagues at the University of Pittsburg. The user would enter a series of clinical findings, including history and examination results and laboratory results. The engine produced a differential diagnosis with probabilities attached. These systems have been shown to improve diagnostic accuracy, but an important drawback is that they disrupt the physician's workflow. The provider has to leave the EHR and reenter data into the expert system. Most physicians perceive themselves as above average diagnosticians and thus see little value for the interruption. INTERNIST-1 had difficulties in arriving at appropriate results for complex patients with multiple comorbid conditions, who are the patients for which physicians need the most help.

MYCIN was developed by Edward "Ted" Shortliffe and colleagues at Stanford University for diagnosis and treatment of infections. A series of questions was asked, and the output was a list of possible bacterial pathogens and recommended antibiotics.

Presently, expert systems with functions like INTERNIST-1 and MYCIN are not widely used in clinical medicine. We do not suspect that this will change in coming years unless these systems are integrated into clinical workflow. The relative lack of availability of specialists and subspecialists, particularly in nonacademic healthcare systems, will make expert systems valuable for creating differential diagnoses and recommending courses of action.

A number of other diagnostic decision-making tools have been developed that allowed for building a differential diagnosis and assisting with subsequent evaluation and management. Most of these were research and educational projects, but some became commercial products. However, market penetrance for these systems has been low, largely because of limited engagement of providers with these sorts of decision support tools.

DXplain is a DSS developed at Massachusetts General Hospital in the 1980s. It was and is used predominantly for research and for education. The provider enters patient data, and the output is a list of differential diagnoses. The input is of clinical data, including patient signs and symptoms and study results. The algorithm considers the relative importance of findings in diagnosing conditions to reach a ranked differential diagnosis list with relative probabilities. On the basis of these results, the system can present possible studies that can be performed to narrow the list of potential diagnoses. Performance of DXplain compares favorably to the performance of experienced clinicians. However, DXplain has not achieved widespread use.

The Quick Medical Reference (QMR) is derived from INTERNIST-1. QMR was developed in the 1980s at the University of Pittsburg, using many of the algorithms of INTERNIST-1. The intent was first to run on microcomputers and second to evolve the approach to decision support. More than 50,000 clinical findings were considered in the knowledge base. More than 750 disorders were in the differential diagnosis of the system. QMR was sunset in 2001.

Isabel is a commercial product developed by Isabel Healthcare. The approach is interactive, with the clinician having the ability and responsibility to narrow the scope and field of the search, responding to feedback from the system. Isabel is integrated with some EHRs, so direct clinical finding entry is not needed. Isabel uses natural language processing (NLP) rather than insisting on standard keywords. There are more than 11,000 diagnoses indexed in the database.

Providers tend not to activate decision support tools. This is likely because of providers' confidence in their own diagnostic abilities and time pressure to provide care and move to the next case. Decision support tools slow the provider down. The future of decision support tools such as these expert systems will likely rely on background analysis and subsequent face-up presentation of suggested diagnoses or management options to the provider.

METHODS OF CLINICAL DECISION SUPPORT

Clinical decision support methods differ somewhat between different EHR systems, but there are some generalities. Methods of decision support include, but are not limited to, the following:

- Embedded information
- Contextual links
- Flow charts
- Rule-based systems
- Likelihood-based systems

Embedded information is probably the simplest clinical decision method. For this, there is text giving a description or advice attached to an orderable or result, and often it is embedded into order sets. For example, an order set for specific type of infection may have attached text indicating to "order one antibiotic from set A and one from set B unless penicillin-allergic."

Contextual links are often embedded into order sets and order sentences and laboratory results. The most common use of contextual links is to give reference information. For example, a link on a medication name may provide approved prescribing information. A link on a laboratory test may give interpretive guidance. This may have the appearance of a hyperlink or an information button.

Flow charts are usually not shown directly in the EHR but are often used when designing CDS events. For example, if a patient is seen for acute ischemic stroke, the patient is 24 hours out from administration of tPA, and there is no hemorrhage on the follow-up brain CT, then an antiplatelet medication is recommended.

Rule-based systems have already been discussed, such as the INTERNIST-1 system.

Probability-based systems use statistics to calculate the relative plausibility of different models that concern a set of data. Then, these probabilities can be matched to threshold levels. For example, if two laboratory tests predict a possible condition (e.g., hepatic damage), then a confirmatory test may be recommended. If the tests indicate a low probability of the condition, then the confirmatory test is probably not needed.

These mechanisms are then used in a variety of designs and methods of user interface to create our decision support tools.

CDS DESIGN

There are numerous possible designs for our CDS tools. Among these are

- Headers
- Links and information button
- Pop-up alerts
- To-do lists
- Lists of results to review
- Hard stop
- Soft stop
- Dashboards
- Gap notification

Headers are embedded into orders and results text in the EHR and give elemental guidance when the indication is fairly narrow. The information is specific to the result or order and not to the patient.

Links and information buttons, as described previously, are most commonly used for reference information that is specific to the attached orderable or result and not specific to the patient.

Pop-up alerts are common and often overused. These appear when a set of conditions appears. A common one in our systems is placing an order for a contrast-enhanced radiological study when the engine detects renal insufficiency. Another is when magnetic resonance imaging (MRI) is ordered on a patient who is coded for a pacemaker or other implanted device. In the latter case, the engine knows that these are potential risks but does not have the knowledge of the specific devices to decide whether the device and its leads are MRI compatible.

To-do lists are groups of decision support alerts and suggestions that are aggregated. Time-critical alerts should not be placed here but should be in a more intrusive format.

Lists of results to review are common in EHRs. Laboratory results always come to our inboxes, but ones with critical results are usually placed in a separate folder and highlighted.

The *hard stop* should seldom be used. One example would be selection of a dose of medication that is widely out of bounds and should not be allowed.

The *soft stop* is similar to a hard stop, but the stop can be overridden.

A *dashboard* is a tool increasingly used by healthcare clinical and business professionals. For clinicians, the dashboard can show admission metrics, such as length of stay and readmission rate, clinical metrics such as care gap rates, and operational metrics such as for documentation completion, query response, and billing level histogram.

A *gap notification* on a particular patient is performed in a variety of ways, but the basic mechanism is the same. If the system detects a care gap, the provider is notified. Common examples are requirements for routine foot and eye examinations in patients who are diabetic. Of course, this can go off track. In one of our hospitals, hospitalists were being notified of the need for diabetic foot exams for patients who were critically ill in the intensive care unit.

Best Design Principles

Basic principles of good CDS design are largely common sense. There can be a fuzzy line between alerting and annoying.

- Intrusive alerts should be used only when the issue must be dealt with immediately.
- Dashboards should be used more because clinicians are influenced by frequent presentation of data. When appropriate, comparison data should be presented.
- Informational links including information buttons need to have current and useful data presented in a manner that fosters clinical utility.

Arden Syntax

Arden syntax is a standard for representing medical data in a form that can be used for decision support. This is presently part of Health Level Seven International (HL7).

A *medical logic module* (MLM) packages the data into categories based on role. The *maintenance category* gives the title, filename, version, unique identifier, responsible institution and author, and fields (slots) for local owners, dates, and validation status.

The *library category* has slots for purpose, explanation, keywords, citations, and institution-specific links.

The *knowledge category* has the medical knowledge base of the module. This has multiple slots, including data, priority, logic, and action, among others. This reads like code with a defined instruction set and syntax.

The knowledge category for an MLM meant to check the diastolic blood pressure is as follows (from Wikipedia).

```
knowledge:
    type: data_driven;;
    data:
    /* read the diastolic blood pressure */
    diastolic_blood_pressure := read last
    {diastolic blood pressure}; /* the value
    in braces is specific to your runtime
    environment */
    /* If the height is lower than height_threshold,
    output a message */
    diastolic_pressure_threshold := 60;
    stdout_dest := destination
    {stdout}
    ;;
    evoke: null_event;;
    logic:
    if (diastolic_blood_pressure is not number) then
    conclude false;
    endif;
    if (diastolic_blood_pressure >= diastolic_pres-
    sure_threshold) then conclude true;
    else
    conclude false
    endif;
    ;;
    action:
    write "Your Diastolic Blood Pressure is too low
    (hypotension)"
    at stdout_dest;
    ;;
```

Arden syntax is not in universal use, but it is a standard used by some.

Design Flaws

Potential design flaws in CDS efforts can be related to the specific item or the context in which the item is executed.

Too Many Alerts: Many facilities have many alerts, which prompt annoyance among the users and a tendency to ignore the alerts without handling them. Intrusive alerts need to be of high importance and infrequent. Only responsible parties need to see the alert. Informatics staff should watch alert numbers, the proportion ignored properly or improperly, and how often the alert changes provider response.

Misfire: The logic of the alert can be complex, so that the alert may fire when it is not intended. An example is the notification to perform a diabetic foot examination on a patient in the neurologic intensive care unit for intracranial hemorrhage.

Wrong Suggested Response: A serious concern is that a course of action is recommended that is inappropriate. An example is a patient who had stroke quality measures activated, and 24 hours after admission, antithrombotic therapy was recommended although the patient had developed an intracranial hemorrhage.

Inadequate Data: A rule may require certain data to be available in order to be activated, so if data are missing, then the rule may not be activated. For example, part of a sepsis rule may require thresholds to be reached for a variety of measurements, including temperature, heart rate, and lactate, among others. If the lactate result has not returned, we do not want the rule to stop but rather to operate with the data it has.

Governance

All enterprises should have a governance structure for decision support. This would be composed of the CMIO; informatics personnel, including decision support staff leadership; medical staff representation; nursing representation; and administration representation. Many decision support elements concern pharmacy, so we include a pharmacy informaticist in this governance structure.

The responsibilities of the governance team would include but not be limited to

- Determine which decision support elements to build and implement
- Determine the type and behavior of decision supports
- Review results of testing of decision supports
- Monitor decision support performance and response of the users
- Assess whether the decision supports have addressed the targeted issues

There is a tendency for individuals to ask for an alert because of a sentinel event. It is the responsibility of decision support governance to ensure that new decision support elements are need, are well designed, and are achieving their goals.

IMPLEMENTATION AND OPERATION OF CDS

Details of implementation and subsequent operation depend on the decision support engines used, and many facilities use more than one because they have different capabilities. Some general guidelines for implementation include the following:

- The suggested CDS elements should be submitted for formalized review.
- The review committee should obtain input from stakeholders and experts regarding the potential benefits and risks of the element. This will include an estimation of the potential firing rate and expected rate of changing the ultimate clinical decision.
- Approved elements may be activated without the alert actually being presented to determine how often it would fire, for which providers, and whether the firing was appropriate.
- Providers are notified immediately prior to a CDS element being turned on, with a statement to report issues with the alert, such as inappropriate firing or aberrant behavior of the engine.
- Firing of the alert and whether the alert changed the clinical decision should be monitored. An alert that is overridden 99% of the time is probably firing too frequently.

There are legal aspects of decision support that are discussed in a separate section that follows, but we need to remember that when we build, alter, and dispense with decision support elements, we are affecting medical care, so patient safety has to remain the most important goal.

Guidelines and Policies

Clinical decision support is an element of Meaningful Use criteria, so most facilities have implemented some sort of DSS. The criteria do not mandate any proof of effectiveness or any specific decision support elements, just that the functionality is present and operational.

The Food and Drug Administration (FDA) has drafted guidance on decision support software for healthcare use.[13] At the time of writing, the final requirements had not been released, but one issue pertains to whether CDS software is considered a device, with different regulatory implications. The FDA is addressing decision support software used not only by the clinician, but also by patients.

Clinical guidelines are commonly used as a knowledge foundation for CDS elements. In general, local policies should provide for local medical staff oversight regarding implementation of guidelines. Guidelines are released by a host of independent societies and work groups, and they can have overlapping clinical arenas and can be conflicting. Not all guidelines will apply in all clinical environments. There is sometimes unintentional or intentional bias in published guidelines.

Challenges in Clinical Decision Support

Many of us believe that CDS should be part of core functionality, including a current and continuously updated best practice knowledge base. Until this expectation is met, we are responsible for the creation, maintenance, and governance of decision support initiatives. Along with these responsibilities comes a host of challenges.

Difficulty Porting to Different Systems: Most enterprises have more than one EHR, usually because of acquisition of other clinics and hospitals and delays in implementing a common enterprise EHR. Therefore, a decision support element needs to be composed and installed in each of the EHRs. Translation of the logic into the different systems is often complex.

Knowledge Management Resources: Clinical guidelines are usually developed by specialty societies and other groups and are not typically given the scope of scrutiny to be considered best practice on a national level. One difficulty is that guidelines for the same condition or issue can differ. Another difficulty is that healthcare systems differ in capabilities, culture, and patient population, so that a guideline created in one context does not necessarily translate into another environment. Some vendors attempt to aid this by presenting protocols and guidelines generally compliant with best practices and evidence-based medicine by respected academic institutions and societies, with the disclaimer that healthcare needs to be individualized. These knowledge resources are helpful because not every healthcare system has a broad distribution of specialty thought leaders. However, the knowledge is often presented in a fashion that can not easily be translated into the format needed by decision support engines. The Agency for Healthcare Research and Quality (AHRQ) is attempting to correct this by evaluating methods to facilitate incorporation of standardized knowledge into EHR decision support, but this effort is just now in development. Finding guidelines can be a challenge because the AHRQ lost funding for the guidelines.gov site in 2018. The American Academy of Pediatrics includes informaticians in guideline development, making them more machine-implementable. More efforts in this realm are needed for all medical specialties.

Evaluation of Decision Support Element Effectiveness: EHR metrics can usually provide data regarding number of times an element has been activated and how many times the provider overrode an alert. Some EHRs can report how often an alert resulted in an order change, indicating an impact on clinical decision-making. However, determining whether the response was appropriate is still a manual task—looking at charts to evaluate the clinical scenario and provider's response.

Pitfalls of CDS

Alert fatigue is common when decision support rules are implemented and the effects are not completely known. Importance of rules is assessed differently by different stakeholders, and we have had some inappropriate CDS requests. Alert fatigue results when many alerts are received such that providers begin to ignore them. This can be reduced by ensuring that interruptive alerts are truly necessary in the present clinical context.

Duplicate firing occurs when multiple providers receive the same alert or a single provider receives an alert repeatedly when inappropriate. An example would be ordering of load and maintenance doses of a seizure medication. It would be appropriate for an alert to fire if a second loading dose was ordered, but a maintenance dose after a load should not trigger an alert. Alternatively, there is risk to the patient if an alert is acted on by more than one provider; an example from one of our facilities is parenteral potassium replacement ordered by two providers who received a hypokalemia alert at about the same time. Luckily, when both ordered replacement, the second provider received a duplicate order alert.

Overreliance on alerts can result in gaps in care. If providers learn to depend on reminders, there is the possibility that they will not remember to do needed tasks on their own. CDS is not a replacement for the careful, thoughtful provider.

LEGAL ASPECTS OF CDS

Legal aspects of CDS are constantly evolving. This is not intended to be a comprehensive discussion. Physician informatics professionals have frequent discussions with enterprise counsel, and specific individuals have varying familiarity with EHR and decision support issues.

There is certainly a risk of using a DSS, and this is most often related to how it is designed and implemented.[14] In general, DSSs should adhere to all of the desirable factors already discussed, but especially be accurate and up to date in knowledge base and recommendations. In addition, the user should not be discouraged from using the system by excessive or clinically irrelevant alerts. However, ultimately, the determination of clinical implications of a CDS event is the responsibility of the clinician. In general, a well-designed CDS system has the potential to reduce malpractice risk.

We would add that the clinician who detects an error or other issue with the CDS system should report this through the appropriate channels, ideally to the CMIO and staff. In 2019, providers, who self-reported errors linked to their EHRs to the state health department, received subpoenas for negligent behavior. Reaching out to the organization in charge of the facility decision support would be a good first step to reporting. Most organization have anonymous reporting hot lines. Escalation to a state agency is appropriate if the organization does not act in good faith to the complaints[1].

There is concern from informatics professionals about liability associated with alerts firing or not firing appropriately. The CDS event fires on the basis of a subset of patient data, so the provider is the only individual who considers the entirety of recorded data.

Most CDS elements are designed locally based on national guidelines and local preferences. While there are certainly local differences in practice patterns, we would argue that for most decision support efforts, there should be general agreement

1. Politico. Rhode Island docs alarmed by subpoenas they link to EHRs. Available online at https://www.politico.com/story/2019/01/30/medical-misconduct-subpoenas-ehr-1107689

across institutions regarding what is expected from the provider. We would even take the recommendations one step further in that the decision support foundation should be part of core functionality for certified EHRs. Unfortunately, there is a general sense that every enterprise has to reinvent the wheel.

Many of the individuals creating the CDS elements are not the ones who have experienced either the alerts or the clinical event that triggered the alert. Also, the question should be asked about whether a particular clinical issue needs an alert.

The healthcare system has a responsibility to monitor and update CDS systems and to ensure that the elements are in keeping with best practices. The healthcare system also has to determine whether the decision support elements achieved the goals and if the elements need editing. This is accomplished through monitoring, as already discussed.

The user has a responsibility to evaluate any CDS notification in the context of the patient's clinical status. Even appropriate decision support tools can result in inappropriate actions. For example, an alert that notifies the provider that a patient does not have a documented creatinine level value prior to performing a contrast-enhanced radiological study should be overridden when the ordered study is for a CT angiogram (CTA) for a patient with acute ischemic stroke; 2018 American Heart Association/American Stroke Association guidelines recommend not delaying the CTA for a creatinine measurement in patients with acute ischemic stroke who might be candidates for endovascular therapy.

The EHR vendor has a responsibility to provide a platform for decision support build and implementation that is reasonably easy to use and monitor.

BUSINESS DECISION SUPPORT

The purpose of this book is to focus on the clinical side of informatics, but business processes must be as streamlined as possible for our healthcare systems to be financially viable.

Among the business decision support tasks are

- Materials management
- Contract management
- Human resources and staffing
- Strategic planning
- Budget management

Information systems staff support the technical side of all of these, although the primary stakeholders are principally involved in selecting the specific application.

Materials management will be tied to billing, so that the appropriate stocks of equipment and supplies are always available.

Contract management is also tied to the billing system because the requirements and conditions for individual vendor and payer contracts are crucial to cost accounting and successful billing and collections.

Human resources and staffing software will depend on clinical load, with not only global needs of the facilities, but also specific needs of the units. For example, overall occupancy may not be high, but full intensive care units require staffing with appropriately qualified staff.

Strategic planning for information systems and for the enterprise requires a frank and accurate assessment of the status of the information systems. Variables to consider include when contracts will be terminated, when equipment will be at the end of life, service contracts, and the need to meet new requirements.

Providers are usually not aware of the importance of business intelligence in this practice. Clinicians' priorities are usually based on patient needs. But, business intelligence and CDS are key to financial sustainability in these increasingly challenging times.

KEY POINTS

- Clinical decision support is a multifaceted approach to improving quality of care.
- Clinical decision support depends on expert knowledge base and an understanding of best practices.
- Clinical decision support elements need to be of a modality appropriate to the urgency of the need.
- Decision support efforts must be evaluated for accuracy and effectiveness.
- There are significant patient safety and legal ramifications to decision support efforts.

Security and Privacy

KARL E. MISULIS AND MARK E. FRISSE ∎

OVERVIEW

Security means the state of being free from threat, and in healthcare means implementation of all of the physical, technical, and administrative safeguards for our systems. *Privacy* in healthcare is the right of an individual to expect his or her records to be protected from unauthorized access, and this includes controls over who has access and for what purpose. Security and privacy have been extensively addressed in guidelines and regulations and are pivotal to the electronic health record (EHR). Informatics professionals should be familiar with security and privacy implications, especially those of the Health Insurance Portability and Accountability Act of 1996 (HIPAA) and Meaningful Use programs, although these are not the limits of regulatory involvement or best practices regarding these issues.

The US government, particularly the US Department of Health and Human Services (HHS), facilitates adherence to best practices of security and privacy through several offices. Among these are the following:

- Centers for Medicare and Medicaid Services (CMS), which governs the Meaningful Use programs
- Office for Civil Rights (OCR), which is responsible for investigation and enforcement of the security and privacy rules, including those pertaining to data breaches

- Office of the National Coordinator for Health Information Technology (ONC), which provides guidance on how to adhere to recommendations and best practices
- National Institute of Standards and Technology (NIST), which sets standards for the security of our computer systems

Among the issues that are commonly dealt with are *data breaches*: unauthorized access to protected health information (PHI). Mechanisms and implications are discussed in this chapter.

The regulatory environment is a changing landscape. The information here was current at the time of composition, but updated and corrected information is available from governmental and other public resources.

First, we consider some key terms in security and privacy.

Covered Entities and Business Associates

The HIPAA rules apply to *covered entities* and *business associates.*

Covered entities are generally the individuals and businesses involved in healthcare or health information management (HIM). These include[1]

- Health plans
  - Health insurance companies
  - Health maintenance organizations (HMOs)
  - Employer-sponsored health plans
  - Governmental programs
    - Medicare
    - Medicaid
  - Military health programs
  - Veterans' health programs
- Healthcare clearinghouses: data-handling entities such as
  - Billing services
  - Community information management systems and networks
- Providers
  - Individual healthcare providers (e.g., physicians)
  - Healthcare provider organizations

Business associates perform functions for a *covered entity* but are not part of the covered entity itself. A common scenario is when our healthcare system contracts with a billing firm. Alternatively, we may use consulting firms to perform analytics. These companies execute business associate agreements (BAAs).

Covered entities can release PHI to business associates, who are then bound by the same privacy and security requirements as the covered entity.

Protected Health Information

Protected health information is individually identifiable health information held by covered entities. The HIPAA Security Rule covers PHI in electronic form, whereas the HIPAA Privacy Rule covers PHI stored or transmitted in any form.[2] The information includes demographic information in addition to information pertaining to physical or mental health of the individual.

What is not individually identifiable information is when, on the basis of the provided information, the identity cannot be deduced. As expected, considering evolving query and analytic techniques, this may be considered to be a moving target and subject to some disagreement, but generally, for information to be not individually identifiable, the following information is removed:

- Names
- Geographic locations smaller than a state, except for the first three digits of a zip code if that includes more than 20,000 people
- Dates other than year for birth, admission, discharge, and death dates
- Data including year or age that would identify a person as age 90 or over
- Phone numbers
- Fax numbers
- Email addresses
- Social Security numbers
- Medical record numbers
- Health plan beneficiary numbers
- Account numbers
- License numbers
- Vehicle license plate numbers
- Medical device identifiers, including serial numbers
- URLs pertaining to the individual
- Biometric identifiers
- Full-face photos and other images
- Any other identifying characteristic or number

A covered entity may assign an identifier to data that are otherwise deidentified for the purpose of reidentification, providing that the following pertain:

- The identifier is not derived from the other identifiable information.
- The covered entity does not use or disclose the methods for reidentification.

For *deidentification*, the data are stored conforming to all of these requirements, but there is a code that is held secure and can be used for *reidentification* if needed. Examples of when this might be appropriate are if examination of a deidentified record might identify a real or potential threat to the individual.

All of these elements are eliminated in *anonymization,* and there is theoretically no reasonable possibility of identifying individual records. Analysis of deidentification and anonymization methods should be performed to ensure that the methods are effective.

There are exceptions to the rules, including those in educational records covered by the Family Educational Right and Privacy Act and health information held by a covered entity as the employer.[3]

Protected health information can be released without authorization to other providers and entities who are participating in the patient's care, including businesses involved in the care. Therefore, providers do not need authorization to discuss information with consultants, laboratories performing studies, or business services performing billing or other administrative tasks requiring this information.[4]

Of course, for immediate patient safety and identification, PHI can be released. When those of us providing healthcare are faced with a medical situation that appears to violate HIPAA, an opinion from administration is certainly valuable, but responsibility to the patient is of paramount importance. In these circumstances, the decision process, including rationale, should be well documented in the patient's records.

LEGISLATION AND REGULATION

Health Insurance Portability and Accountability Act

The *Health Insurance Portability and Accountability Act* was enacted and signed in 1996 and has a number of components that are not topical for this discussion, including protection of health insurance coverage. Here, we discuss the *Security Rule* and the *Privacy Rule.*

HIPAA SECURITY RULE
The HIPAA Security Rule has a number of key provisions. Details are available online, but highlights are presented here.[5]

The Security Rule applies to all covered entities and business associates, pertaining to electronic PHI (e-PHI) as defined previously. General rules include the need for covered entities and business associates to

- ensure the confidentiality, integrity, and availability of all e-PHI they create, receive, maintain, or transmit;
- identify and protect against reasonably anticipated threats to the security or integrity of the information;
- protect against reasonably anticipated, impermissible uses or disclosures; and
- ensure compliance by their workforce.

Confidentiality means that the information is not disclosed or available to unauthorized persons or entities.

Risk analysis must be performed by covered entities. This should include (among other elements) the need for them to

- evaluate likelihood and impact of potential risks to e-PHI;
- implement security measures to address the risks identified in the risk analysis;
- document chosen security measures and, where required, rationale for adopting these measures; and
- maintain continuous, reasonable, and appropriate security protections.

Administrative safeguards include the following:

- *Security management process*: This involves the previously mentioned process to identify and analyze potential risks and implement appropriate measures to reduce the risk.
- *Security personnel*: A security official is designated who is responsible for process development and implementation.
- *Information access management*: There should be processes so that e-PHI is accessed only when appropriate to the user or recipient.
- *Workforce training and management*: Training in security is provided to workers who deal with e-PHI, and sanctions are applied to those who violate the policies.
- *Evaluation*: Periodic assessment is performed as required.

Physical safeguards include the following:

- *Facility access and control*: This is needed to prevent unauthorized access.
- *Workstation and device security*: There must be policies and procedures to ensure proper use and access. Also, this includes policies and procedures for secure transfer, removal, disposal, and reuse of electronic media.

Technical safeguards include the following:

- *Access control*: With these processes, only authorized persons are allowed to access e-PHI.
- *Audit controls*: These implement audit processes for systems dealing with e-PHI.
- *Integrity controls*: These are policies that ensure that e-PHI is not improperly altered or destroyed, including processes to ensure this.
- *Transmission security*: This implements measures that guard against unauthorized access to e-PHI transmitted over a network.

There are additional clauses, but these are most of the essentials.

HIPAA Privacy Rule

The HIPAA Privacy Rule concerns what information is protected, who is covered by the rule, and how PHI can be used or disclosed. The rule is detailed, but some of the highlights are discussed here.[6] This is the source of the regulations on what is PHI. Definitions of many of these terms have already been presented.

Who or what is covered by the rule?

- Health plans
- Healthcare providers
- Healthcare clearinghouses
- Business associates

What information is protected?

- Protected is individually identifiable health information, including demographic information that relates to
  o Individuals' past, present, or future mental or physical health condition
  o Provision of healthcare to the individual
  o Individuals' past, present, or future payment for provision of healthcare

There is no restriction on use or disclosure of deidentified health information. There are principles for use and disclosures:

- A covered entity may not release PHI except as permitted by rule or as the individual or representative authorizes in writing.
- A covered entity is required to disclose PHI if
  o individuals or representatives request access or accounting of disclosures; or
  o HHS requires information for compliance for enforcement investigation.

Permitted uses and disclosures are as follows:

- *To the individual* (may be required under certain circumstances).
- *For treatment, payment, and operations* (TPO).
- *Opportunity to agree or object.*, for example, when the patient or representative can agree or decline to have information disclosure, such as in facility directories, or for notification permissions to family.
- *Incidental use,* for example, brief access of the wrong chart because of a similar name.
- *Public interest.* This is designated in a long list available from HHS, but contains mainly release for public health and legal reasons.
- *Limited data set* for research, public health, or healthcare operations.

TPO includes

- *Treatment*: Provision for healthcare, including consultation with other providers in individual healthcare.
- *Payment*: For financial management of healthcare, including billing, insurance concerns.
- *Operations*: For a variety of healthcare functions, including quality improvement, case management, care coordination, audits, and other activities.

There are many other provisions; a principal one of interest to clinical informatics professionals is the notice of rights, including privacy practices.

- Patients must be notified about privacy practices no later than the time of the first encounter for nonemergent events.
- Notification must be made as soon as practicable in emergency situations.
- There should be posting of privacy practices at sites of healthcare delivery.

We should all have the HHS security and privacy documentation as part of our core reference sets. The summaries are far easier to digest and interpret than the source legislation.[7]

Health Information Technology for Economic and Clinical Health Act

The *Health Information Technology for Economic and Clinical Health Act* (HITECH Act) was part of the 2009 *American Recovery and Reinvestment Act* (ARRA), which created incentives for Health Information Technology (HIT). In this chapter, we focus on the security and privacy implications.

Enforcement of HIPAA was markedly enhanced by HITECH. There are civil penalties for "willful neglect" that escalate with severity and repetition. Breach notification is discussed further in this chapter, but briefly, unauthorized disclosure or use of "unsecured PHI" has reporting requirements and penalties.

Electronic health record access is the requirement that patients be able to obtain their PHI in electronic form if the provider has an EHR. Providers who cannot demonstrate this ability may not qualify for Meaningful Use incentive payments.

Business associate agreements are now governed directly by the HIPAA provisions, whereas previously the BAAs had requirements imposed only by the contracts with covered entities.

SECURITY AND PRIVACY MECHANICS

What Is Reasonable?

Legislation regarding HIT security and privacy uses the term *reasonable* in their language, referring to reasonable precautions and reasonable protection. But, what is reasonable may differ between individuals.

Because the prime purpose of the healthcare system is to deliver healthcare, *reasonable* should mean that the care of patients is not impeded by our efforts. To determine whether this is the case, we need to involve our clinician colleagues in configuring our systems to be compliant.

We can all agree that the following would be examples of what is not reasonable:

- The EHR times out in 5 minutes while the provider is examining a patient.
- The provider must use a prolonged multistep procedure to login to devices when changing rooms or changing patients.
- An administrator's action is required to authorize access and role assignment to a provider at point of care before a patient's records can be accessed.

These examples might sound silly to some readers, but these are from real environments, and we hope that these issues have been revisited.

Clinical informatics cannot be successful without involving clinicians. Intelligent and educated professionals who do not see patients cannot make many pivotal decisions about EHR and access configuration, particularly regarding security. This statement applies equally to physicians who do not practice. We must engage our clinical colleagues.

Clinicians must be able to accept the fact that access to the clinical and business systems is controlled. This means they must

- only access records that they should access, by virtue of position such as provider or peer reviewer;
- not share login credentials;
- not allow others to access devices when the provider is logged in; and
- report any perceived data breach to a security or privacy officer, remembering that incidental access is not a breach.

Security Provisions

Access controls are discussed in Chapter 15. In general, we favor single sign-on access to facilitate convenience of multiple app use. Context matching should also be employed so patient identification is passed between clinical apps.

HARDWARE

Workstations at the healthcare system should be configured so that personal app installs cannot be performed. Staff should depend on personal devices such as phones, tablets, and personal laptops for personal tasks.

More complex is enterprise-owned desktops in provider and administrator offices. Specific applications often need to be installed on those devices, including shared drive access, remote access for work-related files, and office apps, including email, configured for the enterprise and user.

NETWORK ACCESS

Network access is usually restricted. Separate networks are usually provided for medical devices (e.g., pumps and handheld devices), staff, and visitors. Sometimes, there is a specific network for providers, especially because they may need more robust access for cine and other data-rich applications.

Streaming entertainment media services can occupy a large bandwidth, so this should not be allowed on enterprise networks, at least networks that are used for staff productivity and other official activities.

DATA CENTER ACCESS

The data center has restricted access, usually to data center staff and supervisors. The rank-and-file enterprise staff do not need data center access.

SOFTWARE ACCESS

Software security provisions include antivirus and other anti-intrusion solutions. This must be applied not only to web access but also to email access. Configuration is often so that high-risk websites cannot be accessed from the enterprise networks.

PERSONAL DEVICES

Personal phones are often required to be used for work purposes. Personal phones usually need specific work-related apps, including email and secure messaging. Because personal phones may not be on a cellular network that has robust penetrance in the interior of the buildings, Wi-Fi access on a secure network should be arranged. Some larger facilities have cellular repeaters, but these are expensive and cover only specific cellular carriers.

Tablets are often used for professional as well as personal purposes. For phones and tablets, remote wipe apps can usually be installed so that if a provider or employee leaves or otherwise loses authorized access, not only the login can be canceled but also the apps can be remotely removed from the device.

PERSONAL STORAGE

Personal storage devices such as thumb drives, external hard drives, phones, tablets, and other similar devices should not be directly connected to enterprise networks. There are robust solutions for secure data transfer for every platform.

ENCRYPTION

Encryption is encoding data to restrict access only to authorized individuals. No encryption process is perfect, and there are quite a number of algorithmic methods. A commonality of encryption is that there are keys to encrypt and decrypt the data.

Uses of encryption include

- protection of stored data;
- protection of transmitted data;
- digital rights management; and
- ransomware.

Protection of stored data by encryption is especially important on portable devices, including laptops, external storage devices, and thumb drives.

Protection of transmitted data by encryption is common with secure messaging and secure email.

Digital rights management is encryption where only the authorized app with authorization for that piece of media can download or play the media.

Ransomware is where malware encrypts the data of the victim and asks for payment for the decryption key.

The architecture of the encryption as used for data transmission can be *symmetric key* or *asymmetric key*.

- *Symmetric key encryption* consists of both sender and receiver having the same key or perhaps a simple transformation to alter the key. This was common in the first stages of encrypted messaging but is less used now.
- *Asymmetric key encryption* is where the data are encrypted using a public key (the key is not secret), but decrypted by a private-key known only to the recipient. This public-private key pair makes the transmission asymmetric.

Asymmetric key encryption is efficient for relatively small amounts of data, but for large amounts, the math of the algorithms can become complex. Therefore, some transmissions begin as asymmetric, but use of the private key can result in background passing a symmetric key that does the bulk data decryption. The concepts of symmetric and asymmetric methods are sometimes confusing, so the scenarios that follow illustrate this is a very rough way.

Symmetric: If you and I want to share private messages, we can agree on an encryption algorithm and a single key to encrypt and decrypt the messages. We meet and share the algorithm and copies of the key. When we send messages, I encrypt with the algorithm using our key, and you decrypt using the same key and algorithm in reverse. If a person listens to our initial conversation, that person will have our algorithm and keys and will be able to read our messages.

Asymmetric: You and I agree on an encryption algorithm. You generate two keys for the algorithm, one to encrypt and one to decrypt. You send me the encryption key, the public key, meaning I do not have to keep it secret, so you can even send it by email. You keep the decryption key, which is the private key; even I do not know that key. I encrypt a message for you using the public key and send it to you, or I could even post it on the Internet. But, because only you have the private key needed for decryption, only you can read it. Someone else could use the algorithm and public key to encrypt a message but having those does not appreciably help them decrypt a message if they do not have the private key.

AUDIT AND ACCESS LOGS

Audit logs record activity within the medical record. *Access logs* record which user accesses which records. These are considered together in the surveillance process. The purpose is to ensure that access is appropriate and activity is in keeping with appropriate clinical use.

Every EHR has *transaction audit logs*. These are used for a variety of purposes, some of which include user experience and inappropriate access. Audit logs are a regulatory requirement, although many of the parameters regarding their use are not specified. HIPAA and HITECH have requirements regarding the existence of the logs. The logs are maintained for a specified time. The HIPAA Security Rule indicates 6-year retention of reports and documentation of the audits. HITECH requires 6-year retention of disclosure data and 3-year retention of disclosure data through the EHR. Meaningful Use requires 6-year retention, although participation in Meaningful Use is voluntary.

The utility of audit logs can be illustrated by some real-life examples of when they have been used.

- A nurse was found to be accessing charts of multiple patients she was not caring for. Further investigation discovered that she was looking for potential cases for a malpractice attorney.
- A physician was found liable for malpractice after audit logs revealed that he had reviewed but did not address information in the EHR key to the patient's care.
- A physician was found to have simultaneous logins from different locations. He had shared his credentials with his nursing staff.
- A physician was found to be spending time doing clinic notes between 10 PM and 1 AM, after his children had gone to bed, revealing an opportunity to redesign workflow to reduce "pajama time."

Part of the HIPAA mandate is to review information system activity. Sharing this expectation with providers can be a way to warn the staff of the dangers of HIPAA violations yet project the administrative requirement onto regulatory authorities rather than the healthcare system policy.

CYBERSECURITY

Cybersecurity is the mechanisms of ensuring that the requirements of HIPAA are met. This is the compilation of practices to ensure security, privacy, and availability of the data. While media reports tend to consider the focus of cybersecurity to be on malicious threats, in reality, it also should protect against device failures, loss of power, and loss of essential internal and external network connections.

The scope of cybersecurity includes but is not limited to

- protection against intrusion and malware;
- protection against network failure;
- protection against power failure;
- protection against unauthorized user access;
- limiting privileges to those needed by specific users and user groups;
- ensuring integrity of the data; and
- ensuring continuous access to system data.

Some of the mechanisms of facilitating cybersecurity include

- securing the data center from unauthorized access;
- providing uninterruptible power supplies;
- using antimalware and anti-intrusion software;
- providing access controls for all devices that can access the systems;
- avoiding generic logins;
- providing port control for devices where they are not needed (e.g., USB ports disabled);
- testing security measures by friendly intrusion attempts, testing phishing attacks;
- consulting with agencies and companies expert in cybersecurity; and
- making appropriate notification of breaches and development of strategies to avoid similar events.

Expectations of perfect cybersecurity are destined to lead to disappointment. For most enterprises, threats are ongoing, and interference with information systems function is inevitable.

Consultation with agencies can be invaluable, as can attempted intrusions from contracted consulting groups. Some of our affiliated facilities have used consultations with governmental and commercial entities to obtain guidance on improving cybersecurity infrastructure, policies, and procedures and to test defenses.

Security measures should not be so stringent that patient care is impeded. In some of our facilities, nonclinical staff have made a crippling security decision without clinician consultation. Part of our duty is ensuring *availability* of the data, so we must keep that a high priority.[8]

GOVERNANCE AND STEWARDSHIP
Cybersecurity should be a topic discussed at the highest levels of enterprise leadership. The threat to clinical and financial performance is enormous. EHR data unavailable because of ransomware can result in deaths. When leadership is looking to cut the budget, cybersecurity is not an appropriate target. We need to maintain our defenses at state-of-the art levels. We may be able to put off purchasing new beds for a year, but we cannot afford to be a year behind in threat defense and mitigation.

Governance of healthcare system cybersecurity should include representatives from administration, information systems infrastructure leadership, information systems application leadership, and designated dedicated security personnel. Status reports should be made to senior leadership, including near misses and data breaches.

Stewardship of cybersecurity should be shared by all who build, maintain, and use healthcare information systems. We need to educate our clinical and nonclinical users of threats, including new risks. Cybersecurity will only be successful if we all engage in proper practices and methods.

Privacy Provisions

The HIPAA Privacy Rule requires covered healthcare systems and providers to develop and distribute a notice of privacy practices. This is intended to inform the public of privacy issues, which can then foster an understanding of rights of the patient and representatives and responsibilities and rights of the covered providers and entities.

The notice should contain the following information:

- How the covered entity may use and disclose PHI
- Rights the individual may have regarding the information, how to exercise these rights, and how to complain about an issue regarding these rights
- A statement of the responsibility of the entity to protect PHI and that compliance is a legal requirement of the entity
- Date of the notice, which is updated with revisions
- Information on who to contact for further information

Dissemination of the information is physical and electronic. Requirements of providers are that the information availability include the following:

- Notice is made available to anyone who asks for it.
- Notice is posted and also visible prominently on any website of the entity.
- Providers must provide the notice to patients
  - no later than the date of first service delivery except in an emergency situation, in which case the notice is made available when possible; and
  - If the service delivery is electronic, notice is delivered electronically at first request for service, and acknowledgment of receipt should be obtained.

Requirements of organizations include the following:

- More than one notice may be developed, which might depend on type of service.
- Organizations that participate in an organized healthcare arrangement (OHCA) may develop a common notice for use by participants.

Health plans must provide information as follows:

- At the time of enrollment
- Within 60 days after revision of the notice
- At lease every 3 years to remind individuals of the existence and method to access the notice

SECURITY AND PRIVACY OFFICERS

The security and privacy officers are named persons required by the HIPAA Security and Privacy Rules. They can be the same person.

Privacy Officer: A covered entity designates a privacy official who is responsible for development and implementation of the policies and procedures required by the privacy rule.

Security Officer: A covered entity identifies a security officer who is responsible for development and implementation of the policies and procedures required by the security rule.

Security and privacy officers are notified in the event of breaches or other events that place patient information at risk. This includes not only breaches but also events where data are unavailable.

Security officers are often well versed in the technical aspects of cybersecurity and have risen to upper administrative levels. They need excellent understanding of the regulations. They must interface with staff responsible for auditing and defenses, educate users at all levels, and even test the defenses.

Privacy officers are experts in the relevant regulations and may have additional backgrounds in business or law. Many privacy officers come from HIM or similar functions in the enterprise.

BREACHES

A data breach is an unauthorized access of PHI, with a few exceptions:

- Incidental unintentional access, such as when searching for a patient and the wrong chart is briefly accessed;
- disclosure from an authorized person to another authorized individual who otherwise is at the same facility; and
- released data that are not believed to be able to be retained by the unauthorized person who received it.

In the event of a possible breach, a risk assessment is performed. This must assess the nature and extent of the disclosure, including

- nature and extent of PHI involved, including identifiers and likelihood of reidentification;
- the unauthorized person to whom the disclosure was made or who used the data;
- whether the data were actually acquired or viewed; and
- how the risk to PHI has been mitigated.

Breach reporting depends on the specifics of the breach:

- If the breach is felt to be of 500 or more individuals, the breach must be reported to the HHS secretary promptly, at the latest, 60 days from discovery of the breach. This is electronic submission.[9]
- If the breach of PHI affects fewer than 500 individuals, the entity has to notify the HHS secretary within 60 days of the end of the calendar year in which the breach was discovered.

Penalties that can be levied depend on violation categories, which are based on the expectation that the covered entity knew that there was a risk of violation.

- *Level 1—Did Not Know*: The covered entity did not know that a provision had been violated and would not have been expected to know through reasonable diligence.
- *Level 2—Reasonable Cause*: The covered entity should have been aware of the violation but could not have avoided with reasonable care.
- *Level 3—Willful Neglect With Correction*: The covered entity failed to do reasonable diligence but corrected the deficit.
- *Level 4—Willful Neglect Without Correction*: The covered entity failed to do reasonable diligence and did not attempt to correct the deficit.

An unintentional breach may be errantly releasing more PHI than appropriate. Willful neglect might be failure to perform a security assessment and deal with threats.

Penalties for breaches depend on the level and the number of involved individuals. The numbers are the level of breach, penalty for each violation, and maximum for identical violations in a calendar year.

- Level 1: $100–$50,000 each; $1.4 million maximum
- Level 2: $1,000–$50,000 each; $1.5 million maximum
- Level 3: $10,000–$50,000 each; $1.5 million maximum
- Level 4: $50,000 or more each; $1.5 million maximum

Criminal penalties depend on intent and can result in imprisonment:

- Unknowingly or with reasonable cause: Up to 1 year
- Under false pretenses: Up to 5 years
- For personal gain or malicious reasons: Up to 10 years

Key to minimizing the risk is periodic and ongoing risk assessment and reduction initiatives. Education of staff is essential. And, the efforts to protect PHI must be documented so that there is clear evidence of the intent and initiative to protect PHI.

THREATS

Types of threats and brief descriptions are presented in this section.

Malware

Malware is short for malicious software. This is an umbrella term for many of the entities discussed here, including viruses, worms, Trojan horses, and ransomware, among others. This is not a comprehensive list of all potential threats. By definition, malware is harmful. An app that merely reports habits of the user is not necessarily malware.

Reasons for malware creation are as diverse as the individuals who create them. Incentives can be financial, as with ransomware, or merely to be injurious to others, driven by antisocial psychological makeup. Nevertheless, those of us who employ technology for healthcare spend thousands of staff hours and millions of dollars protecting ourselves from these threats.

Viruses

A virus is a small program designed to insert a copy of itself into files on the computer. The virus impairs functioning of the files, whether data or executable. The virus is spread by vulnerabilities in the computer access, which can occur by clicking on a link, opening an email, or opening a file transferred from another computer. The name comes from the similarity of the computer virus to a biologic virus.

Worms

A worm is a small program that replicates itself and spreads from computer to computer. Unlike a virus, the worm does not insert itself into the code of existing programs but does slow computer systems by taking resources from the intended tasks and from communication with the network.

Trojans

A Trojan is also known as a *Trojan horse* because of the similar mechanism of action as the historical reference. The program has an intent far different from that advertised to the target. The user may believe he or she is clicking on a link that will test for viruses, but in fact, a small program will be installed that can allow outsiders to have access to the computer.

A Trojan is one mechanism for ransomware to access systems. Trojans do not generally replicate themselves. They also do not generally insert themselves into the computer code.

Ransomware

Ransomware is a program that either encrypts the files of the target system or sometimes threatens to otherwise compromise the data and demands payment to remove the threat. Often, the ransom is paid using Bitcoin or similar currency, which is difficult or impossible to trace. Often, the ransom is set at a point where paying is more cost effective than trying to work around the damage or engage in the time and expense of an investigation. The ransomware is often delivered by a Trojan.

Spyware

Spyware is an umbrella term for software installed without the user's knowledge and is intended to relay information about the user to a separate party. This can be benign, for the purpose of optimizing the user experience, or malignant, attempting to capture information from the user. Some apparent spyware is produced by commercial vendors and therefore erodes trust in the vendor (e.g., music services). Tracking cookies are considered by some to be a form of spyware.

Phishing

Phishing is an approach to tricking the user to give information, often user IDs and passwords, sometimes credit card numbers. A variety of techniques are used. The most common is an email that appears to be from a trusted source. The email either prompts the reader for information directly or directs the user to a website that looks official. We have received these repeatedly from supposed credit card companies; they often announce a security threat and prompt entry of user credentials to protect against the threat.

The name comes from the similarity to fishing, where an offer of food to a fish is a prelude to the target becoming a meal.

Spear phishing is directed at specific individuals, usually in an organization, rather than broadcast to a number of people. Whaling is targeting senior executives, usually getting attention of the target by presenting a sensitive issue, and prompting the user to enter credentials to view the content or download an app to view the document of concern.

Keylogger

Keyloggers are mechanisms to record the keystrokes on a computer. These are not, by definition, illegal, and often these are used to assess usability. For example, some of the user experience/user interface (UX/UI) designs discussed in Chapter 14 are based on logging keystrokes and mouse clicks recorded during routine clinical use. If a provider takes many clicks and keystrokes to enter a specific order, there is the opportunity for workflow or process improvement.

Keyloggers become illegal when they are designed to steal credentials or other sensitive information.

Back Door

A back door is a method of gaining access to a system by bypassing normal access control. This is not necessarily nefarious. Programmers may leave a back door for troubleshooting or maintenance of a program. Security for access control for the back door is often not as robust as for most users, with credentials that may be able to be guessed. Also, back doors often allow more privileges than routine operational access. For example, with normal user access, a provider can only interact with the data tables through the user interface, which has rules and controls on how and what is entered. A person with back-door access may be able to alter the data tables or program code directly. A back door can be surreptitiously installed.

Botnet

The term *botnet* comes from the words *robot* and *network*. This refers to a network of computers that are infected with malware, which allows them to function as a nefarious network. The purpose of the bots is generally either to gather information from unsuspecting users or to coordinate a denial-of-service attack. For this purpose, the bots communicate with the controller using command-and-control software.

Cookies

Cookies are small pieces of data stored on the user's computer; they help to coordinate the browser experience. Some functions of browsers would be difficult without cookies, so they are not malware.

Cookies are used to tell a website details regarding the user. Among the examples of data stored would be previous products looked at on a store site. Cookies generally do not pose much of a security risk for most applications.

Denial of Service

A denial-of-service (DoS) attack is where a website is swamped with so many nui-sance requests that it cannot address legitimate requests. A form of this is a distrib-uted denial-of-service attack, with the attack coordinated from multiple sources. If the attack is from a single source, that one source can be blocked.

Pharming

Pharming is diverting an Internet address pointer to a different Internet target ad-dress, which is a fraudulent site. Often, the site looks much like the legitimate site. This can be done at the level of the user's computer, the servers that provide the ap-propriate addresses of select addresses (domain name servers), or even at the level of the router.

KEY POINTS

- Security and privacy regulations and best practices apply to healthcare systems, providers, and business associates.
- Regulations governing healthcare security and privacy are among the most sensible in federal legislation.
- Security provisions should be tight, but not so restrictive as to impede medical care.
- Data breaches may need to be reported, depending on the nature, character, and extent of the breach.
- Threats are multiple and expanding. We need to be increasingly vigilant to new threats and keep our defenses at state of the art.

19

Data Science

KARL E. MISULIS AND MARK E. FRISSE ∎

OVERVIEW OF DATA

Data science is a term that has evolved in meaning over the past 50 years. Originally, this was a term used by Danish computer scientist Peter Naur as an alternative for computer science, but it has since morphed to be a term that refers to the field of extraction of knowledge from data. This is taking data analytics to the next level, looking for new relationships that can be applied in disparate situations.

Data scientists are individuals with an understanding of the multiple facets of data science and can design, perform, and interpret the results of their work. Among the assets of the data scientist are a foundational understanding of computer science, statistics, database structure and query, and advanced analytics. In 2012, the *Harvard Business Review* named *data scientist* as the sexiest job of the twenty-first century.[1]

We expect our analysts to produce reports of clinical and business performance of our providers and facilities. We expect our data scientists to use our data and data management structure to discover new relationships. Our analyst may tell us that 25% of our patients admitted with acute ischemic stroke continue to have blood pressures greater than 140/90, and that information may cause us to ask our providers to be more aggressive about blood pressure control in the acute setting. Our data scientist would discover that acutely lowering blood pressure to lower levels results in poorer functional outcome of patients with acute stroke. Patients with acute stroke need their blood pressure to be a little high in order to perfuse surviving neurons in the ischemic brain. Data science has value.

NEEDS

Data science is more than advanced analytics. Identification of new relationships results in new knowledge to help guide medical practice. Among the questions that are asked of data scientists are the following:

- What clinical findings (historical, physical, and laboratory) predict a specific disease? This will help us determine which tests to perform.
- Which treatments are most effective and most cost-effective for a specific disease? These will often not be the same elements (e.g., overuse of antibiotics is partly due to providers ordering medications that should be reserved for resistant organisms or refractory cases). Also, a specific treatment might not be effective in certain clinical cases (e.g., women may not derive the same level of benefit from statins as men).
- Which patients are the best targets for effective chronic disease management to reduce healthcare utilization? Most healthcare systems have identified that a small proportion of patients are responsible for a large proportion of utilization, including emergency department (ED) visits, admissions, and readmissions. Our data scientists may be able to identify which patients and conditions have the clinical characteristics that make them the best targets for our limited disease management resources. This analysis would include assessment for disorders that need enhanced management strategies and that have a reasonable expectation for improvement with intervention.
- Which clinical services are not performing adequately? Every healthcare system component has to be value added, although not necessarily profitable. The Obstetrics hospitalist program at our public hospital will never be profitable, but does meet a need of the community and also reduces complications of pregnancy for the uninsured and underinsured, thereby reducing healthcare and societal costs. On the other hand, a bariatric surgery program might be closed if it is not at least revenue neutral and does not have outcomes that give the program intrinsic nonfinancial value to the community.

In addition to these clinical and operational examples, there are many research applications of data science in an attempt to determine new associations.

Among the tools the data scientist uses are the following:

- *Correlation*: Evaluation of a relationship whether causal or not. One might cause the other, or both factors may be caused by a third element. This is also called *association* and is different from *dependence,* which does indicate a causal relationship of one element on another.

- *Regression Analysis*: A statistical process for looking at relationships between independent and dependent variables. Does the value of one determine the value of another? If not perfectly, are there multiple independent variables that predict the value of the dependent variable?
- *Factor Analysis*: Used to determine the factors contributing to the variability of an association, thereby facilitating targeting of key variables.
- *Time Series Analysis*: A form of analysis where time is the independent variable. Application of time series analysis is to predict the value at a future time by projecting the trend(s) seen during observed time.
- *Data Visualization*: Development of visual representations of data that aid in understanding relationships. For example, one of our healthcare systems developed a map of patient admission and readmission rates related to zip codes. A list of the results might be informative, but visual analysis revealed regions that had insufficient clinics and providers to supply primary care and perform postdischarge follow-up care. The system started clinics in some of these regions.

These and other tools move data science from historical analytics to predictive analytics, by which we can project future trends in disease manifestations. For example, predictive analytics is used for mapping global trends in influenza spread.

The next step is prescriptive analytics: The data analysis tells us what to do. In the influenza example, the analysis tells us which strains of influenza to include in this year's flu vaccine.

USE CASES

Electronic Health Record User Experience

Chapter 14 discusses the design of the user experience for the electronic health record (EHR), including an extensive discussion of the science of user experience. Our goal is to make the EHR easy to use, intuitive, efficient, and a pleasant experience. Also, we want the user experience to be conducive to a balanced and appropriate lifestyle. Let us consider these individually.

Ease of Use: Most clinicians are not excited about the technology of an EHR, a fact that is often a surprise to informatics staff. Providers just want to get through their day providing healthcare. Factors that will adversely affect ease of use include need for more training, difficulty finding data, difficulty with placing orders and performing other tasks, and difficulty creating and editing documents.

Intuitive: This is related to ease of use, but refers specifically to how much user function can be determined intuitively and how much needs training. Training will never cover every task, so the user must be able to figure out task workflows without always calling for help.

Efficient: An EHR interface should be organized so that the user can efficiently find needed information and accomplish required tasks. Hunting through cascading menus is inefficient. Similarly, different users may have different efficiencies. Some of our users leverage order sets and favorites to reduce time and clicks per order. This should be encouraged.

Pleasant Experience: Style is not without value. A pleasant layout and color scheme are essential. The interface should be compact enough to reduce scrolling and navigational clicking, yet not so compact as to be cluttered. An example is an ED tracking board of one of our hospital EHRs. The first iteration was compact but offered limited functionality from the board itself. The second iteration offered markedly enhanced functionality from the board view but was less dense so that only a small fraction of the ED census could be seen at one time. There should be a balance.

Lifestyle: Analysis of an EHR can show if a user is at risk for burnout. Analysis of pajama time (hours in patient charts outside service hours) has shown that some providers are doing documentation late at night, presumably when family schedules allow. This is an opportunity for intervention to improve quality of life for the provider and family.

Fitbit Data

The Fitbit Director of Data Science, Rajiv Bhan, has guided his new employer to use their voluminous data to inform individual users as well as society.

- In cooperation with other fitness apps, Fitbit can assist with improving training of clients and improving results while reducing the risk of injury. And, as more information is contributed, more patterns that contribute to improvement or injury can be revealed.
- Fitbit data have also shown that sleep patterns for most Americans are not in keeping with present recommendations.
- Fitbit data have shown that in patients who are breast cancer survivors and received chemotherapy, those with higher documented activity tended to perform better on cognitive testing.

Further information from Fitbit and other related apps will continue to uncover knowledge to improve occupation and leisure habits of clients that would have been unknowable if not for this technology and client base. This is the tip of the iceberg of knowledge that our data scientists will use to identify opportunities to improve care.

FUTURE OF DATA SCIENCE

Much of the future of data science in healthcare is speculative, but there are some certain targets for data science.

- Reduce spending:
  - Identify patients at risk for increased utilization.

o Identify treatments that are overused or not producing desired outcomes.
o Identify providers who overutilize specific medications or procedures.
- Improve outcomes:
  o Identify best avenues to improve health and reduce utilization (e.g., reduce hospitalization and readmission rates by chronic disease management).
  o Identify management strategies with the best value potential.

The present rate of growth of healthcare costs is not sustainable, and arguably, the present level of healthcare expenditures is not sustainable. One way of reducing expenditures is by not providing care—decreasing availability of healthcare to broad segments of the population. This is not desirable. We believe we can provide healthcare for an affordable price, but limits will have to be placed on what is provided. All members of the healthcare community from patients to providers to healthcare systems, to pharmaceutical companies and other healthcare suppliers will have to be incentivized to be more cost sensitive. Data science not only can help us deliver on those priorities but also can identify methods to reduce healthcare demand.

KEY POINTS

- Data science is able to identify relationships not visible by routine data observation and analysis.
- Data from healthcare systems and from patients and the general public will be used to help improve outcomes and reduce costs.

20

Enabling Technologies

KARL E. MISULIS AND MARK E. FRISSE ■

SPECTRUM OF ENABLING TECHNOLOGIES

Enabling technologies in healthcare are innovations that make significant advancements in process or performance. This is a rapidly expanding field and will influence the direction of primary and specialty care.[1]

The basic concept is generally a device that facilitates some healthcare task that cannot otherwise be accomplished efficiently. Among some of the technologies are

- Medical alarm systems
- Home medical devices
- Home monitoring sensors
- Medication dispensers
- Remote physiologic monitoring
- Telemedicine systems
- Patient portal access

MEDICAL ALARM SYSTEMS

Medical alarms are standard in a hospital setting, but they have been used outside the hospital since the 1970s. There are multiple types, but the commonality is remote notification when a patient needs assistance.

Basic methodology is a personal transmitter with a prominent button worn on the body. When the button is pressed, a short-range radio signal activates a base station, which is in turn connected to telephone lines. Most of these have a sequential protocol so that one or two numbers can be tried, and if there is no human response, then emergency responders are called.

More advanced methodology consists of base stations with direct cellular service or sometimes the personal transmitter with cellular capability. Some of these devices can even be triggered by sensing a fall or other acute event in which the patient may not be able to press the button.

Some of these systems have audio capabilities for one- or two-way communication.

HOME MEDICAL DEVICES

A variety of home devices have provided for home measurements of targeted metrics. These devices often interface with smartphones for patients to track their data and may upload the results to healthcare providers. Among these are devices to measure weight, blood pressure, heart rate and rhythm, glucose, and oxygen saturation.

Some employers either require or incentivize employees to use these technologies if they have appropriate risk factors. For at least one major technology corporation, this has reduced self-insured healthcare expenses more than 30%. However, it is not certain that improved individual health is the sole cause for these savings; employees or prospective employees at risk of financial penalties or disincentives may be electing to work elsewhere.

HOME MONITORING SENSORS

Home sensors can be placed to detect activity and location of individuals in the covered spaces. These can sense if there is no movement in an occupied location or if a fall has occurred. Some advanced sensors use infrared detectors to detect signs of life and distress. These sensors are complementary to the sensors that are becoming standard in the smart home: fire, smoke, carbon monoxide, intrusion, moisture (excess water in a room for any reason), video display of a visitor at the door, temperature (for an automatic thermostat), and others.

MEDICATION REMINDERS

Missing medications is common, especially in the elderly population, but people of all ages may need reminders. There are a host of technologies to remind the user to take the specific medications. Among these are smart pillboxes, monitoring pill bottle caps, dispensers, and reminders.

Many of us first saw use of these medication reminder technologies during drug studies, where the investigators wanted to have some real data to monitor compliance. If a medication has adverse effects, compliance would likely decrease. But, noncompliance is a serious issue even without adverse effects. So, the sponsor would not want a new drug to fail because people did not take it adequately. Subtherapeutic doses of some medications may not only fail to produce anticipated benefits, but also may be worse than not taking the medication at all because of effects of the subtherapeutic dose on the body or target.[?]

REMOTE PHYSIOLOGIC MONITORING

Continuous physiologic monitoring can be performed for electrocardiogram (ECG), oxygen saturation, and other parameters. Some of these have local storage; others feed data to a central location through a wireless connection. A common application of this technology is ECG monitoring of patients being evaluated for possible intermittent arrhythmia. A routine ECG and even a 24- to 48-hour cardiac monitor can miss paroxysmal atrial fibrillation or another concerning arrhythmia. External or implanted monitoring devices can detect arrhythmias over a longer period of recording. Devices that transmit findings in real time have an advantage over those that merely store the data for later analysis.

Home electroencephalographic (EEG) monitoring can be done to look for seizures, but we generally find inpatient extended video monitoring preferable, where the electrophysiological recording can be correlated with the recorded video and audio of the associated behavior.

TELEMEDICINE

Telemedicine is increasingly used especially for specialty services where there are insufficient practitioners in many areas. One arena where telemedicine has been particularly effective is in telestroke.[3] A patient arrives in an outside hospital with symptoms suggesting acute ischemic stroke. Almost every ED can perform the evaluation to determine whether the patient is a candidate for thrombolytic therapy, including computed tomography (CT) of the brain, but many ED physicians want neurology specialist consultation before administering tissue plasminogen activator (tPA), the thrombolytic presently approved for acute ischemic stroke. The time to transfer to a stroke center lessens the effectiveness of thrombolytics and may make the person no longer a candidate by virtue of closure of the time window. Telestroke services can allow the stroke center neurologist to see the patient and participate in assessment by remote staff and aid with the decision-making. Then, whether tPA is given or not, the patient can be emergently transported to the stroke center. A phone call can allow the stroke center specialists to give valuable advice, but the additional information obtained with viewing the patient's examination adds to the value of the consultation.

Other examples of the effectiveness of telemedicine include use for psychiatry, for postoperative follow-up, and for dermatological evaluation.

PATIENT PORTAL

The patient portal is commonly used for checking records or appointment times and communicating with provider offices. Additional functionalities of the portals include uploading clinical information, self-scheduling for some appointments, filling out previsit forms, and payments.

Recent data indicate that patients are more likely to use the portal if they access it through an app on their smartphones rather than from a web interface on their computer.

Portals will only grow in use. As clinical informatics professionals, we can make that happen by ensuring that there is valuable and actionable information for the patient on the portal. Also, we should ensure that the platform for communication with provider's offices is functioning, usable, and used appropriately.

FUTURE DIRECTIONS

Needs of the patients and healthcare systems are aligned in many ways. Among the applications of enabling technologies are processes to do the following:

- *Avoid gaps in care*: Decision support within the EHR can produce alerts for the provider and also for the patient, so that needed assessments and treatments are not missed.
- *Multifacility communication*: Presently, portals are generally for one healthcare system, so we may have a different portal for each clinic and one for our local hospital. While patients can see data from each, they are not aggregated, and providers cannot see each other's data without a separate data-sharing agreement and technology. Technologies are presently in development that will allow the patient not only to see the portal information from multiple providers and facilities in one site or application, but also to allow the patient to authorize providers to share information to help coordinate care.
- *Improve compliance*: Many employers are using home devices that feed data to centralized facilities to monitor blood pressure, glucose, and weight. Compliance improves when the patient knows that the data will be uploaded to his or her provider each day. Similarly, connection with medication storage at the home can remind the patient to take medication.

We will undoubtedly be surprised by the quick success of some enabling technologies and the challenges of others.

KEY POINTS

- Enabling technologies allow for extension of the healthcare system into the home.

- Enabling technologies can be used for a variety of applications, including chronic disease management (diabetes, hypertension); diagnostic monitoring (remote ECG monitoring); senior care (medical alerts, home sensors); and provider visits (telemedicine).
- Enabling technologies are making the transition from niche custom devices to applications on smartphones.
- Enabling technologies, if successful, should improve compliance, improve monitoring of patient status, and engage the patient and family in the disease management process.

Part IV

Application of Informatics in Healthcare

Clinical Teams

MARK E. FRISSE AND KARL E. MISULIS ■

THE IMPORTANCE OF TEAMS

Effective healthcare delivery requires the efforts of a broad array of individuals. Nationally, vast numbers of individuals are involved in healthcare. For every physician who provides care, there are 16 nonphysician workers in the US healthcare system; half of these staff directly support clinical work, and the other half are responsible for administrative activities.[1]

Clinicians work with many different teams. When viewed broadly, the care of every patient requires a unique team. There are common elements, including the primary care clinician and staff, but there are many other elements, including professional care providers, the patients, their family, and others in their environment.

Every team shares a suite of common characteristics. Among these are goals, subgoals, and tasks. These represent a hierarchy of duties responsible for patient healthcare. Goals include the high-level aspirations of improving care of the patient and controlling costs. To accomplish this, there are subgoals, some of which include ensuring the patient is taking his or her medications and getting to the provider for visits. Then, there are tasks within these subgoals, such as medication reminding and transport to the provider.

To feature the common characteristics, we can elaborate:

- **Goals**. Teams share common goals and subgoals, although they differ in roles to accomplish the tasks. For example, the individual who drives a patient to treatment facilities is a critical but often unrecognized member of a care team.

- **Roles**. At times, these roles are defined by licensure, such as the pharmacist who dispenses medications. At other times, they are informal, such as a friend or relative who is available to help a patient stay in his or her house by doing some household tasks.
- **Alignment**. Ideally, team members have incentives aligned to help realize these goals and share a sense of benefit when a goal is achieved.
- **Tasks**. Each member has explicit or implicit roles and tasks. Tasks may be mandatory, sequential, and contingent on the actions of others.
- **Interdependence**. Teams operate with some degree of interdependence. In some instances (e.g., a surgical team or a medication management team), the goals are highly organized. In other situations, goals are more loosely coupled.
- **Resilience**. Teams should have resilience to ensure that if the primary party assigned to a task fails to complete his or her work, a designated backup can take over. A spouse, for example, may be responsible for helping a patient adhere to medication, but if the spouse becomes ill or is unavailable, another relative or friend must know to perform the spouse's task.
- **Awareness**. Team members should know what tasks they need to do and when. They should also be aware of events that may disrupt the standard plan so they can mitigate the disruption.
- **Learning**. Relevant team members should have the opportunity to review processes and outcomes in order to learn how to improve the approach to care.

TEAMS COLLABORATING WITHIN A SINGLE HEALTHCARE SYSTEM

Teamwork is better organized within a single healthcare system than when bridging healthcare systems. Single healthcare systems show the power of teamwork and technology.

The power of teams is evident when examining closed-loop medication management in hospitals. At a minimum, the medication management team consists of a prescribing physician, a dispensing pharmacist, an administering nurse, and the patient. The introduction of computerized physician order entry (CPOE), barcoding technologies, and integrated medication administration systems has closed the loop by keeping track of the status of a needed medication dose from the time of order to the time of administration. The structured automation of this process has also allowed for additional safety checks (e.g., drug interactions, drug dosage errors) and, through analysis of patterns, strategies for timely and coordinated medication administration. These systems lead to fewer prescribing errors yet with no detrimental impact on clinician time.

The power of technology to support teams is evident when examining the impact of electronic health records (EHRs) on referral and consult requests made among clinicians sharing a common EHR. Clinical teams can only be efficient if they are aware of a need and are able to accomplish a requested task within a given time frame. This process begins with a referral (consult request) from one clinician to another. Informatics researchers have studied the effects of implementation of EHR referral management into clinical workflows. The results have shown

- increases in the percentage of referrals in which the specialist note was attached to the referral;
- an increase in the percentage of clinicians who acknowledged the note when it was completed;
- an increase in the percentage of clinicians who communicated the results of the referral to the patient when the note was completed; and
- increased clinician satisfaction with the referral process using the closed-loop process.

TEAMS COLLABORATING ACROSS HEALTHCARE SYSTEMS

Hospital-focused informatics professionals must remember that most clinical and preventive care activities occur in the home, the community, and across an array of ambulatory and other acute care settings. The success of EHRs within hospitals is rarely realized in the more real-world settings of ambulatory and community care.

Consider Medication Administration. After over a decade of concerted effort, e-prescribing and e-reordering prescription drugs (controlled substances excluded) is commonplace; many of the bugs have been worked out, and ambulatory clinicians have almost universally incorporated these technologies into their practice workflows. Similarly, dispensing has become heavily automated with the introduction of pharmacy Web resources that simplify ordering refills. The ability for pharmacy systems and clinician EHRs to transmit prescription-related transactions has made the overall process safer and more efficient. But, the loop is not completely closed because patients encounter great difficulty in both understanding their medication regime and adhering to it. This is particularly true of those who have recently been discharged from a care facility or who have had their medications changed by different providers.

Community clinician-to-clinician referral and communication are problematic; in the absence of a common EHR, electronic referral management and document exchange are clumsy at best and sometimes impossible. Although commercial EHRs have the ability to do direct messaging, the lack of universality of this method and the fact that many clinicians do not read direct-messaged documents makes this avenue unreliable. When a new technology is not broadly dependable, the lowest common technology becomes standard—in this case fax and snail mail.

Community communication beyond the providers is imperfect. While pharmacies take e-prescriptions, communication with patients is often with email, text messaging, or phone calls. There are limitations on what can be transmitted on each of these platforms. Rehab specialists and caseworkers still send snail mail reports and forms for authorizations. Family and friends are often out of the loop altogether, never having direct communication with other healthcare teammates unless they accompany the patient to an appointment. This is particularly problematic for postdischarge care and chronic disease management, for which ongoing treatment, assessment, and self-help interventions are key to success.[2]

ADDRESSING THE CHALLENGES

When looking beyond a hospital or integrated delivery system sharing a common EHR, the current state of affairs can discourage the idealist. Data, even obvious and critical items like an accurate medication list, are often not available; a common and widely available set of actionable clinical data is rarely available to all who play a role in the care of a patient. Of equal concern, a consensual care plan is rarely available and, if available, often cannot be updated as health status and care requirements change. Because clinical data are often updated but rarely repudiated, any view of clinical data is, at worst, simply not current. Care plans can change dramatically; acting on an obsolete care plan can be catastrophic.

On the horizon, the growing recognition of patient engagement, social determinants, and other factors external to the traditional hospital/clinic-focused model present new challenges and opportunities. Facing enormous growth in network connectivity and in entirely new markets like home monitoring, wearable sensors, consumer-based health applications, body monitoring devices, other consumer-focused healthcare, and the *Internet of things*, the clinical informatics professional faces new challenges in reformulating both the purpose and the composition of care teams. Multiple third-party personal information devices, dispersed repositories of patient data, and diversity of medical conditions and people who seek to understand the role of these new technologies present new challenges to the clinical informatics professional.

Professionals must set new priorities to add to their growing list of current obligations. First, they must dispel the notion that all raw data signals will be transmitted to any single EHR. Second, they must not overact to the potential of new analytics systems, interface technologies, and other innovations until they are certain they will demonstrate value to their organization. As ideas, these emerging technologies hold great promise, but as realities, picking a winner before technology matures or picking a technology not suitable for the organization's pressing purposes poses incredible professional and financial risk. One must be patient and let markets mature.

However, a patient approach requires action. The specific technologies and workflows may not be clear, but they will be different. Accordingly, professionals must expand their thinking about care teams and roles. They must understand how a newer array of people, processes, data, and technology can confer across regions the same efficiencies seen in hospitals. They must learn from other institutions and from their professional organizations what might work within their unique organization's mission, culture, and available resources.

Most important, informatics professionals must focus on a limited number of discrete activities of greatest value to their organizations (e.g., postdischarge care management), understand the common infrastructure needs no matter what technologies are introduced, and plan for small pilots to assess the value of targeted interventions. Clinical informatics professionals need to be part of a team both within and across their organizational boundaries to understand the most effective combination of people, processes, data resources, and technologies for both the present and the future.

KEY POINTS

- The composition of teams broadens dramatically when care is extended into the region and into the home.
- Patients and their caregivers also working as formal or informal care teams are equally vital to effective healthcare. Their needs, motivations, and capabilities must be incorporated into informatics solutions.
- Incentives among clinicians, payers, patients, and families are usually not aligned.
- A common medical record is not the same as a common care plan.
- The number of devices collecting data and transmitting data to many different commercial and public resources will grow. Understanding how to integrate these devices and data into actionable care processes is an essential skill.

Patients and Families

KARL E. MISULIS AND MARK E. FRISSE ■

HISTORY OF PROVIDER-PATIENT COMMUNICATION

Traditional provider-patient communication occurred during a clinic visit, by snail mail, or by phone call. Although these were effective, there were challenges, part of which fed the traditional financial structure of the time: a charge for an office visit and sometimes a charge for a phone call. If the provider could not be contacted in a timely fashion, the patient might have to go to the emergency department for a pricey urgent encounter. We made few efforts to prevent medical expenses, partly because that was standard workflow, but partly because we were paid for encounters.

Education for patients and families has traditionally been verbally from the provider, but that is limited by human attention and memory, time, and knowledge base of the provider. Unfortunately, many of our colleagues present inaccurate information for a variety of reasons: failure to recognize one's own limitation of knowledge, hesitancy to admit uncertainty, or a motivation to present information that may guide the patient to decisions that favor the provider, perhaps financially.[1]

Communication methods are changing. Advances in social communication are being applied to medical communication. Also, availability of online information has exploded, with some benefits and some detriments. Many patients and families are surprised to learn that websites and even mainstream press are not peer reviewed. This book was reviewed before, during, and (will be) after release for accuracy, and edits will be made as needed even after release. This process is not in place for most mass media.

NEW AVENUES FOR PATIENT COMMUNICATION AND ENGAGEMENT

The Agency for Healthcare Research and Quality (AHRQ) recommends a number of initiatives for engaging patients and families in healthcare.[2] These include toolkits for educating and engaging patients and families, materials targeted specifically toward hospitalized patients, and materials for office patients. Also, there are some materials focusing on patients in long-term care facilities, ambulatory surgery centers, and staff of the ambulatory surgery centers.

A commonality is a focus on the following:

- For providers and staff:
  - Tools for addressing some of the most important issues in healthcare:
    - Medicine reconciliation
    - Transitions of care
    - Discharge planning
    - Communication
    - Informed consent
  - Patient safety information
  - Laboratory testing process improvement
- For patients and families:
  - Preparatory information for visits
  - Information and preparatory engagement for procedures
  - How to be more involved in personal healthcare
  - How to assemble and ask questions

We touch on some of the methods for patient and family engagement and consider what they bring to the table and how they can affect outcomes.

Email

Email was used for clinical reasons long before HIPAA guidelines were released. Because of security and privacy concerns, email is still used, but there is an added layer of caution to ensure that the communication is appropriate. As with all discussions of security and privacy, up-to-date information should be sought since this is an evolving landscape.

End-to-end encryption is desirable, and some security specialists claim that it is required, but HIPAA does not require encryption, only "reasonable safeguards."[3] This may include ensuring correct email addresses by first exchanging emails to verify the identity of the provider and patient. Also, both provider and patient must ensure that only they can access their emails; family members of each must not have access.

Emails from providers often have an attached statement of appropriate use of the communication, usually with instructions on what to do if the communication was sent to the wrong recipient.

Email capabilities and procedures should be discussed during the visit, including a method to ensure identity when emails are exchanged. We have experienced attempts to gain information inappropriately by an email sender pretending to be the patient.

Email communication should be saved by the provider because this information is used for patient education and clinical management. As such, the email record of exactly what was communicated can be superior to a phone call, for which no transcript usually exists. A disadvantage of email versus a phone call is the lack of immediate responsive dialogue.

Email is not used for urgent communication, and this should be reinforced with the patient. Most providers do not receive immediate notification of a new message.

Portals

Portals are increasingly used, especially because use was incentivized by the Meaningful Use program. Many healthcare systems have portals, although there is great variance in content and effectiveness. While a portal may technically be available and accessible, limitation of posted information and functionality may make the portal little used by patients.

One affiliated healthcare system creates a portal entry on registration, and patients are encouraged to use the portal to view data, communicate with providers, do previsit data entry, and pay bills. Patient-entered health information and scheduling are being deployed.

This portal initially had only laboratory studies and radiology reports, which resulted in sufficient access to qualify for Meaningful Use, but was not optimally useful. Now, provider documentation is on the portal 36 hours after it is finalized. Initiation of this had some pushback from providers, who were concerned about patients seeing their clinical notes, but this objection should be dismissed in our opinion. Patients have been obtaining their records from the health information management (HIM) offices for decades; the patients are reading their charts. Providers need to create clinical notes that are accurate yet appropriate for consumption by the patient as well as other providers. Even psychogenic or behavioral issues can be presented in a diplomatic but clear manner. If a provider has a message to another provider that the provider does not want the patient to see, then the communication should be verbal. Some details of patient portals deserve further discussion:

Portal Content: There are multiple hospitals in the affiliated network just discussed, and specific contents of the portals differ. Some of the criteria for posting information are generally as follows:

- History and physicals (H&Ps) and consult notes: 36 hours after final (when signed)
- Discharge summaries: 36 hours after final
- Provider progress notes: not posted at most facilities
- Laboratory results: 36 hours after final
- Radiology reports: 72 hours after final
- Cardiology reports: 72 hours after final
- Pathology reports: 14 days after final

Patient and Provider Data Review: The EHR inbox should be configured so that laboratory, radiology, and pathology reports appear in the ordering provider's inbox. Therefore, in most instances, the provider will have seen the results substantially prior to the patient seeing them. However, if a provider is slow about checking the inbox or is out of town, the patient may see the data prior to the provider seeing and acting on it. We recommend that our providers clear their inbox daily. If a provider will be unavailable to check the inbox, most EHRs allow the provider to provide proxy access to a covering provider.

Portal Access: Access to most portals is by Web or device app, but there is evidence that there is greater use of the portal if there is a portal app.[54] Part of this is the ubiquitous nature and use of smartphones. Also, mobile apps generally have a more intuitive interface as opposed to Web pages, which may have more complex and confusing functionality.

Portal Users: The peak age group for portal use is in the 30s, but almost all ages use the portal. Teens and those 70 years of age and older are significantly less likely to use a health system portal. Patients commonly access their portal information shortly after a visit, presumptively to view the clinical note for clarification of information and for the results of laboratory data.

Portal Use and Healthcare Quality: There is some evidence that portal use improves compliance with appointments. However, it is very possible that individuals who are predisposed to use the portal may have socioeconomic or behavioral attributes that make them more likely to go to appointments and adhere to provider recommendations.[5] Presently, there are few data showing improved outcomes due to portal use, and there is some evidence supporting absence of effect.[6]

Telehealth Visits

The HHS defines *telehealth* as

> the use of electronic information and telecommunications technologies to support and promote long-distance clinical health care, patient and professional health-related education, public health and health administration.[7]

According to this definition, telehealth includes phone calls, email, and portals, as well as more advanced televisits. In this section, we focus on the televisits and their maturing role in patient and family communication. Telestroke and other contracted acute care telehealth contacts are not included in this discussion.

Scope of Telehealth Visits: Telehealth visits directly with the patients are used for a wide variety of purposes, some of which are as follows:

- Televisit with an established patient, either after hours or if there is no room in the schedule to work in the patient. A video visit can be superior to a phone call.

- Specialty consultation if no qualified providers are local or in a reasonable distance for transportation.
- Postoperative televisit when the patient is at a remote location, preferably in their primary care provider's office. The surgeon can discuss the postoperative course, view the wound(s), and discuss results with the patient without making it necessary for the patient to make a long journey. Because many operative cases involve bundled payments, there is no financial penalty for making a televisit in this circumstance.
- Televisit after stroke discharge. A prompt appointment should be made, but discussion with the patient a few days after discharge can potentially improve compliance with discharge instructions and medications and potentially reduce readmissions.

Telehealth visits could improve provider efficiency and patient convenience, but an obstacle is reimbursement. Many providers are unwilling to not receive compensation for an encounter that has time and other resource demands with a risk of liability exposure. Some payers will compensate for telehealth visits, but many do not. In a liability case, the defense that we did not perform an in-person examination will not insulate the provider from liability; rather, the argument will be made that the encounter should have been in person. That having been said, telehealth visits are expected to dramatically rise in future years.

One of our affiliated healthcare systems has hospitals and employed providers separated by state lines and more than 100 miles. Televisits can dramatically facilitate prompt and efficient care.

Infrastructure for televisits is complex and not without controversy. Generally, the vendor for televisits should sign a business associate agreement (BAA) and meet technical requirements for HIPAA compliance. Use of a commercial telehealth vendor is recommended, and some EHRs offer this service as part of their system. At the time of writing, there were no routine BAAs available for Facetime or Skype, and a BAA with Google only covers chat messaging and not video chat. However, the HIPAA Conduit Exception Rule may apply to some vendors if they are merely the methods of transmission, the data is encrypted end to end, and the vendor cannot decrypt the message. Opinions differ on whether any of these or other commonly used social conference mechanisms meet the conduit exception.

Secure Messaging

Secure messaging is becoming more widely used for clinical communication. In hospitals and large healthcare systems, secure messaging has largely replaced beepers and SMS (Short Messaging Service) between clinicians, mainly because of security and privacy concerns.

Secure messaging can be an independent application, part of the portal, or part of the EHR system. While we presently use an independent system, our plan is ultimately to migrate to one embedded within our EHR.

Low-Technology Mechanisms

Not all communication is high tech. We still make many phone calls, and one of the most common is to discuss critical results of studies or to give updates to families on hospitalization status. Of course, authorizations need to be established before sharing PHI.

An issue may be identification of who is authorized to discuss the clinical situation. One of our healthcare systems uses a password system for patient and family discussions with nursing and providers. A pass phrase is easiest to remember.

We have mentioned that urgent and emergent messages from patients to providers should not be by email or even secure messaging. The same is true for providers: Urgent communication with families or conveyance of sensitive information should be done verbally. For example, a pathology report showing the presence of cancer should preferably be discussed in person, but possibly over the phone. Sending an email or other message is inappropriate unless other avenues have been tried. Allowing the patient to read the report on the portal without being informed ahead of time is not advised.

The argument is made that snail mail is a nonsecure method of communication. However, many people still want to receive a paper copy of their reports. While file cabinets have disappeared from most healthcare systems, they remain in use by our patients as well as our legal colleagues.

Promoting New Methods of Communication

The penetrance of portal use, secure messaging, and other new methods of communication among patients is less than desired, partly because of the method of presentation. Email with a signup link or communication-related literature left in a room or handed to the patient has been virtually ineffective.

We found that enrollment was better with a staff member discussing these issues directly. Enrollment was even better if the provider discussed these methodologies.

Therefore, we recommend that the provider briefly discuss options and expectations for communication with the patient and family at the time of the encounter. This may take only a minute. Then, support staff can give additional information, answer questions, assist signup, and delineate appropriate use. This would include when to use an avenue of communication.

RESPONSIBILITIES OF PATIENTS AND FAMILIES

Responsibilities of the patients and families are to provide accurate and complete pertinent information. Patients and their care partners should

- provide complete and truthful responses to questions;
- ensure they understand instructions and the medical plan;

- reach an agreement with providers of the plan and stick to it as much as possible and appropriate;
- provide feedback to the provider if there are changes that impact patient health or may alter the course of treatment;
- obtain emergency care if needed; and
- adhere to self-help guidelines.

Many of these may seem obvious, but in practice, there is not only errant information transferred from healthcare professionals to the patient and family, but in the reverse direction there is commonly inaccurate and sometimes intentionally misleading data transmitted to the provider. This is particularly true for sensitive data regarding home dynamic or information that might be embarrassing to the patient or family.

Some of the mechanisms of communication discussed are conduits for relaying information to providers, and some of these facilitate the relay of sensitive or embarrassing information. A patient may find it easier to message the provider through the portal that he or she has started smoking again; admission of this under the critical eye of the provider is more difficult. Similarly, a patient may be more able to reveal confidential information, such as a difficult family dynamic, over a messaging system than when all parties are in an examination room. Last, most people should be more likely to be truthful with typed or otherwise digitally stored data because persistence of the record is ensured, whereas verbal communication is believed to be filtered and deniable at a later time.

MEDICAL HOME

The *patient-centered medical home*, or just *medical home*, is a concept best explained by Martin et al. (2004).[8] This product was the result of collaboration between seven organizations as part of the Future of Family Medicine project. Among the conclusions were that a new model of practice should have the following features:

- Patient-centered team approach
- Elimination of barriers to access
- Advanced information systems, including EHRs
- Functional offices
- Focus on quality and outcomes
- Enhanced practice finance

The target for development and rollout would be to multiple audiences, with engagement of all involved in healthcare.

In 2007, the American Academy of Family Physicians, in conjunction with the American Academy of Pediatrics, American College of Physicians, and American Osteopathic Association, released "Joint Principles of the Patient-Centered Medical Home."[9] This consensus statement outlined the need for a medical home that had the following characteristics:

- Personal physician
- Physician-directed medical practice
- Whole-person orientation
- Coordinated or integrated care
- Focus on quality and safety
- Enhanced access
- Payment that reflects the added value to patients

There are details to these items in the citation, which is freely available. As informatics professionals, we are responsible for leveraging information systems, including the EHR, for best practices; reducing medical errors, including gaps; and patient engagement. Whole-person orientation and care coordination/integration are partly managed by us as informatics professionals because we should provide the communication infrastructure and workflow to coordinate care.

The medical home has been implemented in a number of healthcare systems. There are numerous reports of improvements in some quality metrics and outcomes, although there are also reports of costs being higher with improved access and enhanced infrastructure associated with the care coordination. This is not a reason not to move forward with implementation and assessment, but with limited healthcare funds, we need to present these efforts in tandem with mechanisms to reduce inappropriate utilization and make healthcare more efficient.

The next step in this integrated delivery effort will be addition of specialty clinics, hospitals, and other healthcare delivery platforms in the process, sometimes called the *medical neighborhood*.[10] Our part in this will be

- data sharing between providers and healthcare entities;
- communication between providers as well as between providers and patients; and
- knowledge management for the EHRs and for educational information for patients.

It is hoped part of the data sharing will evolve to a real or virtual common data source for problem reconciliation, for medicine reconciliation, and for other facets of care coordination.

KEY POINTS

- Communication needs and conduits have been enhanced in recent years, and we have the expectation that this will continue to evolve.
- Providers have a responsibility to deliver the most accurate and appropriate information to patients and families, and part of our responsibilities as informatics professionals is to facilitate this.

- Patients and families have a responsibility to engage in complete and truthful dialogue with providers, and information systems can help to streamline this process.
- The patient-centered medical home is a concept that highlights the joint responsibilities of the provider and patient in excellence in healthcare.

23

Body, Home, and Community

MARK E. FRISSE AND KARL E. MISULIS ∎

OVERVIEW

The rapid growth of mobile devices that can be worn or integrated into the immediate environment satisfies a need most humans have for connection and convenience. Every day, millions of people experiment with new mobile devices, sensors, and related *Internet of things* technologies in order to develop a richer digital ecosystem. Currently, approximately 50% of the world's population is connected online; Gartner estimated there were 8.4 billion connected devices in 2017, and that by 2020, there will be 20.4 billion devices connected as part of a global service infrastructure.[1] Connected with or in proximity to myriad devices capable of measuring almost every aspect of behavior, individuals are becoming part of an omnipresent and ubiquitous data infrastructure. This infrastructure is organically evolving as individuals and groups understand ways these technologies can meet often previously unimagined needs. Such an understanding evolves over months and years and requires personal experimentation and massive corporate investments. Because it is not possible to precisely predict how these systems will evolve, corporate investors place fortunes at risk chasing their own vision of how the future will unfold.

Similar explorations are taking place in our healthcare system. The potential technologies applicable to healthcare on the person and in the home range from simple watches and other personal devices to complex monitoring systems more commonly seen in hospitals. In many instances, the data from these devices are managed by the device manufacturer; the manufacturer, in turn, must develop data standards, interfaces, and communications methods to bring these data to the attention of appropriate providers. Some devices (e.g., Google's many efforts[2] or the Apple HomeKit[3] and HealthKit[4]) are providing more effective means of integrating data with the electronic health records (EHRs) of traditional healthcare providers.

Many of these technologies are just emerging, and it will be years before care models mature and traditional healthcare providers can be assured of a consistent technological approach. Given the complexities, risks, and costs involved in these endeavors, the cautious and the wise may want to follow consumer health trends closely but not invest time and resources in solutions that may not pan out as technology and consumer culture rapidly evolve. Our cash-strapped healthcare delivery systems, for example, cannot afford to make the risky bets on the scale of Google, Apple, or Microsoft.

Certainly, an explosion of biometric devices, home sensors, and medical devices will generate massive quantities of data that, in their native form, are far too noisy to process and can obscure urgent signals. In raw form, these data would overwhelm any traditional EHR, and because most individuals are cared for by several providers using different EHRs, an EHR-centric repository for data seems unlikely. These realities support the anticipated emergence of personal health record banks capable of storing massive amounts of data and releasing selected portions of data to authorized providers with patient consent. These data could feed analytics programs designed to identify individual health trends and suggest actions. If these data are aggregated from massive numbers of patients and deidentified, machine learning techniques could conceivably be applied to better identify population trends and appropriate care management approaches.

At present, most digital technologies for the person and the home are *not* essential for care in most cases. For home care, a simple log of blood pressure, weight, and blood glucose readings may be far more effective to use than automatic recording systems. Rather than seeking complete interoperability, often home healthcare professionals can do a better job by incorporating results from digital systems into their simpler and more mobile EHRs. These reports, in turn, can be communicated to appropriate care coordinators and providers.

Home digital technologies face challenges one would expect in an environment characterized by rapid technology innovation. Among these are a sluggish and ossified regulatory environment, market dominance by legacy technology products, misaligned incentives, and risk-adverse patients, providers, and payers.

KEY POINTS

- The explosion of data sources on the person and in the home will continue.
- Data from these devices may be capable of identifying health problems.
- These same devices may be able to alert individuals at a "teachable moment" and influence behaviors.
- Many questions need to be answered before a vibrant consumer-focused home care market becomes embedded in our traditional healthcare

delivery culture. Among the people, process, data, and technology issues are the following:

- Data from these many devices are represented differently. Data interoperability will be a challenge.
- Means must be established to transmit data to appropriate caregivers.
- Methods must be developed to allow individuals and their caregivers to act on new data.
- Protecting the privacy and security of personal health information will become a greater challenge as these devices proliferate.
- There is as of yet no generalized financial sustainability model for these new personal and home data infrastructures.

Specialties

KARL E. MISULIS AND MARK E. FRISSE ■

GENERAL CONSIDERATIONS

Electronic health records (EHRs) were generally developed with adult inpatient or ambulatory care as the principal focus. Therefore, the design, functionality, and anticipated workflow serve those arenas well, but serve many other specialties less well. In this chapter, we consider some of the specialties and niche arenas that need additional and altered functionality.

Reasons for the need for special build and configuration can include the following:

- Image capture and incorporation into the report (e.g., radiology, gastroenterology, cardiology, ophthalmology)
- Rapid ordering and documentation. (e.g., emergency department [ED], urgent care)
- Diversity of patient characteristics, such as body growth (e.g., family practice [FP], pediatrics)
- Special templates needed (e.g., obstetrics [OB], ED, pediatrics, ophthalmology)
- Blended inpatient and outpatient care plans (e.g., ED, integrated healthcare system)
- Procedure-based functions (e.g., operating room [OR], gastroenterology, bronchoscopy laboratory, cardiac catheterization laboratory)

The decision has to be made whether the enterprise EHR will be forced into use in a specific arena or whether a specialty system will be used. While use of a specialty system introduces the needs for interfaces, that still might be preferable to provider inefficiency that may be created by not having adequate digital tools. On the other hand, we strive for integration where this can be done efficiently.

The EHRs are making the transition from a transactional focus to a workflow design. For efficiency of practice and for ease of decision support, the workflow design should help all specialties facilitate clinical practice.

GENOMICS

Genomics is already in widespread use, although we may not be completely aware of the present and future implications. Informatics involvement in genomics is in storage, analysis, and presentation of the information. We recommend participation in genomics databases so that the utility of this powerful tool can continue to evolve.

Infectious Disease and Genomics

A wide spectrum of infectious agents are routinely identified using genetic testing. Among these are common causes of meningitis and encephalitis. Results can return within a few hours to assist with rapid confirmation of diagnosis and determination of the best treatment. Similarly, bacterial organisms responsible for sepsis can be specifically identified to accurately target antibiotic therapy based on the hospital's antibiogram.[1]

Cancer Therapy and Genomics

Oncology informatics is discussed in material that follows, but relative to genomics, the genetics of the patient affect prognosis and treatment for a variety of diseases.

The BRCA1 and BRCA2 genes are particularly emblematic of the role of genomics in oncology. These genes code for tumor-suppressor proteins. Mutations in these genes can disrupt the efficiency of action of the proteins, making certain cancers more likely. Most well known are the heightened risks of breast and ovarian cancer, but the likelihoods of some other cancers, such as pancreatic cancer, is increased as well.[2] Not only do females but also males with the gene mutations have an increased cancer risk.

National Comprehensive Cancer Network (NCCN) guidelines use genomics to guide treatment of cancers depending on BRCA1 and BRCA2 mutations.[3] Women with breast cancer who have a gene defect may benefit from bilateral mastectomy because of the high risk of new cancer in residual breast tissue. Chemotherapy for patients with ovarian cancer who have one of these gene defects has new options for management that specifically target DNA repair in the cancer cells.

Tumor DNA sequencing is used particularly commonly in lung and colorectal cancers. Findings from this may be able to be targeted for specific therapy.

Medication Efficacy and Toxicity

Clopidogrel is an antiplatelet agent widely used for patients with vascular disease. The *CY2C19* gene is responsible for metabolism of clopidogrel to an active metabolite. Patients who have two nonfunctioning copies of the gene cannot activate the medication. Testing is not in widespread use because of the low proportion of the population harboring this gene, but it is of value for identifying patients who may not respond to this medication.[4]

The Department of Veterans Affairs has classified several genetic tests as warranted in medication selection.[5] These include HLA-B*15:02 for Stevens-Johnston syndrome evoked by carbamazepine, G6PD for rasburicase-associated hemolytic anemia, and CYP2D6 for codeine toxicity.

The number and utility of genetic tests available that have significant clinical implications are certain to increase dramatically in coming years.

Genetic Testing and Genomic Banks

How do we know the genetics of the patient to determine whether we need to alter therapy? Patients with certain cancers have genetic studies performed on them and sometimes their cancer specimens. This may be routine or part of a research protocol.

In addition to individual genetic analyses of patients, warehouses of genetic information are correlated with clinical information. Only by following patients with disorders and specific genetic profiles will we identify patients at increased or decreased risk for these specific disorders.

ONCOLOGY

Oncology information systems (OISs) should have accommodation for cancer evaluation and monitoring and for chemotherapy and radiation therapy. These have very different clinical requirements and are often not well served by any one application. Methods of ordering as well as documentation are different.

Presently, there is a mix of niche and integrated EHR implementations. As foundational EHR vendors become better in niche applications, we presume that integrated applications will predominate. This will be by acquisition of niche apps with streamlined integration or maturation of the oncology portions of an EHR core.

One of the benefits of a well-designed OIS is the potential for decision support, with standardization of treatment protocols for certain cancers, yet considering specific characteristics of individual patients and their cancer. Changing guidelines necessitate prompt updating of protocols in the system. An ideal OIS would help facilitate this.

Billing for oncology services is complicated, and contract management can be particularly complex. Also, some cancer centers have significant financial impact from the 340B Drug Discount Program, and participation in this requires analytics and reporting.

We consider further informatics issues of medical oncology and radiation oncology next.

Medical Oncology

Medical oncology blends inpatient and outpatient care. The diagnostic component of medical oncology is principally focused on determination of lesion size and geometry and also presence and extent of metastases and cancer staging. As such, close integration with imaging capabilities is essential.

Chemotherapy plans are complicated by multiple medications with different schedules, specifics of pathology, phased treatment plans, and dependencies on clinical data, such as laboratory studies and adverse effects. For example, a common regimen used for breast cancer uses rounds of doxorubicin and cyclophosphamide followed by rounds of paclitaxel. As the patient progresses through therapy, medication doses are adjusted according to tolerability, laboratory studies, including those for white blood cells (WBC), red blood cells (RBC), and renal function, and response to therapy. If a patient has significantly abnormal blood tests, treatment may have to be held, and medications may be given to stimulate bone marrow recovery before another dose is given.

Other requirements of medical oncology apps include accommodation for clinical trials, genomics, compliance with tumor registries, and integration with affiliated cancer centers,

Radiation Oncology

Radiation oncology information systems have to interface with the medical oncology system if not part of an integrated package. Part of this is because many of the requirements are shared, including integration with pathology and imaging results, established protocols with dependencies and contingencies, and reporting.

Radiation therapy protocols are complex, and modern machinery should not only drive but also record treatments, including tracking cumulative doses and geometry.

SURGERY AND ANESTHESIA

Core EHR systems do patient care well, and this should include an efficient and versatile surgical information system, but surgery and anesthesia systems often do not meet hopes and expectations. Basic clinical documentation functionality for surgeons and preanesthesia evaluation is often accomplished by core EHR applications. But, additional functionality is required for the operating rooms.

Operating Room Logistics

Scheduling is the first component. The OR schedule is complex and is usually not amenable to a strictly automated process. Among the complex variables are specific preferences of the surgeon, anticipated duration of preceding procedures; specifics of the case that could affect OR turnaround time (e.g., changing equipment, infection risk); or availability of specific surgical assistants, other surgeons, or others with skill sets (e.g., device vendor staff). Therefore, the schedules for most surgeons are stored in the centralized scheduling system, but entries are dependent on multiple elements of the access and approval process.

Every patient scheduled for a surgical procedure has had a preoperative encounter, whether days before in a surgeon's office, preadmission unit, or the ED shortly before the procedure. The surgery EHR must be able to accommodate documentation imported from other systems, including the history and physical (H&P) and relevant laboratory test results and other reports. Also, the surgery EHR has to allow for digital signing of informed consent documents or allow paper versions or outside electronic versions to be imported. Surgical procedures are generally composed of multiple stages, and keeping track of the encounters can be difficult: Documents and orders need to be placed on the correct encounter. Sometimes, the orders component of this process is facilitated by multiphase order sets.

There are some special considerations for the information systems (IS) infrastructure for the OR:

- Touchscreen devices are often helpful for the OR to facilitate ease of data entry, display manipulation, and ease of cleaning following the procedure.
- Large displays are preferable for the OR because of the amount of physiological monitoring that is standard and because this must remain visible when medications are given or doses adjusted.
- Dual screens are preferable for the surgeon's documentation area because the surgeon may have to consult the picture archiving and communication system (PACS) or another EHR (e.g., office) in composing operative reports.
- Configuration of the EHR, PACS, and associated servers must allow for there being no time-out and for screensavers being disabled for the OR.
- Downtime procedures should include electronic access to not only archived data but also paper surgery and anesthesia forms.

The Surgery

Surgical documentation includes the preoperative note addressing the history, examination, clinical assessment, plan, and rationale for the planned procedure.

Postoperative documentation (the *op note*) is required after the procedure. The mechanism of creation differs between EHRs and surgeons, but in general, there are multiple components. These typically are as follows:

- Patient name
- Date of procedure
- Preoperative diagnosis
- Postoperative diagnosis
- Surgeon name(s)
- Assistant name(s)
- Procedure(s)
- Indications
- Findings
- Complications
- Estimated blood loss
- Specimens obtained
- Details of the procedure

An increasing proportion of surgeons are using templates for individual surgical procedures. These can then be edited to indicate the specifics of the procedure just performed. Also acceptable is to have a description of the basics of the typical procedure and then have a separate text field for entry of specific features of this case.

Postprocedure orders, including medicine reconciliation, are placed before the patient leaves the care of the surgeon.

Anesthesia

Preanesthesia evaluation is usually begun by nurses and completed by anesthesiologists. The result of this is an H&P focused more on readiness for the planned procedure than diagnosis or appropriateness of the planned surgery. Difficulties with previous surgeries or episodes of sedation or anesthesia are documented.

Routine EHRs can do much of this, with the documentation often begun by nursing and then either taken over by the anesthesiologists or supplemented by an anesthesia note.

Among the elements are the following:

- Review of the history, including previous anesthesia
- Review of drug allergies and side effects
- Patient examination
- Assessment of anesthesia risk, often the American Society of Anesthesiologists (ASA) class[6]
- Identification of potential problems (e.g., airway characteristics, intravenous access)
- Plan of anesthesia care, including induction, maintenance, and postoperative care

- Documentation of understanding and agreement to the plan by patient or appropriate representative

Intraoperative function of the anesthesia component of the EHR should include the following functions:

- Documentation of vitals, including blood pressure, heart rate, oxygen saturation
- Streaming view of cardiac rhythm and other biometrics as needed
- Documentation of medication administration, either automatically or through entry by the anesthesiologist or nurse anesthetist
- Notation of which procedures are under way at given times
- Patient position and condition
- Notation of associated procedures (e.g., placing additional arterial or venous catheters)
- Notable events (e.g., cardiopulmonary resuscitation [CPR] required)
- Status of care at completion of operative epoch

CRITICAL CARE

Critical care requirements overlap somewhat with OR requirements. There is a host of physiologic data that is monitored, and while not all of this is in the EHR, at least some of the data should be stored for trending. Workflows in the pre-EHR era included paper charts, bedside physiological monitors with electrocardiogram (ECG) and often respirations and blood oxygen (O_2) saturation. The ECG monitor would spew strips either on demand or when the system detected some significant departure from a normal cardiac rhythm. The strips were cut into segments and taped into the paper chart. Flowcharts of medication administration and vital signs were kept on paper, often susceptible to late entries, errors, and illegibility.

The bedside monitors have evolved, but most of these are not the products of the EHR vendor, although partnerships are common. Ideally, interfaces should allow for storage of select epochs of traces in the permanent record.

With further enhancement of the connectivity of the intensive care unit (ICU), we foresee more extensive use of true connectivity between multiple ICU devices and the EHR, not only for acquisition of physiological recordings of cardiac and respiratory function, but also for driving of pumps, ventilator, temperature management equipment, and other clinical devices.

The ICU workstations for nursing are preferably where the nurse can maintain a view of the patient and the physiological displays. A terminal at a nurses' station is adequate, but even better is a workstation in the patient's room, whether fixed or mobile. If the device is in a fixed location, it should be positioned to allow visualization of the patient while the user is interacting with the EHR.

A computer version of the flowsheet has been hard to design. While the EHR has form capabilities, the best arrangement is a workflow display that shows a combination of interfaced and direct-entered data. Some EHRs offer timeline displays on which elements such as heart rate, blood pressure, and O_2 saturation are shown along with indicators such as vent settings, times of medication administration, and the rates for certain intravenous infusions. The ability to alter the timescale of these displays is of tremendous help for assessing the long and short views of critical care progress.

There are multiple assessment scales developed for diverse clinical purposes, such as SAPS, APACHE II, and NIHSS.[7] There are electronic and paper forms for these. Many of these are optimally shown on the workflow view.

Most patients in the ICU are on intravenous fluids and receive medications with controlled rates. Smart pumps are widely used and in their basic form have algorithms and data that can reduce the chance of errors. The abilities of the smart pump are enhanced when interfaced with the EHR. Then, the settings can usually be pushed through to the pump from the EHR, lessening the possibility of manual programming of the pump with errors. This interoperability also allows for returning data, such as end of infusion, empty fluid supply, or line occlusion. With a visual display of patient metrics, clinical staff can adjust infusions more easily.

Of the errors that are made in medicine, many of them occur in the ICU because of the complexity of care, the multitude of variables for the clinician to consider, and the high-risk patient population. Further maturation of the EHR for critical care use must facilitate advanced critical care decision support to try to avoid as many errors as possible.

EMERGENCY AND URGENT CARE MEDICINE

Emergency and urgent care departments present challenges similar to those in the operating room and critical care units. Evaluation and management must be performed as quickly and efficiently as possible. Because of this, there is usually pressure to use niche ED and urgent care programs. For an urgent care center, this may suffice. But, the difficulty with this in the ED is in care transitions.

Emergency Department

Many hospitals have a unified EHR with somewhat different appearances for the ED and inpatient settings. Some hospitals have different EHRs for the ED and acute care setting, and this presents challenges with potential difficulties for transitions of patients from ED to inpatient status. Orders and notes may not translate adequately from one system to another. Also, as a provider moves between the ED and inpatient floors, having to use a different EHR increases the risk of errors and omissions.

There are few data, but reports have claimed that there is a reduction in ED productivity following EHR implementation.[8] However, this often-cited report was with a custom-developed system, and the changes were only assessed to 1 year, whereas other EHR implementation studies have shown continuous improvement beyond this time.

Desirable features of an ED EHR include the following:

- Efficient system: minimizing time and clicks to find data, create documents, and place orders
- Documentation and order templates driven off provisional diagnoses or chief complaints
- Ease of results review: single source for laboratory results
- Notification of when laboratory and study reports have resulted
- Tracking board for patients in the unit, with indicators of time and clinical progress
- Notification of newly assigned patients and new clinical events
- Embedded communication with other providers (e.g., secure message with hospitalists)
- Ability to store pre-arrival information on incoming patients so that en route and outside-facility information can be stored before registration
- Interface with local and regional health information exchange (HIE) for point-of-care data access to community records
- Dashboards so providers can track their performance metrics
- Scribe-ready implementation

Scribes are used more commonly in medicine, particularly in the ED, where volumes and on-the-fly documentation are particularly suitable for scribe use.

Background configuration for most ED EHRs involves prioritizing orders from the ED. Most orders are tagged as stat by default. Also, some laboratory tests are often performed in a small ED laboratory, while others are performed in the hospital's centralized laboratory. So, the laboratory IS interface must be able to route samples and results appropriately.

Decision support for ED EHRs can be immensely helpful. One example is a sepsis agent, which can alert the provider to a constellation of clinical and laboratory findings that suggest sepsis, thereby hastening further evaluation and management.

Errors occur with all EHRs. Among the errors that occur with particular frequency in the ED are the following:

- *Duplicate orders*: Most commonly, these occur when a provider asks a nurse to give a medication and then enters it electronically, so the patient receives a double dose. Decision support tools should catch this by duplicate order or dose-limiting algorithms.
- *Wrong patient*: Most commonly, this occurs when a provider has multiple charts open and places an order on the wrong one.
- *Ignoring alerts*: A busy ED provider can easily develop alert fatigue.

Alert fatigue is an issue throughout the healthcare system, so there should be evaluation of frequency of firing and efficacy of alerts throughout the system.

Wrong patient data entry and orders have prompted some healthcare systems to restrict EHR interfaces to only one open chart at a time, but this has not been shown to help, largely because there is loss of efficiency and potential for confusion when opening and closing active charts. Present data do not demand restricting the number of open charts.[9] Additional study is needed to compare error rates and provider workflow and efficiency.

Urgent Care

The needs of the urgent care center are similar to those of the ED, but because urgent care centers are less likely to be affiliated with a hospital, there is often more latitude in selection of the EMR. If the urgent care center is affiliated with an outpatient clinic, then that corresponding software might be appropriate, but not all ambulatory systems are efficient in the urgent care arena.

The system requirements are generally similar to the ED systems with tracking board, templates for documents and orders driven by provisional diagnoses and chief complaints, and notification of studies and laboratory test results. Urgent care centers generally do not see acute strokes and cardiac events or major trauma, so capability for dealing with these complex cases is usually not necessary.

Billing is often part of the urgent care EHR system, although it can be done independently.

Many urgent care information systems are cloud based, often with a Web interface. Tablet apps are also common because much of the care and documentation are markedly templated.

Patient educational materials are important for all healthcare encounters but are especially helpful for urgent and emergent care, for which diagnosis-specific instructions are given.

Medication e-prescribing is extremely valuable, as is pharmacy network queries to determine what has been prescribed elsewhere. E-prescribing results in automatic embedding of documentation in the EHR, whereas this does not occur with paper or phoned prescriptions.

ENDOSCOPY: GASTROENTEROLOGY AND PULMONARY

Endoscopic procedures require recording of images as well as a narrative summary. The core EHR does not usually provide an efficient workflow, so a niche system or a bolt-on is often required.

Desired attributes of endoscopic systems include the following:

- Acquisition, editing, and annotation of images from the study
- Incorporation of selected annotated images in the report
- Ease of recording in, out, and event times
- Record findings during the study, including details of observations and sites of biopsy specimens
- Templates for different studies (e.g., various gastrointestinal [GI] procedures
- Quality reporting capability

Documentation by a scribe or other assistant during the procedure minimizes the risk that the findings or details could be forgotten.

OPHTHALMOLOGY

Ophthalmology has been slow to embrace EHRs partly because these practices are often freestanding, not part of large groups that would demand an across-the-board conversion, but mainly because of slowness of development of effective ophthalmology systems. However, by 2016, approximately 72% of ophthalmologists used EHRs[10] at a time when 79% of primary care physicians used EHRs.

As with some other specialties, there is dependency on images and figures, which historically have been photographs and hand drawn. Creation and annotation of images as well as importing of images from devices in the ophthalmology record are required capabilities of EHRs that serve this specialty.[11]

Data entry for ophthalmology is substantial and trends need to be viewed over time. Entering, storing, and viewing these data need to be as efficient as possible.

All specialties are under time pressure to increase service volume and therefore make most efficient use of time, and ophthalmology is higher volume than most specialties, creating a greater potential for dissatisfaction if the EHR is believed to slow the provider.

OBSTETRICS

Obstetrics requires accommodation to high-volume rapid evaluation and management. The trended data differ from much of the data of general medical and surgical practice, so OB usually requires a component customized to this field.

Two major subsets of OB are prenatal visits and delivery. Prenatal visits are usually brief encounters where vital signs are tracked with fetal as well as maternal assessments. Ultrasound measurements and images should be readily viewable. The prenatal documentation and orders should be able to be templated, and as part of the documentation, entered data should result in expected due date calculation and display.

Delivery requires ready access to the prenatal records and additionally needs acquisition and display of fetal-monitoring capabilities.

Many obstetricians have a significant gynecology practice, and this parallels many surgical specialties, where images need to be stored, and also parallels oncology, where staging information and treatment prescription are facilitated.

FAMILY MEDICINE

Family medicine physicians practice in the fields of general medicine, minor surgery, obstetrics, gynecology, pediatrics, and urgent care. Service settings are all facets of acute inpatient, outpatient, ED, urgent care, OB, and long-term care facilities. As such, the providers need to be able to enjoy the efficiencies that the EHR vendors have developed into all of these arenas.

Most major EHRs allow for interface profiles to be switched depending on the clinical venue. This may happen automatically, where the interface changes depending on whether the patient is in the clinic, hospital, or ED. Alternatively, the user may be able to select the interface profile appropriate to where they will be working. Historically, differing locations and clinical roles required separate login credentials, but that is generally not the case now.

PEDIATRICS

Pediatrics has unique challenges in EHR design and implementation. EHRs have been slow to address the complexities of pediatric practice to give the providers the functionality, flexibility, and efficiency of the paper world.

Factors that make pediatrics informatics particularly difficult are

- wide range of patient ages and sizes;
- broad range of age-based needs;
- family practice and some other specialties seeing pediatric patients as well as adult patients;
- requirements for school reporting;
- range of medication selection and dosing requirements that depend on numerous factors, including age and size; and
- challenging clinical decision support because of all of these parametric differences.

We discuss some of the challenges in more detail.

A technical brief was prepared by the Vanderbilt University Evidence-Based Practice Center for the Agency for Healthcare Research and Quality; the brief reported on expectations and requirements for EHRs used in the pediatric setting.[12] While basic core functionality has much in common with the EHR used for adult patients, there are certainly demands that are not being consistently met. This article is freely available and should be in our personal libraries. Among the issues are following:

- *Vaccine Management*: Including recording vaccinations, prompting when vaccines are needed, sharing of data with other systems, viewing of individual elements of combination vaccines.
- *Routine Health Care Maintenance*: Including tracking of child development as well as immunizations, generation of reports for schools and other activities.
- *Family Dynamics*: Including social details, relationships, linking of data between members of a family to recognize patterns of disease or risk.
- *Privacy*: Including providing for privacy requirements with confidential conversations and healthcare, including reproductive and social issues,

allowing access only when appropriate, providing the ability to designate certain EHR items as private.

- *Management of Pediatric Conditions in Vulnerable Populations*: Including special needs for patients with specific disorders, such as genetic, developmental, or acquired disorders.
- *Medications*: Including decision support to ensure right medication, right dose, and right route; accommodation for corrected age; ensuring that alerts intended for adults are not delivered inappropriately to the provider for pediatric patients; ensuring dose rounding is appropriate and correct; and e-prescribing that considers availability of formulations and supply types.
- *Documentation*: Including availability of documentation from other facilities, integration of EHR use into workflow to optimize efficiency and throughput for the office staff as well as the provider.
- *Pediatric-Specific Norms and Growth Charts*: Including normal values for laboratory test results according to age, alerts based on age, flexible displays on growth charts, accommodation for premature infants.

Not all of these will be able to be implemented in the short term, and some of the clinician recommendations in the report were not accompanied by a defined solution. A subset of these will have to be the principal focus.[13] However, we recommend the short-term goal of EHR vendors should be to enhance the following:

- Workflow design and optimization to maximize efficiency
- Single screen for review of data, placing orders, documenting elements of the encounter
- Decision support specific to the age of the patient
- Medication support specific to the age and weight of the patient, flexibility regarding route and dosing, and sensitivity to supply and formulation of stock medications
- Ability of the EHR to record social details important to medical care, coordinate individual access, link records of family members as appropriate, and mediate privacy as determined by age, relationship, and specific medical issue
- Exchange and integrate data from other facilities
- Provide appropriate educational materials

Pediatric Outpatient Clinic

A lower proportion of pediatric clinics use EHRs than adult clinics. All of the factors listed previously are responsible for this, although other factors include

- less interdependency of pediatrics on outside referrals than internal medicine or adult family medicine practice;

- lower reimbursements for childhood care than adult care, resulting in less likely investment in technical infrastructure; and
- high volume with very low margin for loss of efficiency.

MEDICATION SELECTION

Order sets are generally specific to a presentation, presumptive diagnosis, or procedure to be performed. Pediatric management requires that we have order sets with the flexibility to recommend appropriate medications for age and weight. While dose calculators take into account weight of the patient, the weight should be displayed while the provider is ordering.

GROWTH CHARTS

The EHR is adept as drawing growth charts; however, often with transition to a new EHR, previous growth data are not backfilled. Either these data need to be entered so that a complete growth chart can be generated or at least there should be easy ability to review the previously generated growth charts from within the EHR.

In the United States, most parents still want to know height and weight of their child in English measurements. However, most of the rest of the world uses metric units. Also, even in the United States, metric measurement is used for most pharmacy calculations. Display of both English and metric measurements might be desirable, but errors have been made when dose calculations were performed on the wrong metric. Therefore, we recommend that the data in the EHR be entered and displayed in metric units with a metric/English equivalency table available for the provider to tell a patient the measurements. This is complicated by scales in some offices having only English measurements.

Not only different formulations and delivery methods are needed for different ages, but also there are preferences on the part of child and family that affect compliance and ultimately efficacy of a treatment.[14] Our EHR should be able to be flexible about formulations.

Pediatric Hospital Practice

One of the most cited criticisms of the EHR was reported by Han et al. in 2005. Use of computerized physician order entry (CPOE) in a pediatric ICU actually increased mortality.[15] Subsequent studies have not shown that this is a pervasive finding; no worsening in outcome is usually expected.[16,17] However, many informatics professionals expected improvement because of clinical decision support capabilities baked into the EHR. Certainly, initiation of CPOE is disruptive. On paper, the provider is only concentrating on writing down the needed orders. With a new CPOE, the provider is navigating a new system, so their concentration is not devoted entirely to the patient's needs. This is a required learning curve; over time, the provider will find CPOE easier than handwritten orders, especially if they leverage order sets and favorites. But, initially, the learning curve interferes with achieving anticipated potential benefits.

Use of the EHR in pediatric hospital practice does have the potential for improved care, particularly because of clinical decision support aiding medication selection and dosing. Gap analysis for immunizations and other needed interventions can be facilitated by the EHR. This can be a challenge if there is no information sharing, but there should be fewer barriers to this in the future.

A large academic medical system made the transition from a home-grown EHR to a commercial product and initially reported an increase in medication safety reports, but this rate returned to baseline within 3 months.[18] Among the issues that offered challenges to the new EHR were the inability to order half or part doses, difficulty with titration orders, and prescribing medications with off-label administration methods, such as through another route (e.g., intramuscular, rectal).

Issues that we have seen at our large public referral hospital included having to create special methods of attaching barcodes to small syringes and tubes, adjusting rounding conventions, and coordination with the pharmacy to arrange for special pediatric order sentences.

Informatics assistance to create favorite orders for providers has been helpful for most providers, but this is especially helpful for pediatrics, including the neonatal ICU.

Pediatric Emergency Practice

Principal issues for the pediatric ED include efficiency and decision support. Most pediatric EDs often see high volumes in a short period of time. Efficiency is promoted by having workflow pages that give easy visibility for most of the tasks in the ED.

Decision support needs in the pediatric ED are principally to ensure proper medication selection,[19] dosing, and formulation. However, a principal role is also to ensure that critical diagnoses are not missed.[20] This will require clinical decision support design and implementation specific to pediatrics and specific to the ED. This has received insufficient attention so far, and this must be remedied.[21]

Pediatric Subspecialties

Pediatric specialties have many of the same demands as adult specialties. In addition, all of the considerations discussed previously for childhood healthcare apply.

Specialty Referral Management: Provider lists could only include those who see pediatric patients, although this is difficult to implement; for example, a neurology clinic might have mainly neurologists who see adults, but one pediatric neurologist and perhaps one of the neurologists for adults will see patients down to age 12. Also, certain pediatric subspecialists are quite selective, such as a pediatric neurologist who only does epilepsy care. Communication between pediatrician and specialists is key and may be done electronically,[22] but there is no complete substitute for a phone call.

Pediatric Procedure Management: Study and radiology images are stored as for adult patients. OR scheduling has to consider age of the patient because setup and equipment differ depending on age as well as procedure.

KEY POINTS

- Specialties require accommodation to workflows and demands of the specialty.
- Niche systems for specialties may be needed, but if the principal enterprise EHR can reasonably accomplish the task, integration is invaluable.
- Future EHR enhancements will better accommodate specialties, especially those that are impeded in efficiency by having to use a broad-spectrum EHR.

Health Information Exchange in Practice

MARK E. FRISSE AND KARL E. MISULIS ■

THE CONTEXT

Effective collaboration is a prerequisite for effective healthcare delivery. Every clinician and caregiver should share a common clinical record set with a common problem list, medication list, and allergy list and a common listing of laboratory tests and study reports. The patient is a vital component of this collaborative network. Access to common data helps ensure that care is safer and more cost effective. Such sharing simplifies the task of ensuring that drug allergies and duplicate tests are avoided. This same sharing also simplifies quality and performance metric reporting, contracting, and the many other administrative tasks reliant on a complete and accurate clinical and administrative data set.

Healthcare services and healthcare data are highly fragmented. The National Academy of Medicine reported that every year the average elderly patient sees seven doctors across four practices, and that the average surgery patient is seen by 27 different healthcare providers.[1] These metrics do not begin to describe the far larger network of community health professionals, family, and neighbors vital to patient well-being.

From the perspective of many providers, our healthcare delivery system is even more complex. Within most communities and care settings, patients are cared for by different but overlapping networks of clinicians and health plans. In one study, for every 100 Medicare beneficiaries, physicians on average were connected to 26 other physicians.[2] Overall, these physicians may have to communicate with many more direct caregivers as well as patients, family members, informal caregivers, home health providers, pharmacists, a host of other service providers, and a dizzying array of health plans, pharmacy benefits managers, and other parties. Even with the help of accomplished staff and sophisticated electronic health records (EHRs), our ability to communicate and collaborate effectively falls far short of the mark.

The goal of effective *health information exchange* (HIE) is to ensure that care-related data are available to authorized individuals when they are needed (Table 25.1). Prior to the widespread introduction of EHRs, the term *HIE* was associated mainly with specific organizations that combined policies, data standards, and technologies to enhance clinical communication. These organizations were formed as state-sponsored entities, regional alliances, or offshoots of large care delivery networks. More recently, the term *exchange* is more focused on the process of active communication and less on any single approach.

CARE SETTINGS

There are several settings and activities where the need for effective exchange of clinical information is most acute.

Hospitals and Hospital Emergency Departments: Hospital emergency departments (EDs) have been the dominant area of focus because of the likelihood that information from other clinical settings could help in clinical decision-making and because most hospitals adopted EHRs more quickly than ambulatory practices. The emphasis was on the ED's capabilities to receive information; most EDs could not transmit care summaries to providers because most providers lacked both access to a centralized HIE clearinghouse or because neither hospitals nor ambulatory care providers were able to communicate care summaries directly. Although most studies described modest savings due to ordering fewer tests, early benefit was often due to fewer admissions for observation for cases where acuity and past treatment could be clarified by examining clinical data transmitted from external sources.

Ambulatory Clinics: Clinicians often receive updates on clinical status, medications, and other events from other providers, patients, relatives, and institutional data resources. They transmit their own findings and changes to care among the same group of clinicians and family members.

Patients, Families, and Homes: Patients and home caregivers collect and communicate a wide range of clinical information that is essential for maintaining health status and avoiding hospital readmission.

Freestanding Clinics: These clinics can be stand-alone but are frequently affiliated with healthcare provider organizations composed of some combination of hospitals, clinics, retail pharmacies, and health plans. Although the acuity is lower, clinicians and patients expect the same clinical data communications as with ED care.

Rehabilitation, Skilled Nursing Facilities, and Other Care Settings: Interinstitutional transfers of care should be accompanied by exchange of clinical and administrative data. Presently, patients often move from the acute care hospital to rehabilitation or long-term care facilities with limited information and without a previously agreed-on plan.

Table 25.1 SETTINGS WHERE HIE IS OPERATIONAL

Setting	Transmitting to Authorized Clinicians	Receiving (From Other Care Sites)
Hospital ED visit or admission	ADT; comprehensive visit/ discharge summary; comprehensive postdischarge care plan	List of current care providers; laboratory reports; medications; allergies; radiology reports; radiology images; clinic/hospital notes; treatment plans; patient personal health record
Ambulatory visit	Visit summary; medication changes; treatment plan; scheduling and chronic care coordination	Provider lists; problem list; active medications; allergies; recent treatments
Referral request	Referral request for diagnosis, procedures, or treatment recommendations; reason for request; clinical data	Consultation note; encounter summary; active or proposed treatment plan; diagnostic report; procedure report
Prescriptions	Initiate or change a new prescription request Request a prescription refill Medication history request Medication history response Request formulary information	Acknowledge receipt of new, change, or refill request Communicate fill status Medication history request Medication history response Present formulary information
Walk-in clinic	Visit summary	Medications, allergies, and other clinical information as needed
Chronic care	Request for additional services; request for clinical updates	Provider list (professional and patient/family); clinical status report; clinical services requests
Personal care	Health status, including activity, health promotion activities, and preventive care	Access to all care records
Institutional transitions in care	All clinical information required for continuity of care at the receiving institution.	A clear care plan and all other clinical information required for care continuity.
Quality reporting	Clinical and administrative data for quality reporting (or research initiatives)	Quality metric summaries; patient panels; encounter information

Referrals: Referrals are generally a form of ambulatory visits, but requests for diagnosis, procedures, or other treatments sometime involve hospitalization. The referring clinician must provide enough information to set expectations and to facilitate completion of the task. On completion, a summary of the referred work (new diagnoses, recommendations) must be shared among caregivers.

Medication Management: Medication management involves transmission and re-ception of clinical information, including requests for new prescriptions and no-tification of fill status. An incomplete prescription drug history is available from a dispensing pharmacy, but if patients receive prescription medications from mul-tiple sources, a comprehensive prescription drug history can be obtained only if all pharmacies participate in a network like SureScripts. Even that would be incom-plete, however, because pharmacies do not generally maintain records of over-the-counter medications, herbals, supplements, and others.

Quality and Administration: Quality reporting, care improvement efforts, and administrative activities require bidirectional communication. Accountable care organizations, patient-centered medical homes, and myriad other care collabora-tion efforts make effective use of data from populations to compare the care of an individual patient with expected norms for the population. Databases comprising aggregated administrative and clinical data can identify possible gaps in care for in-dividual patients, compare patient status with that of similar patients, and compare practitioner performance with peer practices.

COMMON MESSAGE ATTRIBUTES

Every successfully communicated exchange message has common attributes:

> *Purpose*: Every clinical or administrative communication is driven by one or more implicit or explicit purposes. These may include requesting a referral, assigning a clinical task, transmitting clinical data to one or more current or future providers or caregivers, or communicating information to parties responsible for payment, quality measurement, and other regulatory purposes. Often, the purpose of a communication is implicit, but with respect to referral requests and care coordination tasks, the purpose is made more explicit by the way a message is created and transmitted.

> *Sender and Recipient*: Both the sender and recipient identities must be explicit. At times, either or both will be an organizational unit rather than an individual (e.g., "hematology lab," "renal clinic administrator"). This knowledge can be difficult to obtain. For example, an acute care provider seeking to transmit a care summary may not have an accurate list of referring physicians, primary care providers, or other members of the care team. Some information systems maintain multiple lists (termed *pools*), but these can be contradictory and can remove a sense of individual ownership.

> *Unambiguous Identities*: The identity of every provider and patient must be unambiguous. We must not transmit a message to the wrong provider about the wrong "Mr. John Smith." Resolving ambiguity for providers is simplified through use of the *National Provider Identifier* (NPI), a unique 10-digit identification number issued by the Centers for Medicare and Medicaid Services (CMS). Matching patient names across multiple data sets is more problematic because in the absence of a national unique

identifier, matching records using many and varied attributes is inherently imperfect. Patients may change names (e.g., shortly after birth or with marital changes). Patients may be registered at different sites with name variants (e.g., Jim, Jimmy, James). Dates of birth may be incorrectly entered, and use of Social Security numbers is discouraged. Often, provider institutions have made efforts to create a unique local patient identifier. If an institution requests data and includes their unique local patient identifier, responding while retaining this identifier ensures correct matching. A range of patient-matching algorithms is available; each has slightly different performance characteristics, and some inappropriately matched or *orphan* records may require manual intervention.

Role and Authorization: Every individual or organization plays multiple roles. These differ depending on the care context, so permission to view a communication depends on this context. For example, providers are authorized to access information about patients under their care, but in other instances, the same professionals may be patients themselves or employers. Similarly, a care manager seeking to contact a patient may understand that a family member has been authorized to provide care and should therefore be the target of a message. This is particularly important in the care of children and elderly or disabled adults who rely on others for care and communication.

Content and Representation: The content and representation of each message may differ. At its simplest, the content is a text glob that is transmitted (via messaging or fax) to a recipient who can interpret the content. Common and very useful examples include discharge summaries, radiology reports, and administrative documents. With the appropriate metadata (e.g., patient name, type of report, date), these communications are extremely useful. Indeed, prior to the widespread use of lengthy EHR-generated clinical summaries, dictated hospital discharge summaries and lists of laboratory test results were the most valuable documents to most early HIE participants. While useful to the clinician, these documents are not easily incorporated into medical record systems or databases. With the advent of EHR-generated documents and encoded information, documents can be far more easily incorporated into EHRs and databases, but at times, this value is offset by the difficulties clinicians encounter in searching for information in sometimes overly complex and lengthy computer-generated documents.

COMMON MESSAGING AND EXCHANGE TECHNOLOGY FUNCTIONS

No matter what specific architectural model is employed, messaging and exchange systems have the following characteristics:

Locator Information. Every individual must be associated with one or more means to unambiguously transmit a communication to the right recipient. Clinical professionals associated with one or more provider organization may work in multiple locations using different EHRs. To simplify ensuring that messages reach the right individual or group, they are sometimes sent to a common inbox associated with a practitioner (i.e., "Vanderbilt GI clinic" or "Jones pharmacy at 31st and West End Avenue"). In these circumstances, a staff member will process the message, and often, this level of location is ideal because one is sending a communication to a clinic or pharmacy without knowing the specific individuals who will handle the communication. When transmitting a message to an entity, getting the location right is critical. When sending a communication to an individual, we need to be sure the recipient is available or has backup to review communications when the intended recipient is unavailable. Patient communication also requires locator information. Whether a phone number, an address, an Internet portal account, or a direct message, one must know both identity of the recipient and the best way of contacting the recipient.

Locator Services: A more generalized approach to support clinical data exchange among multiple providers will necessitate a *record locator service* (RLS). These services are essentially tables that map each unique identity (patients, providers) to a set of institutions, each with the institutions' patient or provider identifier numbers and access methods. The RLS may be directly linked with a centralized shared database, or it may consist of a set of *pointers* to the institutions storing the record. In the latter case, authorized requests are sent via the RLS, and the results are returned directly to the requestor. The centralized RLS retains a *transaction log* documenting the exchange. RLSs are susceptible to unwarranted intrusion and could conceivably be a back door to provider databases. Unauthorized access to RLSs may provide intruders with access to protected information. Maintaining RLS security is therefore paramount.

Transmission: Message transmission must be standardized. Their transmission can be either automatic (*push*) or only in response to a valid query (*pull*). Most transmissions employ the Internet's foundational *Transmission Control Protocol and Internet Protocol* (TCP/IP). Along with the basic communication protocol, one employs one of several foundational interoperability standards. Encrypted messages are transmitted through electronic email protocols such as the *Simple Mail Transfer Protocol* (SMTP). Other commonly employed methods include the familiar *Hypertext Transfer Protocol* (HTTP), the *Simple Object Access Protocol* (SOAP), and the related *Representational State Transfer* (REST) approach.

Directory Services and Routing: Given the unambiguous destination of recipient location, exchange and messaging systems must ensure that the message arrives at its intended destination securely and without modification. Maintaining a single logical directory for providers is a challenging job. Even more challenging at times is ensuring that there are lists to inform providers of one another's roles in care. This can be particularly problematic with discharge communications or other situations when the receiving providers are not clearly specified or when a patient has not been referred directly to a specific provider for care.

Matching. A patient record lacking unique identifiers must be matched with other records from the same patient. In some clinical exchange systems, this matching is done with probabilistic algorithms and in others through categorical rules. In some cases, these algorithms can be tuned to specify false-positive/false-negative matches. If one is caring for a patient, matching may be tuned to ensure that every data item is associated with the patient receiving care—even if this identification comes at the expense of not including a few of the patient's records that could not be unambiguously assigned to the unique identifier. If, on the other hand, one is conducting population health research, one may seek to obtain all information about a population, even if a small number of records have data matched with the wrong member of the population.

Terminology Services: After messages are checked for conformance to exchange standards, terminology services are employed to ensure that, when necessary, data are transformed to meet the requirements of recipient systems.

Transaction Logs: Transaction logs are critical components of every database system and every means of communicating information. These logs generally record the identity of sender and recipient, the event time, and at least metadata about the type of information transmitted. Properly designed, transaction logs can support a rapid investigation into possible data breaches or unauthorized use. Data from these logs are also incorporated into machine learning systems to identify anomalous access and other trends. In some instances, the patterns discovered by these inquiries are employed by systems seeking to identify unauthorized access in real time.

Workflow Integration: Perhaps the greatest inhibitor of more effective collaboration is integrating communication into practice workflow. In many instances, the major problem in communication is not transmission of a message but rather ensuring that a message is received by the right party and acted on. Simple transmission of consultation requests, care coordination communication, or clinical information can be hampered if the provider cannot quickly integrate this request into practice workflow. EHR systems are making great strides in both the request of information and its reception, but true workflow integration remains a challenge. When facing disparate practices and seeking to foster communication among providers, great efforts must be expended to ensure that recipients—especially small practices, home caregivers, and patients—can incorporate desired communications into their workflow.

Security: Security refers to prevention of both unauthorized access to data and uncorrupted data translation and transmission. Physical and technical security of every component of an exchange are critical. Stewardship requires an organization to protect its data resources and ensure the integrity of any data exchanged with another party. These efforts are related to but largely distinct from the more complex means of ensuring enforcement of privacy policies.

Governance: Data governance refers to the collaborations, contracts, and oversight necessary to ensure that data are used only in the ways authorized by those who have claim to some degree of data control. Writ large, governance may include many managerial and business processes. In this context, governance encompasses development and enforcement of privacy policies and necessary managerial and clinical rules to ensure trust among all stakeholders.

COMMUNICATION AND EXCHANGE MODELS

There are many different ways to exchange data with other systems. The approach taken should be driven by the availability of technical options and both clinical and administrative needs. Despite the advances in technologies and adoption, fax transmission is, at times, the only realistic option.

EHR-Centered Systems

As a few large EHR vendors gain market share, institutions using one of these vendors can often send and receive information without leaving the EHR encounter. These vendors search across multiple institutions using the same EHR vendor, integrate data received, and present a single merged document integrated into the patient record.

To foster collaborations among clinicians, schedulers, and other administrators, patient scheduling is another area where common vendors can collaborate.[3] Some approaches allow patients to grant access to their data to any providers who have Internet access, even if they do not have EHRs. This approach lets the provider access patient information on a Web browser and may also allow upload of encounter notes to improve continuity of care.

Alliances

Dedicated third-party alliances can also facilitate data transmission and reception across different clinical systems.

Carequality: Working across the entire healthcare industry, the Sequoia Project's Carequality provides a national-level, consensus-built, common interoperability framework that enables exchange among health data–sharing networks. Created initially as the Nationwide Health Information Network (NHIN), Carequality's three areas of emphasis are in the provision of well-defined technical specifications, common governance rules, and a uniform provider directory containing network addresses and roles. In some instances, Carequality can send updated provider directory information as well as requested clinical information. These systems are also designed to exchange information with the Department of Veterans Affairs (VA) and the Department of Defense (DoD) medical records systems. (As the VA and the DoD adopt new commercial EHR systems, their ability to share information will increase.)

The CommonWell Health Alliance: Members of this alliance share standardized ways of enrolling patients; managing consent; identifying patients; linking records from the same patient; locating records; retrieving records; and ensuring authorized provider and patient access. Most, but not all, of the major EHR vendors participate in the CommonWell Alliance. This alliance supports Integrating the Health Enterprise (IHE) profiles, REST-base services like Fast Healthcare Interoperability Resources (FHIR) and Health Level Seven International (HL7) Argonaut, as well as many other transaction types.

Direct Messaging: Direct is an encrypted, point-to-point communication method capable of sending almost any communication. Direct has been used successfully primarily for referral communications and at times for discharge communications and other purposes. This approach was introduced as a substitute for the HIE requirements of the Health Information Technology for Economic and Clinical Health (HITECH) Act. Simply put, Direct is a means of sending any digital item through secure email-like protocols employing public key encryption (public key infrastructure, PKI). A successful Direct implementation requires a reliable health information service provider (HISP) to route messages securely and adhere to standardized methods of representing communications, often using the CCD (continuity-of-care document) format. As a critical mass of providers develops, sending a message via Direct through an EHR becomes more straightforward; the greatest challenge is in understanding the most effective way to receive a Direct message and to integrate the communication into practice workflow.

Regional and State Exchanges: Some of the earliest exchange efforts were developed by state or regional organizations. Created prior to widespread adoption of data standards, these organizations often had to develop their own technologies and rules. Many of the early regional exchanges failed because of technical costs, mistrust, workflow issues, and, in the absence of capitated payments, an inadequate financially sustainable business model. But, some notable examples continue to thrive, including organizations in Maine, Maryland, Colorado, Kansas, New York, Ohio, and Indiana. Generally, they adapt to regional or state priorities but adopt common data standards and exchange techniques. As the marginal cost of exchange drops with EHR-based methods and other means of standards-based communication emerge, these exchange organizations continually innovate to maintain a sustainable business model. These exchanges can contain a single centralized database, or they may contain only pointers to primary data available from systems where the care is delivered.

ADT Messaging

Admission, discharge, and transfer (ADT) messages, encoded using the HL7 standard, are typically initiated by a registration application to inform ancillary systems that a patient has been admitted, discharged, transferred, or has had some other event. They also can include provider information.

More recently, selected ADT messages have been employed by health information organizations and hospital associations to unite primary care providers, payers, and others accountable for coordinating care for patients by providing secure messages in real time. Providers can then access appropriate systems to obtain additional information.

These systems are simple, inexpensive, secure, and accessible through many secure messaging services. One can expect more extensive data exchange organizations to incorporate these technologies.

Blue Button

Blue Button, a government-initiated branding and community engagement effort, is focused on encouraging provider organizations to give consumers access to their own health data. Blue Button provides a way for patients to download their data from the VA My HealtheVet Portal, Medicare (MyMedicare.gov), and other systems. By selecting the BlueButton icon on a Web portal, all data are downloaded into a standard format that can be integrated into a growing number of apps or viewed through a Web browser. The system is simple, secure, and comprehensive. Blue Button 2.0 from CMS, for example, makes available 4 years of Medicare Part A, B, and D data for 53 million Medicare beneficiaries.

PATIENT-DRIVEN HEALTH REPOSITORIES

Personal health records are becoming a valuable element of any HIE strategy. A decade ago, PHRs were considered curiosities, and most commercial PHR efforts had not met expectations. This may be changing for several reasons. First, a far greater amount of actionable health data is collected from the person or in the home. Examples include the growing number of mobile applications linked to smartwatches and other body sensors. Apple's HealthKit is one of several examples that unite both EHR data and personally collected information. Second, many cloud-based companies, such as Amazon, Google, and Microsoft, are collaborating with consumer products and EHR vendors to create a more expansive view of a PHR.

Many of these data are not easily accessed by commercial EHRs, partly because the volume of data is such that integrating all recorded data into an EHR makes little sense. Most clinicians want summary reports and notification of trends but not every data item; often, these data are managed by third-party consumer firms not traditionally a part of our conventional healthcare delivery system. Not every datum from continuous positive airway pressure (CPAP) device activity monitors, dietary intake recorders, connected scales, and blood glucose–monitoring devices is needed in the EHR. Finally, these comprehensive patient-controlled PHRs may foster more comprehensive pragmatic patient-centered outcomes research efforts.

These and other trends suggest that, for many patients, a far greater collection of data from EHRs, monitoring devices, and other products will be stored in cloud-based repositories under the control of the individual patient or their delegates. Significant analytics will be performed on the individual data to identify trends, relationships, and health events. Access then becomes a matter of authorization, abstraction of key data elements, and incorporation into EHRs or other clinical care systems. Mandl and Kohane suggested that these new systems will "effectively become a health information exchange of one."[4]

INFORMATION BLOCKING

For many years, providers have expressed legitimate concerns about practices employed by EHR vendors, providers, or other parties that prohibited affordable, efficient, and secure HIE. These practices include contracts that exclude data sharing, interface creation, or data transmission fees that make exchange financially prohibitive, implementations that employ nonstandardized exchange approaches, and misleading privacy concerns. Each can conceivably prevent exchange of data to other provider organizations or among providers using EHRs from competing vendors.

The 21st Century Cures Act[5,6] defined *information blocking* as practices employed by providers or vendors to "knowingly and unreasonably interfere with the exchange or use of electronic health information." Information blocking is said to occur if there is interference with the ability to exchange or use information; when the party responsible should know that their activities create such an interference; and when there is no reasonable justification for their practices.[7]

Whether formally or informally defined, information blocking does thwart both direct clinical care and the ability to advance toward a learning healthcare system. This is a serious problem because it prevents timely access to information required to manage patients' health conditions and to coordinate their care.

INTEROPERABILITY

The term *interoperability* is frequently associated with HIE because exchange of information does require assurances that information sent from one source can be acted on by the recipient. But, there are many different levels to interoperability. At the most primitive level, the transmission of a dictated discharge summary in simple text meets a simplistic view of interoperability because a message is sent by one machine to another in a way that can be understood by the recipient. In this case, the document is essentially a digital facsimile with minimal data standards (ASCII [American Standard Code for Information Interchange] data format), and it lacks any other standardized document structure, grammar, or syntax. These documents have been the mainstay of medical practice for decades, and, in many circumstances today, the transmission of vital documents in this manner still meets many acute care needs. A few writers have called this simple transmission "narrative interoperability."[8,9]

The Potential

More effective means of sending and receiving health information suggest potential far greater than that achieved by unstructured text documents. Laboratory tests, if represented in the LOINC (Logical Observation Identifiers Names and Codes) standard, can be transmitted from one system and incorporated into and used by the clinical decision support rules of another. Similarly, standardized medication information can be received by clinical information systems to generate an aggregated medication list. Virtually every clinical and administrative message can be, and often has been, standardized to enhance clinical care.

Standardization and exchange also allow data to be aggregated to support work in public health, population health management, administration, and research. This ability to aggregate data, analyze it, and act on it is vital to policy, improvements to care quality and cost, and ambitious large-scale research projects combining genetic and clinical data, like the National Institutes of Health's (NIH's) All of Us program.

Interoperability Levels

The value of data to clinicians and other stakeholders is very much determined by the extent to which data are standardized. A clinician in an urgent care setting may only need to scan a summary text report, or, with greater degrees of standardization, may want to create an integrated medication list or incorporate external reports into a standardized clinical report. To clarify how exchange of data can be used, three different levels of interoperability have been described[10]:

- *Foundational Interoperability*: This is simply the ability to communicate data through standardized communication protocols. These include the previously described SMTP, HTTP, SOAP, and REST approaches.
- *Structural (Syntactic) Interoperability*: This is the exchange of information according to consensus on data standards, message formats, and document structure. Syntactic interoperability seeks to standardize the structure of a message and both its essential and optional elements. A laboratory report, for example, may require number of elements (e.g., patient name, date, laboratory test, result) arranged in a certain order, and it may allow optional fields (e.g., comments) as well.

- *Semantic Interoperability*: This level seeks to provide context and meaning to messages so that they can be automatically processed by recipient systems. These semantics are communicated by representing data in ways that explicitly relate concepts with one another. An explicit declaration of terms and their relationships is called an *ontology*. Although publications attempt to make clear distinctions between syntactic and semantic interoperability, the boundaries may seem blurred. Historically, message formats of necessity rely on standardized approaches to both syntax and semantics.

CONTENT STANDARDS

Health Level Seven International

Health Level Seven International is an international not-for-profit, standards development organization (SDO) accredited by the American National Standards Institute (ANSI); it defines a comprehensive framework and related standards. They are the source of the most widely used medical data standard in the world (HL7 Version 2), but they are involved in many other standards for exchange, integration, sharing, and retrieval of electronic health information, including specifications for Version 3 messaging, Clinical Document Architecture (CDA), CCD, FHIR, and the Arden Syntax. Many find the HL7 site inscrutable, and those wanting to learn more are advised to consult focused texts and published reviews on this topic.

HL7 Version 2: HL7 Version 2 is the most commonly used transaction standard in healthcare. Each message is represented as a sequence of fields delimited by vertical line (|) characters and ending with a carriage return. Each message begins with a message subject heading (MSH), which in turn defines the syntax of the remainder of the message. Further structure is defined within the message by other specified characters (e.g., ^, &, #). Its inconsistent data models and somewhat arbitrary interpretations (often depending on different use cases) led to a decade-long effort to create HL7 Version 3.

HL7 Version 3: HL7 Version 3 is a more ambitious and complex standard based on object-oriented principles and a standard *reference information model* (RIM). The RIM expresses the data content needed in a specific clinical or administrative context and provides an explicit representation of the semantic and lexical connections that exist between the information carried in the fields of HL7 messages. HL7 Version 3 is expressed in eXtensible Markup Language (XML). Its extreme complexity has discouraged widespread adoption.

Fast Healthcare Interoperability Resources: FHIR was created in part as reaction to the overly complex HL7 Version 3 specification. The emphasis of FHIR is on simple application programming interfaces (APIs) based on concepts commonly used in clinical care (e.g., medication prescription, diagnosis, procedure, growth chart). It relies heavily on common approaches like HTTP, XML, and JavaScript Object Notation (JSON). FHIR is usually associated with the *Substitutable Medical Applications and Reusable Technologies* (SMART) initiative. SMART is an open platform for *substitutable*[11] third-party apps that can be integrated with EHRs and other systems. A *SMART on FHIR system* is a health information technology system that has implemented the SMART on FHIR specification and is capable of running SMART apps. A *SMART on FHIR app* runs against a SMART on a FHIR system, extending its functionality through the use of clinical and contextual data.[12] SMART on FHIR apps have three attributes: a data access layer based on FHIR; a security layer that provides narrowly scoped authorization to specific portions of a patient's record; and a single-sign-on layer.[13] The ease with which SMART on FHIR apps can be developed and integrated into EHRs facilitates more widespread use. The HL7 *Argonaut Project* is a private-sector initiative seeking to rapidly develop FHIR-based API and core data services specifications to enable expanded information sharing for EHRs and other health information technology based on Internet standards and architectural patterns and styles.

National Council of Prescription Drug Programs Script: Like HL7, the *National Council of Prescription Drug Programs* (NCPDP) is an ANSI-accredited SDO that focuses on prescription drug standards. The NCPDP telecommunication standard specifies the structure of pharmacy claims records, and its SCRIPT standards support a range of processes concerned with prescription medications, including e-prescribing and medication history services. The standard for representing medication information in an EHR is *RxNorm*, not SCRIPT. RxNorm, produced by the National Library of Medicine (NLM), supports semantic interoperability by normalizing drug terminologies for generic and branded drugs.

Digital Imaging and Communications in Medicine: The *Digital Imaging and Communications in Medicine* (DICOM) standard is the worldwide standard for storing and transmitting medical images. Every DICOM data object includes multiple metadata elements describing the image and one element for the digital image data itself.

Clinical Document Architecture (CDA): The HL7 CDA is an XML-based markup standard capable of specifying and encoding the structure and semantics of any clinical document. XML is a highly flexible representation that can be parsed by machines and read by the human eye. XML is the basis for many Web-based implementations; hence, its use is becoming widespread in data standards. Because of its extreme flexibility, federal data standards emphasize a more streamlined set of standards called the *Consolidated CDA* (C-CDA). The C-CDA brings together disparate approaches and adopts the CCD's approach of incorporation of rules defining its components through a set of predefined attributes (e.g., title, document number, text name) by means of a *document type definition* (DTD).[14] These attributes can range from highly unstructured data to rigorously structured data elements. C-CDA implementations have harmonized significantly since their federal mandate in 2012; extensive technical support resources are available, and, through "connect-a-thons," vendors have collaborated to harmonize their approaches to a more significant degree.

Integrating the Health Enterprise (IHE): IHE is a collaboration providing a common technical framework to address a wide range of clinical integration needs. Driven by use cases, IHE Profiles describe how standards can be incorporated into workflows in meaningful ways. Each use case leads to one or more Integration Profiles that define the systems involved, the specific standards used, and the details needed to implement the solution. Each profile has been reviewed and tested by industry partners. These profiles are widely used in EHR systems to meet a host of clinical and administrative needs. Examples of profiles include the following:

- *Cross-Enterprise Document Sharing* (XDS): These profiles facilitate the registration, distribution and access across health enterprises of patient EHRs. There are multiple XDS profiles for various specific needs.
- *Cross-Enterprise Document Reliable Interchange* (XDR): This profile is used for point-to-point communication through push notification.
- *Cross-Enterprise Document Media Interchange* (XDM): This profile supports environments with minimal technical capabilities. It is the standard used by the Direct Project.
- *Cross-Community Access for Imaging* (XCA): This profile supports query and retrieval of medical imaging data held by other communities.
- *Patient Demographics Query* (PDQ): This profile is used to retrieve patient demographic information from a shared directory to improve patient matching.
- *Patient Identifier Cross Referencing* (PIX): This profile is used to simplify access of information across multiple care sites through an RLS.

Terminologies and Ontologies

A number of standard terminologies form the backbone for representing medical or administrative concepts. Many times, these terminologies either represent an underlying relationship among concepts or can be incorporated into ontologies that provide more comprehensive mappings. Collectively, these systems constitute components of a terminology service.

Common terminologies include:

International Classification of Diseases, Ninth Revision, Clinical Modification (ICD-9-CM): The ICD-9-CM had been the mainstay of administrative coding for several decades. There are approximately 13,000 ICD-9-CM codes, each three to five characters long. Several good reasons were advanced to abandon ICD-9. First, although the potential number of codes was not exhausted, some segments of ICD-9's structural hierarchy were complete, and related codes had to be assigned to topically unrelated chapters. Second, code-based medical billing required detail beyond the limits of ICD-9. Third, biomedical research based on ICD-9 billing codes alone suffered from serious limitations. Finally, the World Health Organization no longer supported ICD-9, and most of the world had already adopted ICD-10.

The *International Classification of Diseases, Tenth Revision, Clinical Modification* (ICD-10-CM): ICD-10-CM represents encounter diagnoses and a range of other concepts. Developed by the World Health Organization and in use in over 100 countries, *ICD-10* contains over 68,000 billing codes; each is represented in three to seven alphanumeric characters. Like *ICD-9*, *ICD-10* also has procedure codes (*ICD-10-PCS* [Procedure Coding System] codes), but these are employed only for inpatient billing. *ICD-10* has deeper semantic relationships than *ICD-9* and in principle should be more helpful to represent clinical status through claims data. In practice, the system is extraordinarily complex, and its idiosyncratic degree of detail has at times been the butt of humor (e.g., W55.41XA: Bitten by pig, initial encounter; V97.33XD: Sucked into jet engine, subsequent encounter; V00.01XD: Pedestrian on foot injured in collision with roller skater, subsequent encounter). More significantly, the use of *ICD-10* as the federal standard for the United States differs dramatically from its use by other countries; most other countries employing this standard are not as reliant on *ICD-10* for medical billing and payment, and their healthcare payment infrastructure is far less complex. Although the true cost of conversion from *ICD-9* to *ICD-10* is not known, if one includes training, certification, technology, and administrative costs, one can question the cost-benefit of this major policy change. *ICD-10* certainly challenges manual coders because effective coding requires a deep understanding of anatomy, physiology, medical terminology, and disease processes. But, it is a fait accompli.

Current Procedural Terminology (*CPT*): The *CPT* is a medical code set maintained by the American Medical Association. It describes medical, surgical, and diagnostic services from the perspective of services rendered rather than diagnosis. *CPT* is employed by physicians, coders, patients, accreditation organizations, and payers for administrative, financial, and analytical purposes.

LOINC: LOINC identifiers are used to express laboratory results but can be applied to many other settings as well. LOINC encoding is mandated through EHR certification criteria.

RxNorm: RxNorm expresses drug semantics by providing a set of names and relationships based on the drug vocabularies commonly used in pharmacy management and drug interaction software. Different clinical information systems employ different commercial pharmacy management and drug interaction software (e.g., First Databank, Micromedex, Gold Standard Drug Database, Multum). RxNorm provides links between these vocabularies and fosters interoperability between systems employing different vocabularies.

Systematized Nomenclature of Medicine—Clinical Terms (SNOMED CT): SNOMED CT is a set of comprehensive and precise health terminologies used worldwide to foster semantic interoperability. SNOMED CT supports the many federal EHR certification standard requirements, including maintaining a problem list of current and active diagnoses, family history, vital signs, smoking status, and cancer registry information. It also maps from *ICD-9* to *ICD-10*.

Unified Medical Language System (UMLS): The UMLS is a major
ontology resource linking medical vocabularies and standards. It has
three components: a meta-thesaurus containing terms and codes
from *CPT, ICD-10-CM,* LOINC, MeSH (Medical Subject Headings),
RxNorm, SNOMED CT, and other vocabularies; a semantic network
composed of semantic types and relations; and a set of natural language
processing tools.

KEY POINTS

- Effective coordination of care requires sharing of information among
  clinicians, patients, family members, and other parties providing or paying
  for care.
- Health information exchange (HIE) is a general term used to describe
  such sharing. It is usually a verb and a process, not a noun describing a
  specific organizational form.
- There are many different ways to transmit and receive information
  securely; choices depend on technologies and clinical workflows.
- As is the case with all personal information, methods must be employed to
  ensure that privacy principles and preferences are maintained.

Population Health Management

MARK E. FRISSE AND KARL E. MISULIS ■

OVERVIEW

A mastery of population health management is a challenging, but critical, clinical informatics skill. The challenges and opportunities are many:

- Data standards and terminologies are inconsistent.
- Many different disciplines make use of population health data for different purposes.
- Sources of clinical, social, and environmental data are proliferating.
- New incentive structures are being developed to align clinician and patient behaviors.
- New collaboration technologies are continually changing expectations.
- Proliferating quality and payment metrics often require far more data than what is necessary for routine clinical care.

As a term, *population health management* often overlaps with the terms *population health* and *public health*. The *health* component also varies. Recognizing that health and disease are a continuum, some have dispensed with the term *disease management* or restricted its use to specific chronic conditions. Recognizing the same health-disease continuum, some health plans have favored the term *population management*. An examination of search term frequencies demonstrated these changing trends. Until recently, *population health management* and *population health* have been used differently. Use of the term *population health* has been constant for many years and is used more frequently in Canada and Australia than the United States. The inclusion of *management* is primarily an American phenomenon emerging in parallel with a growing emphasis on new payment structures (e.g., capitated care) and new types of delivery organizations (e.g., managed care organizations [MCOs]).

Effective population health management requires an understanding of the many reasons why different professionals seek population health data. Public health professionals employed by municipalities, states, and the federal government monitor, study, and report community, regional, or national health outcomes in order to create more effective public policy. Examples include infectious disease reporting, immunization data resource creation, and syndromic surveillance. Traditionally, the data available to these professionals are limited by legislative mandates requiring submission by clinicians and other groups. The data are therefore sometimes incomplete, and their receipt can be a significant time after an event has taken place.

Payers are focused on the health and cost-effective care of their members. Rather than directly seeking the long-term health of communities, payers of necessity must focus on the clinical and financial outcomes realized through the health or illness of those covered in their health plans. Because they are financially responsible, health plans ultimately receive the data for every billed patient care event no matter who the provider is. Providers have a financial incentive to submit data in a timely manner, but often all data are not clean and resolved for many weeks.

Managed care organizations and other integrated delivery practices are focused on the well-being of the patients, and cost and quality of their healthcare determines payment. With a few exceptions, these MCOs are paid for patient care by many different health plans and payment approaches. Although MCOs may be financially responsible for outcomes, their immediate picture of patient data is strikingly incomplete. Their only immediate access to information is through the clinical data in their electronic records, clinical data obtained from other providers, or claims submitted to (but not yet adjudicated by) payers. Although a trend to real-time claims access is growing, most generally adjudicated claim files are typically only updated monthly, quarterly, or annually.

Clinical providers, on the front line of care and critical to managing the health of individuals and populations, seldom have timely access to all of the data they believe they need for care. Even if they share a common electronic health record (EHR) with a large system, they often find that their patients seek care across many institutions employing different technologies that make clinical data sharing challenging. Also, because of pricing and financial concerns, administrative claims data sharing is almost impossible. Except for clinicians in unique payer-provider alliances or those treating populations with draconian penalties for out-of-network care, the notion of a closed network borders on mythology.

Fortunately, our collective ability to measure, analyze, and manage the care of individuals and populations is changing with the availability of more real-time data, newer means of identifying critical care needs, and better methods for technology-enabled patient communication and care team coordination. Most of these changes are indirectly the result of a broader societal alignment toward reducing healthcare expenditures. As traditional fee-for-service wanes and patients are paying for a greater proportion of their care, there emerges a greater societal collective effort to lower costs; incentives are becoming more aligned. Fortunately, technology costs are also dropping as data standards truly become standardized and as vendors also realize that information blocking is no longer a viable strategy. Finally, patients, families, and care teams all have at their disposal a range of professional and consumer technologies to communicate, influence behavior, measure task performance, and report on health status.

This convergence is becoming apparent in every sector—even in public/population health. The Air Louisville project, for example, demonstrates the potential of integrating real-time data sources and empowering patients, clinicians, payers, and government to pursue better collective improvements to health. Air Louisville is seeking new solutions to asthma care through a collaboration with the Louisville metro government, a nonprofit institute, and a technology company providing asthma medication inhalers with GPS (Global Positioning System) capabilities. In the spirit of a public health initiative, early investigations showed that crowdsourced real-world data on inhaler use, when combined with environmental data, could both suggest better urban environmental policies and be used as the basis for a community-wide asthma hazard notification system.[1]

THE CLINICIAN PERSPECTIVE

The primary goal of population health management technologies is to improve the delivery of important and actionable data as part of care delivery. All too often, these few and fairly straightforward task-focused items are obscured by a cascade of data items that may drive reimbursement but often come at the expense of efficient and effective care. Although clinicians need to evaluate their performance relative to peers, guidelines, and standards, their ongoing primary concern should be focused on the patient before them. The generation of population-level quality metrics are a byproduct of care; their collection should never intrude on care.

CLINICAL DASHBOARDS

Dashboards are a popular method to manage populations and Web-based systems integrating data from disparate sources. Many care managers and other professionals rely on these systems both to improve care of individuals and to report on organizational performance in the care of populations. Ideally, these systems allow health care professionals to

- view composite and individual measures for population and individual patients;
- summarize care for all patients as well as for common conditions like cardiovascular disease (cholesterol, blood pressure, oral antiplatelet therapy), diabetes (hemoglobin A1C, foot examinations), and mental health

- apply filters to select specific populations based on provider, service location, medical condition, age, plan coverage, or other factors; ; and
- characterize specific risk factors (e.g., smoking, alcohol, opioids).

Although attractive in principle, dashboards do not realize their potential unless they can be integrated into provider EHRs. The primary challenge for any dashboard is to bring to the primary care provider's attention only critical and actionable items in the course of a clinical encounter. An EHR-enabled quick overview of clinical status, essential screenings, risk factors, and related items is often a part of the more comprehensive overview that includes the problem list, medication history, allergies, and recent medical events. Other data collection tasks (for quality reporting and payment) and secondary care management activities may better be performed by support staff who use the same EHR or more comprehensive dashboard or care coordination systems. All too often, systems designers fail to differentiate what is essential for immediate care from what is arguably more important for reporting of care quality and care intensity.

QUALITY REPORTING

Clinical practitioners are often burdened with care interruptions required only to simplify, for others, reporting of quality metrics. Quality metric reporting is critical; the primary concern is how to report data accurately at the lowest possible cost to providers and to their organizations. This is part of a broader national concern over the sincere but collectively mindless proliferation of additional metrics whose rationale has no evidentiary base. Providers are trapped in a *measurement-industrial complex* that often revises metrics before early versions have been incorporated into training, workflows, and technologies. Furthermore, although regulators demand reporting of only a subset of the many metrics available, technologists and informaticians must be able to accommodate whatever choices are made from a long metric menu. A policy offering an "or" specifying only a subset of metrics becomes an "and" to the persons who must design and implement them into care systems that accommodate all choices.

Quality and performance metrics are usually placed in one of the following categories:

- Quality measures
- Performance improvement measures
- Technical measures (e.g., interoperability)
- Financial measures

Within each category are many candidates that require varying degrees of manual reporting and intervention. Each metric can be reported through a number of means. Submissions can be made directly through electronic records, via federally qualified data registries, or through a Web interface. Other metrics originate from consumer surveys and adjudicated claims. Understanding the best fit for a practice or organization requires a deep understanding of the true costs and benefits of each incentive program, each approach to reporting, and the true total organizational cost of measuring and reporting. The temptation is often to hurl significant financial and personnel resources at these problems before the appropriate degree of critical thinking and planning has been done at the organizational level. As always, focusing on the fundamentals is an important practice.

KEY POINTS

Clinical informaticians should address the following issues when thinking though an approach to population health management:

- Most comprehensive population health management systems cost more than expected, disrupt workflows of providers, and fail to realize major economic benefit. All technology and payment trends suggest a bright future for more comprehensive and integrated population health management, but the path from the present to a bright future is costly and usually disappointing.
- Seek a quick win; do not "boil the ocean." Identify one intervention for which a better approach to collection, analysis, and intervention can be clearly demonstrated and be perceived of value to practitioners and every other involved party.
- Be mindful of the real value of data and ensure the data required to intervene are available or can be made available at low cost in terms of both organizational investment and clinician time. If presented with a choice between two different immediate, popular, and actionable courses, begin with the approach that is simplest.
- Many of the most important and actionable immediate population health management initiatives can be addressed with a fairly basic set of claims and clinical data.
- Emphasize the quality of data that will populate data warehouses; do not seek to automate more complex data collection processes until one is certain of success.
- Plan for a more comprehensive solution and a more robust data infrastructure, but do not invest excessively in technologies and disruptive workflow changes before all stakeholders are invested in the effort and until one is certain that others have achieved realized gains from similar approaches.
- Follow the industry. EHR systems are evolving to support greater degrees of population health management, and many vendors are promoting more ambitious data warehouses within their own platforms. Leveraging comprehensive EHR systems may be a wise initial step.

- At the same time, do not think in silos or always try to go it alone. Be mindful that major efforts to forge new partnerships between payers and providers will lead to new approaches to data sharing and data use. Providers, MCOs, payers, public health officials, and quality reporting organizations all have different needs, but over time, a robust data warehouse and a common approach to data management and stewardship will simplify the tasks.

Researchers

MARK E. FRISSE AND KARL E. MISULIS ∎

OVERVIEW

Every healthcare professional can incorporate the spirit of research into his or her professional life. Ideally, every clinical or administrative action should be informed by the best knowledge and evidence, and every outcome or experience should contribute to a richer evidentiary base and a deeper collective wisdom. Clinical informatics professionals play a vital role in ensuring that their colleagues can realize these ambitious aspirations. This chapter does not address how to do research, what questions to ask, what technologies to use, or what methods to apply. The focus is on ensuring that those asking questions have availability to the right data in representations that allow for the pursuit of answers.

EVERYONE IS A RESEARCHER

Researchers are people who seek evidence to establish facts and to reach new conclusions. Research, and researchers, can be informal or formal. In an informal sense, the simple observation and transmission of new information that leads to a deeper understanding and a local improvement in care is performing research. Under this broad and informal umbrella, individuals who encounter workflow barriers or suggest even modest improvements to clinical decision support are, at the least, informal researchers. Under ideal circumstances, every clinician and support staff whose care is informed by the best possible evidence and whose system contributes new data to improve understanding of healthcare contributes to the research activities and hence plays a critical role as the member of a research team.

An Example Is Illustrative: Often, clinical decision support rules do not perform as expected. In particular, they may cry "wolf" to such a degree that vital messages are drowned out by a barrage of extraneous alerts and notifications. Providers will indeed express their concerns. Sometimes, these concerns are idiosyncratic or minor. At other times, they may reflect fundamental opportunities to improve a clinical system or workflow to produce better performance. Given the many concerns raised by clinicians, clinical informatics leaders must identify which concerns are of the highest priority and warrant a more systematic study.

The Role of Pioneers and Pilot Studies: Ideally, a concern can be addressed by limited quantitative assessments carried out by one or at most a handful of clinicians who are most affected by the potential problem. The evaluation process could begin by simply asking these clinicians to document on paper the times that an event takes place. They could count, for example, how many times a clinical decision support alert fires and document the number of instances when the alert is appropriate or inappropriate. A simple list providing the date, time, patient, alert, and result will allow others to review the system in an effort to understand the clinical context.

WHAT FORMAL RESEARCH CAN DO

Formal research efforts are managed by trained professionals pursuing systematic investigations seeking improvements based on more rigorous data. These systematic processes may be entirely local, or they may extend to include regional, national, or even international collaborations. These activities may not be formal clinical trials suitable for publication. Often, they are more straightforward efforts to improve care at a specific enterprise through analysis. Among the range of activities are the following:

- Improving the quality and effectiveness of local care
- Improving the efficiency of care through more effective integration of technology with clinical and administrative workflows and processes
- Contributing data to one or more research consortia
- Participating in formal clinical trials
- Conducting population health research designed to inform policymaking

WHAT TO LOOK FOR FROM DATA SETS

Research efforts relying on data warehouses can be constrained by many factors. First, one may lack the "big picture" necessary to study a specific problem. If patients seek care at many facilities in addition to the system managed by the researcher, unless these data are somehow incorporated into the database, the picture is grossly incomplete; in these circumstances, collaboration among providers and payers can be fruitful.

Second, even a comprehensive data resource does not contain all of the data elements necessary to address most pressing research questions. This is often the case if one seeks to ask questions about events that take place in the home or community. Social determinants of care, for example, are vital for readmissions, but even some of the most critical elements such as housing status, solitude, and economic means are lacking. Similarly, more sophisticated means of measuring nonadherence to medication therapy may increase predictive value, but unless one can couple data with meaningful action, the effort is futile. Clinical informatics professionals should aggressively weigh in on studies lacking data required for action. More sophisticated analyses of the "wrong" data will not improve the outcome.

Third, the data fields may be present in the schema, but the fields often are not populated by complete entries from individual local systems. One can think of a data warehouse for clinical research as a repository for the impressions of hundreds or thousands of different healthcare professionals, each with different interpretations of events and the ways they record events. Many clinicians, each with their own style and time constraints, often have insufficient incentive to record data with the scope and granularity required for secondary research.

Fourth, the contents of a data warehouse are the product of a complex representation and transformation *pipeline* where many different and sometimes arbitrary decisions can alter the interpretation of data. Logical Observation Identifiers Names and Codes (LOINC) encoding of laboratory tests serves as an example. Studying 49 million laboratory results from across five hospitals, investigators found that results were represented by more than 4000 laboratory observation codes. Investigators found that 80% of the total tests from all institutions could be accounted for by only 80 codes, and that 99% could be accounted for by only 784 codes.[1] What is concealed beneath the study is the enormous efforts a centralized entity took to map local codes to standardized LOINC. One institution may use the nonstandard term *CBC2* to represent the complete cell blood count with differential panel and *WBC* for a single element in a differential count. Others may have even more arbitrary codes. Each institution, laboratory, laboratory vendor, or electronic health record (EHR) vendor must take these codes and, to meet federal EHR certification requirements, map these to LOINC. The codes of LOINC for white cells include "leukocytes in blood" (26464-8), "leukocytes in blood by automated count (6690-2)," and "leukocytes in blood by manual count (804-5)." Similarly, the CBC term can be mapped to at least eight different codes. Where diagnoses and problems are concerned, the *International Classification of Diseases, Tenth Revision (ICD-10)* and SNOMED CT (Systematized Nomenclature of Medicine—Clinical Terms) also allow for many different valid representations. Accordingly, even if data are encoded by standards, analyses should include the appropriate degree of groupers to associate common terms that clearly relate to the same type of data under study but that might be coded with an excessive degree of granularity.

Finally, circumstances often necessitate accurate linking of an individual's clinical data across multiple sites. Any linking algorithm is imperfect. Bayes theorem applies. One must be aware of the linkage methods used and, depending on the study, ensure that the degree of both inappropriately linked records and records that should be linked is within expected bounds.

WHAT TO DO WITH DATA SETS

Clinical informatics professionals must play a role ensuring that data warehouses are secure and that personal and organizational health information are used only as laws, regulations, and policies allow. Technical, policy, and procedural safeguards must be in place and stress-tested to ensure they perform according to expectations. Policies, for example, cannot just be recorded on paper; policy principles and practices should be embedded into organizational culture. Transaction logs cannot simply be created; their performance should be assessed periodically to ensure they can be used when questions are raised about data access and use. Often, informatics professionals must play an important educational role to ensure that personal health information and other confidential materials are not transmitted to unsafe settings or used in unanticipated ways. Clinical informatics professionals should ensure that the data used by researchers can be trusted to answer the questions they ask and that lessons learned be applied whenever possible.

KEY POINTS

- Research can be informal or formal.
- No matter what the scope and depth of a research endeavor, one must ask the right questions, have the right analytics expertise, and, most important, have availability of the data necessary to create actionable change.
- One must have access to all required data sources.
- Data resources must include the right data elements.
- The data elements, often arising from many sources, must be complete, coherent, and standardized.
- One must understand the data representation and transformation methods employed from collection through analysis to use.
- Patient data from multiple sources must be linked accurately.
- Effective data use requires policies, procedures, and technologies necessary to retain confidentiality and ensure public trust.

Part V

Future Trends

On the Horizon

KARL E. MISULIS AND MARK E. FRISSE ■

OVERVIEW

Healthcare faces an uncertain future. Demographic trends, financial pressures, and rapidly changing technologies will lead to new promise and peril. New approaches may foster dramatic changes in how care can be personalized and supported across a continuum. At the same time, proliferating data sources place new pressures on those responsible for integrating data for care and for those who are entrusted with the privacy and security of healthcare information. But adapting people, processes, and technologies to change generally takes years and not months. Accordingly, clinical informatics professionals must do more than speculate on their future actions, they must take actions **today** in anticipation of the tomorrows ahead. For hospital and clinic-based professionals, one central question will be the extent to which their current EHR technology will evolve with sufficient rapidity and to what extent a different or supplemental data infrastructure will be required.

Why are we interested in the future? The future is our roadmap into the unknown. Rather than blindly allowing events to unfold, we should have a live-updated map of the future, increasingly less precise with distant time. If we leverage our efforts and resources, we will write the future.

NEAR FUTURE

Among the events that we want for the near future are:

- use of large data sets to answer clinical questions;
- transition from a focus of Informatics on implementation to a focus on optimization;
- more connections and interoperability to communicate with additional systems;
- more effective processes and systems to impact outcomes and costs;
- improved access of disparate patient information sources through a single interface; and
- improved use of data for improvement and for development of the learning health system.

Large Data Sets: Large data sets reside not only in increasingly large healthcare systems, but also in repositories of health information exchanges, payers, consumer devices, and government entities. These data sets not only allow for greater data access across the continuum of care but also allow for generation of new knowledge that would be undiscoverable with smaller data sets. We have already seen some of this with data sets of the Department of Veterans Affairs, contracted research databases, and even corporate data sets. In 2004, the results of an analysis of patients with migraine and stroke showed one expected result, that patients with migraine were 67% more likely to suffer stroke than those without migraine. Further analysis of this data set showed that patients who received triptans for their migraine were no more likely to have stroke than those who did not, whereas patient who received ergots for migraine did have a higher incidence of stroke, by 49%. This study was performed on records of more than 130,000 patients from United Healthcare.[1] A study of this size and power would not have been possible by a single clinic or university. The power of large data sets cannot be underestimated.

Transition to Optimization: We look forward to the transition of informatics efforts from less implementation to more optimization. Vendors have focused heavily on function of the EHRs and only recently have spent more effort and resources on improving usability. While some of us embraced the digital transformation of medicine, most clinicians and support personnel just want to accomplish their jobs. Any change is disruptive. Every EHR transition at least temporarily reduces productivity of a healthcare system.[2] Some enterprises will change systems, often in response to acquisition or other forms of consolidation, but these changes should slow down so we can then focus on the best use of whichever tools we have selected for our healthcare enterprises.

Connections: We expect more connections. Some of these connections will be between EHRs and between EHRs and information systems for payers and patients. Improved interoperability should be demanded by the public as well as the healthcare community. Any efforts to use protectionism or price to suppress the free flow of information should be firmly denounced. There should be more standardization of interfaces. Part of this should be greater standardization of interfaces of medical devices, but part would be more robust performance of interface engines. Similarly, there will be more connected devices, particularly patient-monitoring equipment for a broad range of purposes, including monitoring of glucose, blood pressure, oxygen, activity, weight, and other metrics. Devices can now monitor compliance with medications, and this technology should expand.

Focus on Outcomes and Costs: Many clinical informatics professionals' responsibilities have been focused primarily on EHR implementation and adoption. Increasingly the focus must transition to effective use of data to impact clinical outcomes and costs. We have spent billions of dollars on the technical hardware and software and human resources to implement our information systems. These investments will only be returned if care becomes more efficient, more patient-centered, of higher quality, and at lower cost.

Patient Access: Patients' access to information should be easier. Presently, patients often have multiple portals, one for each clinic and hospital, and each of these has limited and differing functionality. No technological breakthroughs are required for portal access to be consolidated, and this will allow for additional functionality. Ideally, patients will be able to view results from multiple clinics and healthcare systems using a single user interface. Messages should be able to be transferred between the patients and all participants in their care from within this user interface. Scheduling of appointments and procedures should be available across these enterprises from the single portal interface. Patients should be able to control data flow between enterprises and clinicians from their portal.

Learning Health System: The learning health system will need to be expanded and refined so that it is no longer a cutting-edge concept but rather the status quo.

FAR FUTURE

Among the advancements anticipated further into the future could be

- centralized data access replacing individual database access;
- improved translation of knowledge from bench to bedside;
- delivery of knowledge always in the right format to the right people at the right time; and
- full implementation of the learning health system.

Centralized data access could be manifest by clinicians having all data they are authorized to see available in one display. If data have to be searched for in multiple locations, some busy clinicians will not make the effort; any impediment to data availability will result in care being given with an incomplete data set. It is hoped the concept of each clinic and hospital having an insular database will fade. While enterprise data may be stored locally or remotely in specific locales, this separation should be invisible to the clinician who needs clinical data from multiple enterprises.

Translation of medical research from bench to bedside is a pivotal role of the medical research community. The role of clinical informatics is to facilitate not only the translation, but the deployment of learned data to healthcare facilities. We have an uneven consensus in healthcare with many facilities and providers being slow to adopt new proven protocols or methodologies. If we fully implemented the informatics in knowledge management, this would be less likely.

The mission of the national intelligence community is to *get the right information to the right people at the right time*. This needs to be the mission of clinical information systems. And, the data needs to be delivered in the right format, so that the data can be seen easily and up front and integrated within the workflow of the clinician.

All of these elements are woven into the *learning health system*. With available data and analytics, we should be able to discover and refine new avenues of healthcare delivery, dispensing with the obsolete or inefficient.

THREATS

- Abandonment of government efforts to coordinate healthcare informatics.
- Demise of support for the uninsured, which will jeopardize informatics advances for all but the wealthiest and most selective healthcare systems.
- Loss of quality-based incentives for providers and systems.
- Resistance to unique identifiers.
- Security threats with broad multisystem targets.

Governmental Involvement in Developing Informatics: We have made progress in expansion of clinical informatics largely because of government policy in incentives and regulation, as detailed in Chapter 5. However, a backlash has developed concerning intrusion of government in the practice of medicine and in society in general. If the incentives change so that the balance is in favor of protectionism and isolationism, then much of the data sharing we anticipate will not occur. Even now, those of us involved in data sharing across a clinically integrated network have healthcare enterprises that are more than happy to view the data from other enterprises, but do not share their data with others in the network. This lack of data sharing places the health and lives of our and their patients at risk. If we believed our claim that our principal focus is on the patient, there would be no hesitation to share data.

Uninsured: In the United States, legislation had resulted in a reduction in the uninsured population, with the claimed goal of providing healthcare coverage for all. We have backtracked substantially on this effort. Our politicians forget that almost all patients will receive the care, just that those without healthcare insurance will mainly receive emergency and late-stage disease interventions and not take advantage of the much cheaper and more effective preventive care. Also, we physicians have been rightfully unwilling to allow patients to die without care, so many of our hospitals have proportions of uninsured that are unsustainable financially. Meanwhile, many hospitals dump uninsured patients on public and university hospitals. As one hospital physician said at a party: "If a patient has no insurance, they are too tough a case for me." Informatics requires significant resource investment in equipment, personnel, and engagement by users and administrators. If the monies to poorer healthcare systems disappear, so will informatics programs; these healthcare systems will have to spend their precious resources in the operating room, emergency room, and intensive care units and not on information systems.

Quality-Based Incentives: Alternative payment models have been rolled out and might be rolled back. The impetus was to pay for quality rather than volume. Realistically, we need to have volume as a significant component of compensation so there is incentive to see more than a minimum number of patients. However, the incentives should also be designed so that a significant component of provider reimbursement is based on quality and efficiency of care. If we backtrack on quality-based reimbursement, we will return to the days of more unnecessary procedures. Informatics and analytics are the backbones of quality-based incentives. These could become obsolete.

Unique Identifiers: Unique identifiers are used in many countries for healthcare. There has been pushback by a vocal and it is hoped small contingent of the US population because of concerns over privacy and identity theft. However, the absence of unique identifiers is a patient care quality and safety issue, in addition to a large administrative burden. Many computer algorithms and humans are involved in patient matching, and with unique identifiers, much of this could be obviated. Lack of these identifiers will continue to result in difficulty with patient matching in healthcare systems and clinically integrated networks.

Security Threats: Security threats are likely to become more aggressive and more sophisticated. We will need better centralization and standardization of threat identification and mitigation. Healthcare systems do not have the personnel and resources to give the kind of protection that will be needed for advanced attacks. Data connections between healthcare systems do produce a wider target for cyberattacks, but, they also allow for a level of security that small systems could not provide. We must ensure that we have downtime plans in the event of a disabling attack. Such an attack would historically be the product of a small group of nefarious but gifted computer specialists. The next generation of attacks may be a component of national cyberwar, with nations using these capabilities to gain political and economic advantage.

KEY POINTS

- The future of clinical informatics is likely to produce larger data sets due to enterprise consolidation and integration.
- More connections between health information systems and between systems and payers is expected, as there is a common interest in streamlining administrative processes.
- We should increase our focus on outcomes and costs for the sake of the patients and of the national budget.
- We should leverage our EHRs and knowledge systems to make every health information system a learning health system.
- Security threats will become more sophisticated. We must ensure that each of our systems have state-of-the-art defense.

Staying Current

KARL E. MISULIS AND MARK E. FRISSE ■

GENERAL APPROACH

The approach to keeping current depends on the stage of one's education, stage of career, and anticipated career trajectory. These issues are decided on the basis of interests and what skills and credentials will be needed.

We presume that those entering the field of clinical informatics come from a spectrum of backgrounds. Most will have a clinical background in medicine, nursing, pharmacy, or other medical field. Others will come from technical backgrounds, applying their skills to healthcare.

Opportunities for education include degree programs, fellowships, and certificate programs. We consider avenues to achieve each of these.

FORMAL EDUCATION

Few entering medical students know what clinical informatics is, let alone have it as a career goal. But, for the few who have developed an interest through either primary or secondary exposure, combined MD and PhD programs should be considered. There is value to learning clinical informatics in parallel with basic and clinical science. In addition, many MD, PhD programs have financial support, lessening the financial burden of medical school.

Interest in informatics often develops during residency, when the benefits of decision support are evident, and the power of analytics is appreciated. For these individuals, informatics training during graduate medical education (GME) often saves a bit of time because GME and informatics training can overlap.

The PhD programs in biomedical or clinical informatics are of most use for those who anticipate roles in academics or high-level data science. We expect that a PhD degree will be an almost required academic credential, especially for top-tier departments, even for those with MD degrees. The informational content and learned skills in research and project management obtained in graduate school offer a background that is hard to obtain with experience alone.

Master's programs are useful especially for physicians, nurses, pharmacists, and technical professionals who plan to be operational informatics practitioners, working for healthcare systems or industry. The master's programs complement the clinical training experience, giving the practitioner a combined clinical medicine and clinical informatics knowledge base that is difficult to reproduce without clinical education. PhD researchers and data scientists are essential members of the clinical informatics team, but those who expect to be effective chief medical informatics officer (CMIOs), chief nursing informatics officers (CNIOs), or similar need clinical credentials.

Nondegree programs, including some fellowships, are valuable for clinicians who expect to make clinical informatics a significant part of their career but do not necessarily aspire to be academics or data scientists. Nondegree students typically have other terminal credentials, such as MD, DO, or DNP, and are not necessarily looking for more initials after their name but need to learn the content.

As of the time of this writing, board certification in clinical informatics could be obtained by physicians who had obtained their informatics training purely by practice experience, growing to be CMIOs or industry equivalents. This opportunity will and should expire. The value of formal informatics training to the practice of applied clinical informatics cannot be overstated. For nonphysicians, there are excellent certification programs from societies that have a focus on health information and informatics. Similar programs exist or are emerging in other clinical disciplines as well.

MEDIA

Most media relevant to clinical informatics are either electronic or paper print products. Texts are best suited to introduce the reader to the field, as with this book, or to provide focus on a specific area, such as analytics or decision support. When searching for media, one is advised to consult literature from computer science, clinical care, policy, finance, and related disciplines.

Periodicals are an essential resource for clinical informatics professionals. Among the most popular is the *Journal of the American Medical Informatics Association* (JAMIA), which has both research and practical applied informatics information. There are many more, and a Wikipedia page is devoted to this topic.[1]

In general, periodicals are a good resource for tightly focused information, although topical reviews are published in some informatics journals. We recommend looking through the tables of contents of informatics journals and selecting high-impact or high-interest articles for further consumption. Of course, original research articles are unlikely to change practice without at least some additional supporting data.

The Office of the National Coordinator for Health Information Technology (ONC) has developed an extensive set of instructional materials that provide an introduction to most of the important arenas of clinical informatics.[2] While this is not a substitute for other educational opportunities discussed here, it is a good introduction. These materials are a combination of electronic print media, slides, and narrated slide shows. These are free to download.

CONFERENCES

Societies

There are multiple societies, but among the most prominent are

- AMIA—American Medical Informatics Association
- AHIMA—American Health Information Management Association
- HIMSS—Healthcare Information and Management Systems Society

Most society meetings offer minicourses in addition to platform presentations, and many offer poster presentations. The minicourses are particularly valuable for assistance with local timely issues, such as installation of a new application or optimization. Poster presentations are particularly useful because of the opportunity to talk with presenters for questions and for making future networking contacts.

Vendors

Vendor conferences are particularly valuable for addressing issues with the vendor applications or interfaces. Knowledge leaders from the vendors are usually at these meetings. They can be much more helpful than salespeople at addressing strengths, limitations, and troubleshooting of issues.

Vendor conferences often have minicourses regarding specific applications, and these are valuable. Among the programs we have found helpful are physician architect and analytics courses.

Shopping for applications at a vendor convention can be problematic because of the lack of comparison shopping. However, if users of the applications are present, we can usually get straightforward information about the product.

Workshops and Minicourses

Many universities have workshops and minicourses in addition to their formal degree programs and fellowships. Some of the offerings that we have noted include the following:

- Programming of a specific language
- Analytics
- Decision support methods
- Best practices for a specific condition or specialty

Short courses should be of interest to informatics professionals and should include those related to

- communication skills;
- presentation skills;
- influencing others;
- negotiation skills; and
- crisis management skills.

These learning opportunities broaden perspectives, challenge conventional thinking, and complement on-the-job experience.

PROFESSIONAL NETWORKS

Professional networking with other informatics professionals and with those in related fields is essential. Among the most important reasons for this networking are the following:

- Consultation for determining informatics strategy
- Consultation for addressing shared problems
- Advice on developing new skills
- Exposure to new career opportunities

Many institutions share common applied clinical informatics challenges. Although we commonly discuss these challenges with others sharing similar software solutions, much is to be gained by understanding how professionals employing different systems have dealt with the issues. Each vendor and each approach has strengths and weaknesses. One can learn from others.

Networking is also essential to address any dearth of expertise in some areas of practice. Few communities have all of the expertise required and collaborations are often essential.

The careers of clinical informaticists evolve over time; most professionals will hold several positions during their career. Connections made with others help explore when and how to make career transitions.

Conscious effort must be applied to develop and maintain professional networks. Many can be fostered through some of the following avenues:

- Professional conferences regarding informatics or our medical specialty
- Vendor events, including conferences and courses
- Meetings within clinically integrated networks and health information exchanges
- Local, regional, and national committees

We recommend maintaining contact with individuals at all levels of the healthcare system. We recommend having some reason to touch base occasionally to foster the relationships and to focus conversation on areas of common interest or need.

EXPERIENCE

Many practicing clinical informatics professionals were trained on the job. Some clinicians without formal informatics training had prior training in computers, electronics, or research and used that background as a foundation for exploring their roles in applied clinical informatics. While we advocate strongly for a formal educational program, we also recognize that there is great value to operational experience. This value applies also to those who have had formal education in informatics. Clinical informatics is a rapidly evolving field, and without experience, the skills are lost or become obsolete.

We recommend that those who have CMIO as a career target not only obtain additional formal informatics training but also work as an assistant CMIO in a clinically busy environment. There are advantages and disadvantages to both academic and nonacademic facilities, being markedly different environments, but experience in both is valuable. This first part of the career must have substantial real responsibility. At this stage, the assistant CMIO is mentored into the job by the CMIO and other leaders as well as nonclinical colleagues. We learn a lot from our database administrators, interface engineers, pharmacy and radiology informaticists, nurse informaticists, and analysts. The assistant CMIO not only must learn the clinical application of knowledge management, decision support, and user issues but also must learn project management from needs assessment all the way to post-launch assessment and optimization.

An alternative path is to go directly from training to be CMIO at a smaller healthcare facility or perhaps a clinic. This can work, but we do not recommend this path. There is a lot to learn about people, process, and technology even after completing formal training, and all it may take is one unfortunate project outcome to put an early end to an otherwise-promising clinical informatics career.

Corporate experience with a vendor or other industry such as analytics can be a valuable stage of a career. In general, the most effective corporate clinical informatics professionals have had clinical medicine and applied clinical informatics experience. If the corporate informatics professional then does switch into a CMIO position or similar spot, the corporate experience can be a significant advantage, especially in understanding the priorities, interests, and abilities of the vendor. Developing new data analytics skills will be essential.

Last, those with clinical training can be most effective if they are at least somewhat clinically active during their informatics careers. Physician and nurse informatics professionals who are divorced from clinical medicine risk losing experience with using our systems and frankly losing the focus that we all need to have on the patient. An author of two chapters in this book, Dr. Doug Dickey, is a senior executive of a leading EHR vendor yet carves out time to see patients in clinic every week.

No matter what our role is in informatics, in the end, the goal is the same: improve patient care. It is all about the patient. We need to keep up and keep our focus on the patient.

KEY POINTS

- Foundational training depends on the background and interests of the future professional. Clinicians with terminal degrees of MD, DO, MBBS, DNP, PharmD, or similar can benefit from informatics doctorate training, but master's training will likely meet their needs.
- Obtaining a PhD in biomedical informatics provides the background to excel in data science and foundational informatics research. Partnering with clinicians makes for a powerful combination.
- The informatics knowledge base is growing so quickly that we need to make a continuous effort to keep up.
- Corporate work experience can be quite valuable for informatics professionals.
- Networking with individuals at other institutions is extremely valuable. Many problems we encounter in clinical informatics have been encountered elsewhere.

Part VI

Appendices

Case Discussions

KARL E. MISULIS, JEFFREY G. FRIELING, AND MARK E. FRISSE ■

OVERVIEW

These cases studies are written as hypothetical scenarios but are all based on our personal experiences practicing informatics in a variety of healthcare settings. Details have been altered to allow the educational purpose of the case presentations be clearer, and also for anonymization. As with healthcare systems in general, events are more complex than they may seem, and no system or person is perfect. Especially with clinical informatics, there is seldom a single cause to any event.

INSTALLATIONS AND UPGRADES

Management of a mature healthcare information system is challenging enough, but when we are performing new installations and major upgrades on top of the day-to-day duties, there is the potential for further stress to our staff, our budgets, and ourselves. Issues can occur at multiple levels, from project management to technical issues.

Project Management Challenges

Cost Overrun

Cost overruns are common in projects, not isolated only to information systems. In this vignette, we are in the midst of an installation of a new niche application for the gastroenterology laboratory. This will have to interface with our electronic health record (EHR) as well as the equipment in all of our endoscopy laboratories. As a large healthcare system, we have more than one type of endoscope. But the anesthesia system is the same throughout our organization.

During the project, we learn during testing that the images from the endoscopes are not flowing into the new niche gastrointestinal (GI) reporting system. We subsequently learn that the reports are not transferring seamlessly into the EHR for storage and transmission to referring providers.

We need to buy an interface engine to bridge the image translation from one set of endoscopes to the niche system. Specifications had indicated that an interface with one type of scope was part of the basic negotiated build, but the interface with the other is now needed and was not part of the contract. We task an interface engineer with connecting the interface engine and ensuring that the data flows correctly.

The next step is tasking an interface engineer and informatics staff with ensuring that the GI system delivers the reports to the EHR, and that the reports subsequently are delivered to the referring provider via the appropriate method. Referring providers who use our EHR have the report sent to their electronic inbox. Those who receive and view direct messages have the reports sent via Direct. Those without capability of electronic receipt have the report faxed from within the EHR. We have to keep track of which method of communication works for which referring provider.

All of these added needs result in cost overruns, which can be a substantial fraction of the overall budget. To reduce the likelihood of cost overrun, we should try to anticipate as many of the resources needed as possible and consider use cases, scenarios that are likely to be encountered. Also, building a bit of extra funding into the budget can help mitigate some of the financial impact of overruns.

The most common reasons for overruns are unexpected equipment needs and additional people-hours needed for the tasks. Also, because of the three different methods that referring providers use to get reports, we will have to create a system for ensuring that each referral source receives the reports in the format they can consume. Unfortunately, an easy way to circumvent this issue is to fall to the lowest level of technology and fax reports to everyone. Until there is a new standard expected of every healthcare system and provider, this can occur.

Delay in Build and Implementation

We are adding an ambulatory extension to our acute care EHR, which is expected to facilitate continuity of care and especially benefit care transitions. The ambulatory clinics are using a legacy EHR, which is expected to be retired by a specified date.

The system is designed and built in a BUILD domain. Then, the project enters system testing, where the system itself is tested to ensure that it meets agreed-on requirements. This testing goes well. The next phase is integration testing, where the system is tested for data flow between components of the ambulatory environment. There is failure of some of the interfaces between the clinical and business components of the system. Charge capture and submission of clean claims are jeopardized. Additional interface personnel have to be tasked to fix these issues. As is typical with complex builds, there is not one reason for all failures, but rather a host of issues that need to be fixed individually. Integration testing and comprehensive charge testing take 1 month longer than anticipated, pushing back the date of launch. But, the project is back on track.

During the final phase of the build, we discover that the printers used by our legacy system in all of our clinics will not work with the new system; new equipment with enhanced capabilities is required. This not only adds to costs but also delays rollout because the clinics cannot begin to transition to the new system until compatible printers are online. The monies are requested and the orders placed, but the launch is delayed another 2 months.

The downstream effects of these delays are multiple. Not only do the resources cost money, but also we have to continue to pay maintenance fees for the legacy EHR system and continue to task personnel to support the system. By this time, the system is beyond the end-of-life (EOL) date, so if the system crashes, there will be nothing other than local support unless we contract, at additional expense, with a third party for ongoing support. Also, by the time of the printer issue, providers had already built a 25% reduction in clinic load into their schedule. Now, the clinics are scrambling to fill those slots and free slots for when the system will go live.

Delays can be particularly difficult to avoid. In our experience, the most common cause of delays is failures during integration testing. During project planning, we typically allow more time on the Gantt chart for testing than we expect and often schedule an additional phase of testing, which we hope will not be needed. Budgeting for this ahead of time allows for fewer surprises.

Inadequate Physician Adoption

User adoption begins with engagement of future users in the selection and design of the system. This not only ensures that the system will meet the users' needs and expectations, but also gives the users a sense of ownership, making them more engaged in optimizing performance and often generally having a better attitude about the new system than if they were uninvolved.

Our healthcare system acquires a primary care clinic that has been using paper records; they have never had an EHR. After onboarding of the providers and staff of the clinic, we assess the clinic for needs. Among our discoveries are the needs for robust network connections within and outside the building, the need for space redesign for workstations, and the unencouraging mutterings of providers and staff.

We ask two of the providers and select representative staff from billing, scheduling, nursing, medical assistants, and laboratory to assist with the implementation. The only consensus is that they do not want to make the conversion. They arrived in this decade without an EHR and do not want it now. We have no choice but to insist that this transition is an understood requirement for the acquisition. Reluctantly, some of them participate with our staff in the implementation.

Two months later, we go live with our ambulatory EHR, and there is plenty of at-the-elbow support. The office staff are required to use the system. The providers use the system but retain the capability of dictating notes, principally for when they are behind in clinic.

Two months later, our informatics nurses assess the clinic workflow. Almost all providers are dictating every note and are giving verbal orders to nurses. We explain that without directly entered data, the provider is likely to miss metrics and decision support alerts, but this falls on polite but deaf ears. We then explain that unless they meet computerized physician order entry (CPOE) and clinical documentation requirements, they will have lower personal reimbursement for their work, in accordance with healthcare system compensation policy. Our informatics nurses return a few weeks later and observe that nurses are placing orders logged in as the provider. Providers who used to dictate their notes each day now are weeks behind on electronic clinical documentation.

There is no technical solution to this problem. The clinic has had a culture of self-governance, having made it to this year without an EHR, forgoing Meaningful Use incentive payments. Also, there is a culture of the providers being able to press the staff to perform tasks that are unsafe and illegal. This is bad medicine, and administration has to enforce proper behavior and protocols for their new acquisition. This cannot be allowed.

With less severe adoption issues, we advocate a multiprong approach. Engaging the provider in the EHR process is best, but if the provider joins after the EHR implementation is mature, then we require training before starting work. We should require periodic updates in training, and with guidance of medical staff leadership, we have a requirement for particular EHR metrics to maintain clinical privileges and receive compensation. Illegal activity is not permitted and is dealt with swiftly and appropriately.

Peer governance is one key to dealing with the multilayer behavioral issues that this case demonstrates. An office manager can make threats towards noncompliant personnel, but we have had the best success when the physician informatics professionals work with physicians, nurse informaticists work with nurses, and experienced informatics technical staff work with clinic support staff. If a physician is resistant to change, the chief medical informatics officer should intervene. However, at the end of the day, we have to be prepared to release staff, both clinical and nonclinical, and even physicians, for bad behavior or nonparticipation in the team.

EHR Upgrade Issues

SOFTWARE REGRESSION

Our healthcare system EHR is upgrading to a new code level. This is incremental and does not require downtime; rather, a rolling install is used, so at the most, the user will have to logout and login again to hit another server that is already updated.

Shortly after the upgrade, providers report to the help desk that the dosing calculators do not work. Many medications are given based on weight and other parameters, and the type of calculation depends on the medication. Some may be based on lean body mass, others on total mass. Many medications have dosing dependent on renal function, so they are adjusted for creatinine clearance. Clinicians were trained to order the medications, and the calculator would make these calculations, at least they did until this particular morning.

Our staff consults with our EHR vendor, and apparently between the times we purchased the code upgrade and the installation, a patch was released for the calculators. But, because the upgrade had not been installed, there was no prompt to install the patch. Your staff installs the patch, and the calculators are functioning again.

Software regression is where a previous function of the EHR is broken with an installation, upgrade, or patch. These are usually unforeseen, but then can usually be patched, with installation of small bits of code that fix the break.

Users should be aware of the possibility of regression and report suspected events as soon as possible to the help desk. In this case, our clinical staff had to abandon the calculators for the several days required to fix the issue. Pharmacy performed and double-checked doses, performing the calculations, using a system that was integrated with the EHR but not directly a component of it.

CHANGE IN USER INTERFACE

There are phases to adoption of an EHR. Initially, there is some excitement and perhaps a bit of fear about use of a new system. Users can become frustrated trying to find information or accomplish some task. This tends to abate when they have gained experience with the system, with the user improving in efficiency. The user often discovers or is taught additional capabilities of the system. Eventually, a user who spends much time using the system becomes quite facile.

Then, the cognitive neuroscientist working for our EHR vendor comes up with a new user interface that arranges information, data entry fields, and buttons in a more logical and intuitive manor—at least more intuitive for the new user. The previous user now has another phase of searching for buttons and learning the new tree arrangement of menus. This new interface is installed, and the productivity and efficiency of our providers fall, and the voiced frustrations grow.

Significant changes to the user interface must be rare. When a significant redesign is to be rolled out, there must be training for the users almost as if it is a new EHR. The small book *Who Moved My Cheese?* (by S. Johnson. New York, NY: Putnam; 1998) should be in our library.

Replacement of an EHR

Replacement of a functioning EHR can be more disruptive than the first installation. While those who are still using paper may resist conversion to an EHR, those who have even a marginally functioning EHR often resist conversion; they are not interested in what is new but rather in what works.

Determining Need for Replacement

Our clinic has merged with another large clinic. The combined information systems staff is not happy with either EHR. Our clinic EHR is EOL, expected to have support terminated in about a year. The larger clinic uses an EHR that is still viable but is not meeting needs, particularly analytics for quality and population health. Jointly, we decide on a new EHR for the combined clinic enterprise.

What are the factors that affected our decisions? Without question, the EOL EHR had to be replaced. But, one option would have been to extend the instance of the larger clinic to the smaller clinic. As we are moving into population health, the capabilities of the EHR in that arena are limited. A third-party program would have to be installed on top of that EHR. Also, a consideration is the EHR selections of the local hospital. The principal hospital serving the clinics is part of a consortium that can interface some EHRs better than other EHRs.

After submitting requests for information to four vendors, then soliciting requests for proposals from the two vendors who seemed to be able to meet our expectations, we negotiate the best price for the one we conclude is our first choice, an EHR which can accomplish our tasks and interface with the hospital at an affordable price.

As informatics professionals, we have to carefully consider the reports of a system not meeting needs and expectations. We have too often seen users complain that an EHR is incapable of doing X or Y function when it can; they just do not know how to do it. So, in addition to evaluating alternative apps, the conversion to which could be very disruptive, we ensure that we are leveraging the complete functionality of a system already in place.

Issues With Transition

Changing an EHR is traumatic. When changing from paper to electronic EHRs, previous records have to be imported, usually by scanning a certain historical epoch, such as 2 years. When records older than that are required, the paper records will have to be retrieved from secure storage.

In our clinic merger where both clinics were already using EHRs, we agree on a record transition plan. Providers need to see the previous records of their clinic patients. We agree to import the last 2 years of records from both systems into the new EHR. Because these are mainly primary care clinics, the records of all patients are brought in because patients generally have ongoing care with our providers. If these were specialty clinics, perhaps we would only bring in records on an encounter-occurrence basis because long-term follow-up is not as likely.

Efficiency and productivity are adversely affected with launch of the new EHR, because of both the new operational details of the system and the need to look at historical records in a fashion typical for most EHRs, where there are living lists of diagnoses, problems, medications, and events.

Change in an EHR system should be done with careful consideration. There is risk of significant loss of provider efficiency and productivity until use of the new system becomes the new norm.

SYSTEM PERFORMANCE

Unexpected Downtime

Downtime is expected with any EHR. There are methods to reduce downtime, but with major installations and upgrades, some downtime is expected. Sometimes, the downtime can be minimized by cycling servers, so that the user may have to log off and then back on to another server, but in this example, we discuss unexpected downtime.

Our 500-bed regional referral hospital has a mature EHR functioning well and has fairly good adoption by users. The system has been well maintained and configured, and all reasonable measures to reduce downtime have been implemented.

On this day, a new security guard is making rounds through one of the data centers. As is common in this facility, there are red circular buttons that, in conjunction with a radio-frequency identification (RFID) badge, allow for certain secure doors to open electronically. However, the new guard passes his badge over the RFID reader and instead of hitting the circular button next to the door, presses the large square red button on the opposite wall. This kills power to the data center and sounds an alarm.

This data center is primary for the EHR, so users are immediately kicked offline throughout the hospital and in the affiliated clinics. An announcement is made over the public address system and called to the clinics about the EHR failure. At this point, the cause has not been diagnosed. Within minutes, response to the alarm in the data center identifies the power failure, and discussion with the terrified security guard diagnoses the issue.

Users open envelopes taped to the back of the computer monitor that contain downtime instructions. They follow the instructions to login to the downtime servers, which contain 48 hours of read-only data. The users use paper forms, which are printed in the clinical units for notes and orders until power is restored and the EHR servers rebooted. After the EHR has been restored, the paper orders and notes are scanned into the system.

The downtime event is discussed by information systems staff and leadership, and the causes and effects are reported to users as well as to enterprise leadership. A plan is made to change the appearance and labeling of the kill switch.

In this story, based on a real event, downtime was for about 1 hour, which was surprisingly short considering that it would take about 20 minutes for the servers to reboot and for user access to be restored. If the downtime had been longer, then laboratory and radiology reports would be sent to the clinical units by tube or courier.

Downtime information, in this case, was read-only from every workstation, including users' personal devices because the network was not affected. Also, 48 hours of downtime information was stored in a secondary data center. If the network had failed, the computers at the hospital clinical stations have 48 hours of data for patients on that unit only. Personal devices would not have access. Clinics have read-only access to the charts of patients scheduled to be seen that day.

Slow Response Time

It is 2:00 PM on a Tuesday, and users are complaining about slow response time. There is a perceptible lag between the time that a button is clicked and the response. There is a lag in the entry of typed data into fields.

We consult our system engineers, who report that system response time had risen abruptly just minutes prior to the first user complaints to the help desk. Over the subsequent hour, our staff determine that the slow response time was because of a demanding query that a clinical analyst had unleashed on the system in prime time. The query is terminated, and response time is restored.

Slow response times can develop for a wide variety of reasons, including unexpected user load, server failure, or unexpected demands on the system.

Historically, computer programs would terminate when encountering an error. However, termination of an EHR system has tremendous patient safety and care efficiency implications. If a program can do a workaround and continue to accomplish most tasks without terminating, that is preferable. This is *fault tolerance*. Fault-tolerant systems are less likely to crash, but the programming that makes them fault tolerant can make them much slower during a problem phase.

Most searches would not slow the system perceptibly, but some can be so intensive that they can occupy significant resources. Because of this, queries during the day are minimized; rather, they are run after midnight when system load is less. Also, most healthcare systems have enterprise data warehouses (EDWs), which extract key data that is most likely needed for clinical analytics. Search of the EDWs does not affect response time of the clinical system. In full disclosure, this episode occurred some time ago, and modern EHR and database systems should be more tolerant of episodes of high server load.

DATA BREACH

A data breach is a fear for all systems, clinical and nonclinical. Nonclinical information is a target especially for those who plan identity theft. Clinical data are a target for those who might be searching for potential malpractice cases or for curiosity regarding the health and healthcare of someone of interest. Luckily, large data breaches are uncommon. But, the posture of any enterprise is not to wonder *whether* a data breach will occur but rather to wonder *when* it will occur.

Incidental Access

Incidental access is a common occurrence in clinical medicine. An outside hospital wants to transfer a patient to the referral hospital for a higher level of care. As the receiving physician, you search your EHR to see if the patient already has a record. You are given the first and last name and date of birth. Use of the search routine reveals no results. Because the patient is female and the last name might have changed with marital status, you search for the first name and date of birth, leaving the last-name field empty. Three patients are found, all with multiple encounters. To determine which is the correct patient, you open the three charts in order and ultimately identify which one is the patient to be transferred.

Is this is breach? No, it is not according to the breach rule. This states that access of a chart is not a breach when it is "unintentional acquisition, access, or use of protected health information by a workforce member or person acting under the authority of a covered entity or business associate, if such acquisition, access, or use was made in good faith and within the scope of authority."

No notification of the other two patients is needed, and no Department of Health and Human Services (HHS) reporting is needed.

Intentional Breaches

Most healthcare facilities have ongoing security surveillance, searching for unauthorized access. One algorithm includes a search for patterns that suggest inappropriate access. In the course of our data review, we are alerted to a suspicious pattern. The login of a nurse on one of the clinical units indicates someone is reviewing charts of patients seemingly at random. Interspersed with access of the unit patients, the nurse has reviewed charts generally of patients who are in their senior years.

Further investigation and ultimately discussion with the nurse reveals that he had accessed the data of 47 patients and passed the information to a friend, who planned to use the information for identity theft. Police were notified, and the legal process unfolded.

Data breach reporting requirements mandated that we notify the individuals whose data were compromised; we provided a brief statement of what happened, what data were released, the steps they should do to deal with even the early stages of identity theft, and what our enterprise is doing to investigate and prevent further breaches. The notification of the patients has to be within 60 days from detection, although preferably, it should be as soon as the data are available so that measures to protect further data use are limited.

At the end of the year, a description of this breach must be reported to the secretary of HHS, which can be done online. Because the number of affected individuals was less than 500, the report need not be made immediately but rather within 60 days after the end of the calendar year in aggregate with any other breaches. Similarly, no media notification is needed, such as a press release, because the number of individuals affected was less than 500.

KEY POINTS

- Issues and problems will occur in every healthcare information system. Our jobs will never be without surprises, and most of them are not pleasant surprises.

- We should have a structure for dealing with problems; the structure includes
  - rapid assessment and engagement of individuals who can deal with the issue;
  - notification of leadership;
  - notification of users of any disruption in service or functionality; and
  - notification of users when the issue has been solved.
- Subsequently, discussions between information systems staff and leadership should
  - review the case;
  - identify causes;
  - describe the immediate mitigation strategies;
  - describe the fixes; and
  - identify changes to policies, processes, or infrastructure that might prevent further vulnerabilities.
- The focus for any issue is not, *Who is to blame?* but, *What is the solution?*

Self-Assessment

KARL E. MISULIS AND MARK E. FRISSE ■

Question: True/false: The United States spends the most of Organization for Economic Cooperation and Development (OECD) countries but is only at the 50th percentile in health outcomes.

Answer: False. The United States does spend the most of OECD countries on healthcare per capita but is last of this group in health outcomes.

Question: True/false: The healthcare team is composed of both formal healthcare workers and people who give informal care from the community

Answer: True. The extent of the healthcare team we must consider is extensive, involving both formal and informal workers.

Question: True/false: Most hospitals use certified electronic health records (EHRs), but most ambulatory clinics do not.

Answer: False. While penetrance of certified EHRs is greater in hospitals than in clinics, the Centers for Disease Control and Prevention (CDC) estimated that 87% of clinics use EHRs.

Question: Which of the following statements about data, information, and knowledge is true?
A. Data are values.
B. Information is data in a context to be meaningful and actionable.
C. Knowledge is a structured compilation of information to guide decision-making.
D. All are correct.

Answer: D. All are correct. However, the definition of knowledge is somewhat controversial and dependent on the point of view of the individual

Question: Data that are true or false with no other possibilities are termed
A. Discrete
B. Boolean
C. String

Answer: B. Boolean is true or false, with no other possibilities, even null. The datum has to be set to one or the other.

Question: Which would be applications of data arrays?

A. Radiology images
B. Text-based clinical documents
C. Both
D. Neither

Answer: C. Radiology images are stored in arrays of data, representing the pixels of the images. Clinical documents are stored in string arrays.

Question: Which of the following are reasons for data errors?
A. Patient providing incorrect information
B. Entering data into the wrong field
C. Misunderstanding the patient
D. Entry of data into the record of the wrong patient
E. All of the above

Answer: E. All of these are common reasons for data errors and occur commonly in healthcare systems. None are completely avoidable.

Question: True/false: Order sets should be created for specific diagnoses and be based on best practices.

Answer: True. Part of the job of informatics leadership is to coordinate with medical leadership and ensure that order sets are based on best practices and evidence-based medicine.

Question: Routine duties of the chief medical informatics officer (CMIO) include all of the following except

A. Interface with senior leadership on information systems and provider issues
B. Participate in leadership of clinical decision support efforts
C. Build interfaces for new software applications.

Answer: C. the CMIO may participate in design and subsequent testing, but the skills of the CMIO are not best served by writing code except for perhaps guidance to the programming process.

Question: True/false: Informatics staff should largely be generalists, avoiding personnel with focus on specific specialties, to ensure seeing the big picture.

Answer: False. While generalist informatics staff is most common, specialty informatics professionals are needed especially for larger enterprises and specialties with unique information systems needs and challenges.

Question: The Security Rule and Privacy Rule are part of which legislation?

A. HITECH (Health Information Technology for Economic and Clinical Health) Act
B. HIPAA (Health Insurance Portability and Accountability Act)
C. FDASIA (Food and Drug Administration Safety and Innovation Act)

Answer: B. These rules were part of the HIPAA of 1996. Some later modifications were made.

Question: What was the principal informatics implication of FDASIA?

A. Expansion of FDA authority to regulate EHRs and decision support functions
B. Prohibition of cooperation on decision support efforts
C. Release of guidelines for release of deidentified medical information

Answer: A. The FDASIA of 2012 expanded the regulatory responsibility of the FDA, but in practice, it has not so far significantly affected commercial EHRs and collaborative systems.

Question: HIPAA's business associate agreement (BAA) does which of the following?

A. Absolves businesses associated with liability relating to covered entities
B. Promotes joint ventures between vendors and covered entities
C. Establishes a relationship between covered entities and vendors that extends obligations to comply with HIPAA regulations

Answer: C. Familiarity with the BAA is core for informatics professionals. A principal role is to extend HIPAA obligations.

Question: HITECH was part of which legislation?

A. American Recovery and Reinvestment Act
B. HIPAA
C. Patient Protection and Affordable Care Act

Answer: A. HITECH was part of the American Recovery and Reinvestment Act of 2009.

Question: Removal of preexisting illness exclusions was part of which legislation?
A. HIPAA
B. Patient Protection and Affordable Care Act (ACA)
C. Sherman Act

Answer: B. The ACA removed these exclusions, although this provision has been weakened by subsequent legislation.

Question: The Office of the National Coordinator of Health Information Technology (ONC) was mandated by which legislation?
A. ACA
B. HIPAA
C. HITECH

Answer: C. ONC was mandated by the HITECH Act of the American Recovery and Reinvestment Act of 2009. However, the position had been created previously by executive order by President George W Bush.

Question: True/False: The learning health system (LHS) is integral to all certified EHR technologies.

Answer: False. LHS is not an application available from a vendor but rather is a process within a healthcare system to improve care using available technologies, requiring participation of the spectrum from providers to leadership, to analytics, to knowledge sources, to community, and to patients.

Question: Which data are easiest to search for actionable results?
A. Structured
B. Unstructured
C. Both are equally easy to search

Answer: A. Structured data are easiest to search; we can find what we are looking for by a structured query. Unstructured data are particularly difficult to search. If we search for "diabetes," an unstructured data set would return with "diabetes" in the context of "diabetes type 1," "diabetes type 2," and even "no evidence of diabetes."

Question: Match the term with the definition: 1. Data representation 2. Data modeling
A. Turning the data into a format that the computer can understand.
B. Design of the data organization that we use for the enterprise.
C. Neither is appropriate.

Answer: 1. A. All data are ultimately represented by bits. We must turn everything from laboratory values to radiology images into bits. 2. B. We use a model for data organization, starting with conceptual, then logical components.

Question: Which of the following statements regarding database models is correct?
A. Providers using EHRs with hierarchical databases notice much quicker response time.

B. Providers using relational database structures have substantially longer times for patient lookup.

C. A database model is largely transparent to the clinical provider.

Answer: C. Both models are so fast and responsive that the provider would not know by response time which model was being used. In fact, often the clinician is looking at information from more than one database and therefore likely more than one database model.

Question: What is the function of the arithmetic logic unit (ALU) of a computer's central processing unit (CPU)?

A. Determine whether statements are true

B. Perform calculations

C. Keep track of where in the instruction set the CPU is

D. A and B

E. All of the above

Answer: D. Choice A is the logic task and is a computation to determine whether one numeric value is greater, less, or equal to another. Choice B is the arithmetic task and accomplishes not only number crunching but also calculations for even string handling. Choice C is a function of the pointer in a small area of memory in the CPU: keeping note of where the CPU is in the stack of instructions.

Question: Which is the binary sum of 00000001 + 00001001

A. 00001002

B. 00001011

C. 00001010

Answer: C. $1 + 9 = 10$

Question: Which of the following is true about firmware?

A. Software responsible for low-level functions of the computer

B. Hardware on which the software runs

C. Solid-state external media used for data transport

Answer: A. Firmware is software used to perform low-level functions such as interaction of applications with device hardware.

Question: Match the type of memory with usual purpose.

1. RAM (random access memory)
2. ROM (read-only memory)
3. EEPROM (electrically erasable programmable read-only memory)
4. Virtual memory

A. Flash drives for transport of data

B. Media storage reconfigured for use as memory for memory-intensive functions

C. Main memory used for executing programs

D. Nonvolatile memory used for firmware

Answer: 1 = C; 2 = D; 3 = A; 4 = B.

Question: What is pseudocode?
A. Language used to write malware
B. Fake programming language used for design or educational purposes
C. Instructions created by a compiler

Answer: B. Pseudocode looks like a very readable type of computer language, but there is no interpreter or compiler for it.

Question: What is the difference between an interpreter and a compiler?
A. A compiler turns program code into an instruction set for later execution.
B. An interpreter executes lines of code individually without requiring a compiler.
C. All computer languages are amenable to both compiling and interpreting.
D. A and B are true
E. All are true.

Answer: D. Not all languages are amenable to interpreting.

Question: True/false: CMIOs and chief nursing informatics officers (CNIOs) need to have advanced familiarity with Python and C++ at a minimum.

Answer: False. At least in the opinion of the authors, healthcare enterprises are not well served tasking the valuable time of these informatics executives with computer programming.

Question: Match the following devices with their purpose.
1. Hub
2. Router
3. Bridge

A. Connects multiple networks so they can behave as one
B. Connects a number of devices on a network
C. Connection between different networks

Answer: 1 = B; 2 = C; 3 = A.

Question: What is the difference between a wireless access point (WAP) and a repeater?
A. The WAP has a wired connection with the network, whereas the repeater has a wireless connection with the network.
B. The WAP connects wirelessly between both the network and the user devices, whereas the repeater connects one user device to another.
C. The WAP allows user devices to bypass the network and directly communicate with servers, whereas a repeater sends user information to security servers for analytics.

Answer: A. Both serve as connections to a network for wireless devices. The difference is how they, themselves, are connected to the network. The repeater depends on a WAP for signal source.

Question: Which of the following statements are true of server virtualization?

A. Virtual servers may have different operating systems.

B. Virtual servers may have different versions of the same operating system.

C. Virtual servers may have different installed apps.

D. All are true.

E. None are true.

Answer: D. All of these are valid applications of virtual server technology.

Question: Match the use case with the most appropriate device.

1. Picture archiving and communication system (PACS) workstation
2. Rounding device
3. Nursing unit workstation

A. Desktop workstation, thick client
B. Thin client workstation
C. Mobile tablet

Answer: 1 = A; 2 = C; 3 = B.

Question: MUMPS is an example of which database model?

A. Relational

B. Hierarchical

C. Neither

Answer: B. MUMPS is a hierarchical database.

Question: In the ACID database rules, which one refers to the requirement that if part of a transaction fails, the database is left as it was before the change was attempted.

A. Atomicity

B. Consistency

C. Isolation

D. Durability

Answer: A. Atomicity is as described. The change is all or none.

Question: Which of the following is a valid SQL (Structured Query Language) query?

A. INNER JOIN FIrstName, LastName FROM Patients;

B. OUTER JOIN FirstName, LastName FROM Patients;

C. SELECT FIrstName, LastName FROM Patients;

Answer: C. JOIN commands refer to query of data from more than one table, so they would need that reference.

Question: Which would not be a realistically valid reason for having to initiate downtime procedures?

A. Software update

B. Network server crash

C. Failure of communication with remote data center
D. Power failure
E. All are valid reasons

Answer: E. All of these are valid possibilities. Updates would be planned, but the others would be unplanned.

Question: Which of the following statements regarding sensitivity is true?
A. Sensitivity is the true positive rate.
B. Sensitivity is the reciprocal of specificity.
C. Sensitivity for an ideal test would be 0.

Answer: A. Sensitivity is the true positive rate. It is the rate at which people with disease have a positive test.

Question: Which of the following is a correct statement regarding specificity?
A. Specificity is equal to 1 – sensitivity.
B. Specificity is the best indicator of the ability of a test to identify patients with disease.
C. Specificity is the true negative rate.

Answer: C. Specificity is the true negative rate. It is the rate at which patients without disease have a negative test.

Question: Which formula is correct for calculating positive predictive value?
A. True positive / (True positives + False negatives)
B. True positive / (True positives + False positives)
C. (True positives + True negatives) / (False positives + False negatives)

Answer: B. The positive predictive value (PPV) is the ratio of all positives to all who tested positive. This is an indication of what value to place on a positive test. Contrast with sensitivity.

Question: Which of the following is NOT a valid method of calculating the positive likelihood ratio (LR+)?
A. Sensitivity / (1 – Specificity)
B. True-positive rate / False-positive rate
C. False-negative rate / True-negative rate

Answer: C. This selection is the formula for the negative likelihood ratio.

Question: Which is a correct interpretation of relative risk of 2 of exposure to a chemical and development of disease?
A. Patients who were exposed were twice as likely to develop the disease.
B. Patients who were exposed were half as likely to develop the disease.
C. Patients who were exposed were likely to develop the disease twice.

Answer: A. Patients are twice as likely to develop the disease.

Question: A study is done comparing a new drug and an old drug for a particular type of cancer. The odds ratio comparing the two arms of the study is greater than 0 but less than 1. What is the correct interpretation?
A. The new treatment is equally effective as standard therapy.
B. The new treatment is effective but only slightly better than the standard treatment.
C. Outcome with the new treatment is worse than with standard therapy.

Answer: C. The outcome is worse with the new therapy than the standard therapy. An odds ratio of less than 0 cannot occur; it is a ratio and cannot be negative.

Question: Which is the correct method to calculate number needed to treat (NNT)?
A. NNT = Control event rate - Experimental event rate
B. NNT = 1/Absolute risk reduction
C. NNT = 1 - Relative risk

Answer: B. NNT is the reciprocal of the absolute risk reduction. Control event rate – experimental event rate (CER - EER) is the absolute risk reduction; 1 – Relative risk is the relative risk reduction.

Question: What is the correct interpretation of NNT?
A. The size of the study group that would be required to achieve significance, on the basis of pilot study data
B. The number of patients who respond to treatment
C. Expected number of patients who would have to be treated to achieve one positive response to treatment

Answer: C. NNT is the expected number of patients who would have to be treated to achieve one positive response to treatment.

Question: In Bayes theorem, what is the meaning of $P_{A|B}$?
A. Probability that A is true given that B is true
B. Probability that A is true given that B is false
C. Probability that both A and B are both true

Answer: A. $P_{A|B}$ is the probability that A is true given that B is true.

Question: In Bayes theorem, what are P_A and P_B?
A. Probabilities of patients in groups A and B having clinical events
B. Probabilities of condition A and condition B in the population, respectively
C. Probability of patients having both condition A and condition B

Answer: B. Probabilities of condition A and condition B in the population, respectively

Question: Which is the correct formula for Bayes theorem?

A. $P_{A|B} = \dfrac{P_{B|A} \times P_A}{P_B}$

B. $P_A = \dfrac{P_B \times P_A}{P_B}$

C. $P_{A|B} = \dfrac{P_{A|B} \times P_B}{P_A}$

Answer: A. This is the classic Bayes theorem formula.

Question: In decision tree analysis, what is the meaning of life-year?
A. A measure of the probability of living 1 year
B. A quantity of living for 1 year
C. A quantity of living for 1 year with good health status
    Answer: B. Quantity of a patient living for 1 year, irrespective of quality of life.

Question: What is the meaning of quality-adjusted life-year?
A. A life-year adjusted for conditions that reduce the value of the year
B. A life-year adjusted for whether the patient received control or experimental therapy
C. A life-year adjusted for whether patients are continuing with therapy
    Answer: A. Residual disease or complications of treatment can reduce the value of a life-year.

Question: Which is the correct formula for incremental the cost-effectiveness ratio?

A. $Incremental\ Cost\text{-}Effectiveness\ Ratio = \dfrac{\left(benefit\ new - benefit\ old\right)}{\left(cost\ new - cost\ old\right)}$

B. $Incremental\ Cost\text{-}Effectiveness\ Ratio = \dfrac{\left(cost\ new - cost\ old\right)}{\left(benefit\ new - benefit\ old\right)}$

C. $Incremental\ Cost\text{-}Effectiveness\ Ratio = \dfrac{\left(cost\ new - benefit\ new\right)}{\left(cost\ old - benefit\ old\right)}$

Answer: B. Incremental costs over the incremental benefit.

Question: Which of the following is NOT a reasonable approach to resource management in project planning?
A. Allow some additional funding for extra resources if needed
B. Allocate monies into a hidden fund for incidentals
C. Schedule an extra phase of testing that might not ultimately be needed

Answer: B. This would not be ethical. C is a common approach and is valid because sometimes additional testing is needed.

Question: In informatics projects, system testing is which of the following?
A. Testing of the functions of the new application
B. Testing of data flow between components of the environment
C. Testing of the new application in the production domain

Answer: A. This is testing of the new system in isolation.

Question: In informatics projects, integration testing is which of the following?
A. Testing of the functions of the new application
B. Testing of data flow between components of the environment
C. Testing of the new application in the production domain

Answer: B. This is testing of the new system passing data between systems emulating the environment in which it will be functioning. But, this is not done in the production domain.

Question: What is software regression?
A. A previous element of a system no longer works appropriately after an upgrade or update
B. Reversion to a previous version of an application because of failure of an implementation
C. Implementation of a legacy version of an operating system in a server set to accommodate a legacy application

Answer: A. Regression is never intentional. The typical story is that an upgrade fixes many of the issues it was intended to address, but there is a break in some other functionality.

Question: Which of the following are common challenges for pediatric practice with system EHRs?
A. System EHRs are not capable of doing weight-based dosing.
B. System EHRs cannot accommodate pediatric and adult order sets.
C. System EHRs are unable to participate in immunization reporting.
D. All are issues.
E. None are issues.

Answer: E. Although there are multiple issues with system EHRs making pediatric practice inefficient, most EHRs are capable of all of the tasks listed in A–C.

Question: Match the threat with the description.
1. Ransomware
2. Trojan
3. Worm
4. Virus

A. Small program that copies itself and inserts itself into files on a computer, impairing function
B. Small program that replicates and consumes resources of the computer without inserting itself into resident code
C. Program that encrypts computer files and demands payment for a decryption key
D. Program that allows outsiders to have access to the afflicted computer

Answer: 1 = C; 2 = D; 3 = B; 4 = A.

Reference Data

KARL E. MISULIS AND MARK E. FRISSE ■

INFORMATICS CONCEPTS

This section presents concepts key to informatics with an expanded definition. Brief definitions of other terms are in the subsequent section.

Alternative payment model (APM): Provider payment structure that considers quality measures for reimbursement. APMs are part of a larger and complicated structure to change incentives for providers from purely volume based to more based on quality and efficiency of care.

Antitrust: Refers to a series of US laws that seek to promote fair competition. The ultimate goal is to protect consumers from collusion.

Application: Set of instructions, including one or more programs, that performs a task for a user. *Application suite* is a group of applications with a common or entangled interface. This is as opposed to a program which performs one or more tasks on a computer. Healthcare applications such as most EHRs and nonmedical applications such as LibreOffice look to the user like one program, but rather are multiple programs accessed through a common interface.

Architecture: In computer systems, the high-level structure of the system.

Back door: Method of accessing a system without going through standard access controls. May be nefarious but often is used for system development.

Best practices: Procedures or practices that are generally agreed on by research or experience as having the best outcomes.

Bluetooth: Short-range wireless (UHF [ultrahigh-frequency] radio, ~ 2.4 GHz) communication used especially for connecting nearby devices.

Board certification: Demonstration of mastery of a field by meeting specified requirements. The requirements are usually a combination of successful educational qualifications and passing examination(s). Certification in clinical informatics is offered for a physician by the American Board of Preventative Medicine (ABPM) and the American Board of Pathology (ABP). These are subspecialty certifications, meaning that the candidate must already be board certified in one of the American Board of Medical Specialties (ABMS) specialties before applying for this subspecialty certification.

Bolt-on: Software that is an add-on to a larger system, typically to accomplish a specific task that the foundation system does not do or does not do well.

Boolean: An element that has a value of true or false, without other possibilities.

Botnet: Network of computers with malware linked to function as a nefarious network. The purpose is denial of service or gathering information.

Breach: See *Data breach*.

Bridge: In networking, connects multiple networks so they can act as a single network.

Build: Software construction and configuration ultimately resulting in an application or suite of applications. This is a combination of writing code plus integrating objects or modules to produce the resulting application.

C (programming language): Extensively used programming language that has been the foundation for other languages. Source code can be read by humans fairly easily, yet it generates efficient machine code when compiled.

Center for Medicare and Medicaid Services (CMS): An agency of the US Department of Health and Human Services that administers the Medicare system and works with states on administration of the Medicaid system.

Client: Computer equipment that communicates to servers for function. Clients often have some independent computing power but are designed to work with networked servers.

Client-server model: Computer systems where there are centralized servers that serve client devices.

Clinical decision support (CDS): Assistance with clinical decisions, which can be through EHR functionality, such as embedded knowledge in order sets, reminders, and alerts, but also includes access to best practice and other clinical guidelines.

Clinical Document Architecture (CDA): XML-based format standard for clinical documents intended for electronic exchange. Developed by HL7.

Clinical informatics: Information science and engineering applied to healthcare. Also called health informatics.

Compiler: Software that translates computer code from one language to another, usually from a human-friendly language in which the program is written to a language that can be executed by the computer system. Source code is the original language. Target language is the output of the compiler.

Context sensitive: In healthcare, this is the ability of applications to share configuration information, specifically so that applications are showing data from the same patient (e.g., EMR and PACS).

Continuity-of-care document: Electronic document with patient information needed for medical care; used often as a standard in the United States.

Cookie: A small file that usually stores information relevant to a website. Typically not malicious, this is a method of websites tracking our preferences.

Correlation: A mutual relationship between variables that is not necessarily causative.

Cost-effectiveness ratio: Used to compare the costs and results of differing courses of actions, for example, what the cost of a treatment is that would increase life expectancy by a year. Because there are options compared to a standard practice, an *incremental cost-effectiveness ratio* is most commonly employed.

Credentials: In informatics, refers to the information needed to access a particular system. I may have credentials as a medical staff provider. Being a medical staff provider then gives me privileges, which are the specific capabilities that I have when using the system.

Data breach: Release of protected health information or other confidential information to an unauthorized user. CMS has specific definitions of what information release constitutes a data breach and what to do in case of a breach. (Chapter 18)

Data lake: Large repository of data stored in its natural format, not processed as it would be in a data warehouse or data mart.

Data mart: Subset of data stored in database format for a specific purpose. For example, we have a data mart for tracking parameters of glucose control to identify possible new diabetics or uncontrolled diabetes in our hospital and ED.

Data mining: Process of analyzing large data sets for the purpose of discovering patterns and correlations that could reveal new valuable information—building knowledge.

Data modeling: Steps in the development of databases beginning with a conceptual model (organizational entities, attributes, relationships), then a logical model (structure and logical relationships), then a physical model (implementation using a specific database management system and physical infrastructure). For example, for an EMR, the conceptual model defines the care sites, providers, patients, and relationships between them. The logical model defines the structure of the data elements, such as fields for patient name and demographics or provider name and license number. This includes relationship structure, such as data to indicate which providers have seen which patient, what privileges a specific provider has.

Data representation: How data are structured digitally for databases. There are many different variable types, and representation indicates how specific data are manifest in the data arrays.

Data visualization: Placing data in a visual context, which can reveal relationships that are not evident from inspection of a tabular display.

Data warehouse: Database pulling together select data, often from multiple data sources. The focus is on aggregation of important data and analysis rather than on transactions, which would be the purpose of the native database.

Data, information, knowledge: In information theory, this is a layered conceptual framework. *Data* are values, such as a creatinine level. *Information* is where the data are in context giving meaningful utility, such as creatinine of 3.7 having different implications depending on whether the patient is on hemodialysis or was thought to have normal renal function . *Knowledge* has multiple definitions, but here we refer to distilled information, such as protocols for management of renal insufficiency in different clinical scenarios.

Database: An organized set of data, facilitating storage and retrieval. Common types of databases include relational and hierarchical. (Chapter 7)

Decision support: A system that supports clinical, business, or organizational decision-making. Usually used in the context of computer-mediated decision support, but the term can also refer to a human-mediated process. (Chapter 17)

Decision tree: Tool with a tree-like appearance for examining options and potential outcomes of clinical or business decisions.

Denial of service: Threat to a system where a host is overwhelmed by nonsense connections and cannot accomplish intended tasks.

Direct messaging: Sending clinical records using a national encryption standard for secure transmission.

Downtime: Period of lack of function of all or part of an information system, usually planned (e.g., for upgrades or new installations) but sometimes unplanned (server crash or network failure).

Electronic health record (EHR): The definition of EHR according to HealthIT. gov is "a digital version of a patient's paper chart. " Our definition goes far beyond that of the paper chart, with capabilities of communication with other systems and facilities, analytics, and clinical decision support.

Electronic medical record (EMR): Digital equivalent of the paper medical record. When data not pertaining to just medical care are incorporated or when data from more than one healthcare delivery site are included, the term *electronic health record* is used.

Encryption: Process of conversion of data into a code that cannot be read without a digital key. Used to prevent unauthorized access to the information.

Evidence-based medicine (EBM): Medical practice that relies on evidence from well-designed experimental studies. Quality of evidence is considered in assessment of the determination of best practices.

Factor analysis: Statistical method to determine determinants of variability, especially of two or more correlated variables.

Firmware: Computer code that tells the hardware how to handle instructions, whether from software or with the firmware of other devices.

Foreign key: Field in a database table that has an identifier that points to the primary key in a field of a different table.

Gantt chart: Chart for project scheduling comprised of horizontal bars, representing components of a project whether activities or subprojects.

Genomics: Study of the structure, function, and mapping of genetic code. In healthcare, refers to study or practice of inclusion of genetic data into clinical decision-making.

Go live: Common term for the activation of a new application or program system. Typically includes copying the code from the build environment to the production environment and turning on the system. Go live includes the initial phases of troubleshooting.

Health information exchange (HIE): System that facilitates exchange of information between healthcare systems. The term can refer to the technical infrastructure of the exchange or the organization performing the exchange.

Heuristics: Information and problem-solving methods learned through experimentation, experience, and observation.

Hierarchical database: Database organized in a tree-like structure with parent-child relationships.

Host: In networks, a computer or other device connected to the network, which may have resources or functions useful to other devices on the network.

Hosting strategy: Where our servers are. Could be local (in our facility data center), remote (in a vendor server farm), or a mixture, with some apps locally hosted and others remote.

Hub: In networking, a node with multiple connections.

Informatics: The science behind information systems. This includes research as well as clinical components.

Information blocking: Unreasonable constraint placed on exchange of information, accomplished by policy, intentional technical constraints, or unreasonable financial limitation.

Information systems: Term for the compilation of people and technology that governs and provides information management services to an organization. Also sometimes used to refer to the specific technical infrastructures.

Information technology: Technical infrastructure of information management systems. Includes database storage, servers, networks, applications, and all of the other components of the system.

Integration: Sharing of information between systems. Integration is usually intended to accomplish a series of tasks that no one system can accomplish well alone.

Integration testing: Phase of application testing where individual components are tested as a group. This tests the functions of the components in the setting of dependencies and interfaces between elements.

Interface: Connection between two components of a system. The components may be separate software applications or hardware devices or between an application and a device. The term also applies to interfaces with humans for user interaction (input/output) or data sharing, and interfaces with other systems, as in an information exchange.

Interoperability: The ability of systems to exchange data and otherwise communicate to accomplish a shared task. Systems should have standardized interfaces such that little or no custom work is needed to move information between the systems.

Issue: Reported events with an application or system that need to be addressed. May be problems with the system or potentially user error.

Joint Commission: Organization that accredits hospitals and healthcare organizations. Effectively sets standards for performance of systems in a number of areas.

Keylogger: Surveillance software that records keystrokes and other direct interactions with the system. Not always nefarious, but can be. Keyloggers not only can steal user IDs and passwords but also can monitor efficiency of use of an EHR.

Knowledge base: The compilation of information available to draw on for a specific task. This includes knowledge of the human user, embedded information in the system, and foundational information for decision support systems.

Knowledge management: The general concept of handling information and resources by a healthcare system.

Launch: Activation of a system for production use by the users. Strictly speaking, this term does not apply to upgrades because the term implies first revelation to the public.

Learning health system: Health system that integrates internal data with external evidence to improve healthcare. This is not a computer program but rather a system-wide commitment.

Logical operator: A symbol representing a logic function, such as AND or NAND.

Malware: Malicious software—includes viruses, worms, Trojans, ransomware, and others.

Markov model: Model for predicting transitions in a system where there are probabilities of a transition, such as between three states of well, sick, and dead.

Markup: Entries in a document that give nonprinting commands, such as a style.

Master patient index (MPI): Index of patients for a healthcare system. An enterprise master patient index (EMPI) accomplishes the task for a wider enterprise and is more robust about matching patients in different information systems.

Meaningful Use: Program for incentives to meet minimum government standards for using EHRs.

Medical home: Model of primary care that is patient-centric, coordinated, high quality, and accessible.

Network: In information systems, a group of affiliated devices to share resources with the connection infrastructure. Sometimes used to indicate just the connections and not the connected devices.

Node: In networking, devices in a network which can receive, transmit, or relay data. May be a connection point such as a hub or an operational deice such as a computer, server, or printer.

Object-oriented programming: Programs are built with procedures that handle data with fields and internal processes (objects) rather than writing all processes. Objects can be reused elsewhere in the same program or in different programs.

Operating system: Software that is foundational to system hardware and applications, providing the mechanisms for the applications to use the computer resources and accomplish basic tasks.

Optimization: In information systems, a process of improving use and performance of a healthcare information system, involving both user training and system improvement.

Patch: Changes or updates to a computer program that fix an issue or enhances some function.

Payer: An individual or organization providing compensation for services. This can be the patient or the insurance company.

Personal health record: System where patients can manage their own health information.

Pharming: Directing users to a fraudulent website that resembles a legitimate site for the purpose of obtaining credentials or other personal information.

Phishing: Sending emails that appear to be from legitimate sources but have the purpose of capturing user credentials.

Pointer: In programming, a pointer is a piece of data that stores the location of a specific memory address, essentially placing a bookmark for a place to go to when needed.

Population health: Broadly defined as the health of a group of individuals. Term is often used as an initiative within a healthcare system to manage and improve the health of the population.

Portal: Mechanism for users to access a specific healthcare system, with credentials and functionality appropriate to the user. We think of patient portals, but there are also portals for other users.

Predictive analytics: Statistical method of analyzing data and using findings to predict future events.

Primary key: The principal index key for a particular table in a database. A foreign key in another table points to this primary key.

Privacy: In information systems, the concept of classifying what data can be shared, especially with third parties.

Privacy rule: HIPAA rule that establishes standards to protect medical records and personal health information.

Private key: A cryptographic key that can decrypt a message, yet is specific to a user or group. The key itself is a small piece of code that is paired with the public key.

Protected health information (PHI): Information about an individual related to health, healthcare, or payment for healthcare. The definition is specific, pertaining to HIPAA regulatory guidelines.

Protocol orders: Orders that are executed in response to the status of a particular patient. For example, a protocol order may be executed if a patient has a reaction to contrast dye administered in a computed tomography suite; contact with a provider to get an order is not needed. As opposed to a *standing order*.

Pseudocode: In programming, a hypothetical programming language for design or educational purposes.

Public key: A cryptographic key that can be used by anyone to encrypt a message. A second user-specific key is required to decrypt the message (private key). Keys are small sets of code.

Python: Programming language that is high level, meaning that it is closer to the written language of the programmer and far different from the machine language used to execute instructions. Execution requires an interpreter (line-by-line execution) or compiler (program conversion to instructions that the computer and operating system can understand).

Query: Can refer to a computer programming language that facilitates searching within databases or refer to an actual programmed search.

Ransomware: Program that encrypts or otherwise threatens the files of a system, with a demand for compensation to remove the threat.

Record locator service: Healthcare system or health information exchange service that allows clinical staff to find records across more than one information system.

Regression: Loss of or error in function of a computer program, usually as an unexpected consequence of an upgrade or patch.

Relational database: Database structure that features categories for data elements with indexed relations between items.

Repeater: In networking, a device that extends the range of your wireless network by receiving and retransmitting data to and from devices and your network.

Request for information (RFI): In beginning a project, after identifying the need and what solution(s) may be needed, an RFI is sent to a number of vendors or other potential suppliers to determine principally capabilities of what they have to offer. The RFI contains information on the need and related present technical infrastructure. The desired information is whether the vendor can meet the needs and to obtain a preliminary assessment of how resource intensive and disruptive the solution might be. The information obtained helps to determine whether the vendor will be asked to submit a proposal.

Request for proposal (RFP): The RFP usually follows the RFI and assessment of responses. A few select vendors will be chosen to submit a proposal. The RFP includes specifics of the requirements of the solution and additional details about related local infrastructure. If the vendor responds with a proposal, it will contain specifics of the ability to meet the requested specifications, estimates of resource needs for implementation and operation, and estimated costs for acquisition, build, installation, operation, and maintenance. Usually, additional numbers are supplied regarding the costs of adding users or otherwise expanding use of the application. In the present climate, healthcare systems have to plan for the possibility of acquisition of other healthcare facilities and providers.

Router: In networking, a connection between different networks but the networks remain distinct, and the router controls data transfer between them.

Secure messaging: Mechanism of communication using transmission methods that are HIPAA compliant.

Security: In healthcare information systems, security is the methods to protect not only patient data but also the information systems themselves from various threats, both physical and electronic. This also includes provisions for providing access when there are issues with the infrastructure, such as power outages.

Security rule: HIPAA requirement to use appropriate administrative, physical, and technical safeguards to ensure confidentiality, integrity, and availability of protected health information.

Semantics: In programming, function of the commands, what they mean.

Sensitivity: Ability of a test to correctly identify those who have a disease. Mathematically, this is the proportion of patients with a disease who have a positive test, the true positive rate.

Server: Combination of software and hardware that provides a platform for running of programs on other device-program units, termed *clients*.

Server virtualization: Partitioning of a server into multiple virtual servers that can run different operating systems, configurations, or applications.

Single sign on: A mechanism whereby users can log in to a single interface and launch individual apps without having to log in to each one.

Smart client: Type of client that uses HTTP connections rather than having applications installed on the client. Leverages many benefits of thin clients (local installation and updates not required) and thick clients (more robust performance than thin clients).

Software regression: Where a system may lose one or more functions after update or upgrade. The intended improvement may have accomplished its goals but broke other previously working functions unintentionally.

Specificity: Rate at which patients without disease have a negative test. Mathematically, this is the proportion of patients who do not have a disease having a negative test, the true negative rate.

Spyware: Software installed without the user's knowledge and intended to pass information to a third party.

SQL: Structured Query Language, a standard language for query and manipulation of data from a relational database.

Standing orders: Orders given as part of a standard set. For example, standing orders may be available for all patients during intake for a surgical procedure.

Subroutine: In programming, code set that is part of a larger program for a defined function.

Syntax: In programming, the set of rules to which the language adheres, such as commands and structure.

System testing: Stage of development at which the testing is to determine whether the specific system meets specifications regarding performance and functionality.

Table: A set of data in a flat tabular arrangement. Often, the columns are categories (e.g., date of birth, name, medical record number), and the rows are individual elements (e.g., patients or encounters or lab tests).

Table space: Storage locations for a database. The term does not specify the type or organization of the data, just the allocated space on the physical media.

Thick client: Client devices in a client-server architecture that are fully functioning computers, capable of executing productivity applications locally with data passed to the servers.

Thin client: Client devices in a client-server architecture that pass data to and from the servers where the principal computing is done.

Transaction: A single operation that cannot be divided into multiple operations. A transaction must be complete or fail completely.

Trojan: Small program that allows outside parties access to a computer.

21st Century Cures Act: Among other elements, grants safe harbor for many collaborative use cases.

Value equation: One of a variety of equations that is best defined as presented by Harvard's Michael Porter: $Value = \dfrac{Outcomes}{Costs}$. There are variations on this, but this is the foundation.

Virtual private network (VPN): A VPN is when a system allows an enterprise private network to be accessed from a public network, outside the system.

Virtual server: Combination of hardware and software that functions as a server for a front-end application. However, the actual servers may host multiple virtual servers with differing operating systems, operating system versions, or specifications.

Virus: Small program that inserts a copy of itself onto a computer.

Wi-Fi: Wireless networking technology using radio connection. Short for wireless fidelity.

Wireless access point (WAP): In networking, extends the wired connections to wireless connections by radio communication.

Worm: Small program that replicates and spreads from computer to computer. Differentiated from a virus by not inserting itself into the code of existing programs.

Zero client: Client in a client-server architecture where there is no storage or significant computing power on the client. Has communication capabilities but lacks the operating system of a thin client.

ABBREVIATIONS

ABMS	American Board of Medical Specialties
ABP	American Board of Pathology
ABPM	American Board of Preventive Medicine
ACA	Affordable Care Act, also known as the PPACA
ACR	American College of Radiology
ADT	Admit, discharge, transfer. A type of data set
AHIMA	American Health Information Management Association
AMIA	American Medical Informatics Association
API	Application programming interface
APM	Alternative payment model
Cath	Catheterization (e.g., cardiac cath)
CBC	Complete blood cell count
CCD	Continuity-of-care document
C-CDA	Consolidated Clinical Document Architecture
CCOW	Clinical Context Object Workgroup
CDA	Clinical Document Architecture
CDC	Centers for Disease Control and Prevention
CDS	Clinical decision support
CIO	Chief information officer
CMIO	Chief medical information/informatics officer
CMP	Comprehensive metabolic panel
CMS	Centers for Medicare and Medicaid Services
CPT	*Current Procedural Terminology*
CPU	Central processing unit
CT	Computed tomography
DICOM	Digital Imaging and Communications in Medicine
DIK	Data-information-knowledge organization
DoD	Department of Defense
EBM	Evidence-based medicine
ECG	Electrocardiogram (variant of EKG)
Echo	Echocardiogram
ED	Emergency department
EHR	Electronic health record
EKG	Electrocardiogram (variant of ECG)
EMR	Electronic medical record
EOL	End of life
ETL	Extract, transform, and load
FDA	Food and Drug Administration
FDASIA	Food and Drug Administration Safety and Innovation Act of 2012
FHIR	Fast Healthcare Interoperability Resources
HHS	Health and Human Services (Department of)
HIE	Health information exchange
HIMSS	Healthcare Information and Management Systems Society
HIPAA	Health Insurance Portability and Accountability Act (1996)
HIT	Health Information Technology

HITECH	Health Information Technology for Economic and Clinical Health (Act)
HL7	Health Level Seven International
ICD	*International Classification of Diseases*
ICU	Intensive care unit
JAMIA	Journal of the American Medical Informatics Association
JSON	JavaScript Object Notation
LDAP	Lightweight Directory Access protocol
LIS	Laboratory information system
LOINC	Logical Observation Identifiers Names and Codes
MACRA	Medicare Access and CHIP Reauthorization Act
MIPS	Merit-Based Incentive Payment System
MPI	Master patient index
MRI	Magnetic resonance imaging
MeSH	Medical subject headings
OECD	Organization for Economic Cooperation and Development
OIS	Oncology information system
ONC	Office of the National Coordinator for Health Information Technology
OT	Occupational therapy
PACS	Picture archiving and communication system
PCORI	Patient-Centered Outcomes Research Institute
PHI	Protected health information
PHR	Personal health record
PPACA	Patient Protection and Affordable Care Act
PT	Physical therapy or prothrombin time
QALY	Quality-adjusted life-year
RFI	Request for information
RFID	Radio-frequency identification
RFP	Request for proposal
RIS	Radiology information system
SMART	Substitutable Medical Applications and Reusable Technologies
SMS	Short message service
SNOMED CT	Systematized Nomenclature of Medicine—Clinical Terms
SQL	Structured Query Language
SSO	Single sign on
UI	User interface
UMLS	Unified Medical Language System, an ontology service for medical vocabularies, including a meta-thesaurus with codes from other ontologies, including SNOMED, *CPT, ICD-10,* LOINC
UX	User experience
VA	Department of Veterans Affairs
WHO	World Health Organization

NOTES AND REFERENCES

CHAPTER 1

1. Smith M, Saunders R, Stuckhardt L, et al., eds. *Best Care at Lower Cost: The Path to Continuously Learning Health Care in America.* Washington, DC: Institute of Medicine; 2013. http://www.nap.edu/catalog/13444/best-care-at-lower-cost-the-path-to-continuously-learning

2. Schneider EC, Sarnak DO, Squires D, et al. *Mirror, Mirror 2017: International Comparison Reflects Flaws and Opportunities for Better US Health Care.* New York, NY: Commonwealth Fund; 2017. http://www.commonwealthfund.org/interactives/2017/july/mirror-mirror/

3. Verghese A. How tech can turn doctors into clerical workers. *New York Times Magazine.* May 16, 2018. https://www.nytimes.com/interactive/2018/05/16/magazine/health-issue-what-we-lose-with-data-driven-medicine.html

4. Remington PL, Catlin BB, Gennuso KP. The county health rankings: rationale and methods. *Popul Health Metr.* 2015;13:11. https://www.ncbi.nlm.nih.gov/pubmed/25931988. Although one sees variants of the included figure in many publications, the relative contributions are the result of a regression analysis of 400 counties and are "empirically derived." See the associated white paper: http://www.countyhealthrankings.org/sites/default/files/differentPerspectivesForAssigningWeightsToDeterminantsOfHealth.pdf

5. Figure 3-1 in Smith M, et al., *Best Care.* http://www.nap.edu/catalog/13444/best-care-at-lower-cost-the-path-to-continuously-learning

6. Pham HH, O'Malley AS, Bach PB, et al. Primary care physicians' links to other physicians through Medicare patients: the scope of care coordination. *Ann Intern Med.* 2009;150(4):236–242. http://www.ncbi.nlm.nih.gov/pubmed/19221375

CHAPTER 2

1. https://www.healthit.gov/providers-professionals/meaningful-use-definition-objectives

2. https://dashboard.healthit.gov/quickstats/quickstats.php

3. https://www.cdc.gov/nchs/fastats/electronic-medical-records.htm

4. Nakamura MM, Harper MB, Castro AV, Yu FB Jr, Jha AK. Impact of the meaningful use incentive program on electronic health record adoption by US children's hospitals. *J Am Med Inform Assoc.* 2015;22(2):390–398.

5. Nakamura MM, Harper MB, Jha AK. Change in adoption of electronic health records by US children's hospitals. *Pediatrics.* 2013;131(5):e1563–e1575.

CHAPTER 3

1. Kidney Disease Improving Global Outcomes program.
2. Dutta E, Kar A. A case-control study identifying the characteristics of patients providing incorrect contact information at registration for DOTS in Pune, India. *Indian J Tuberc.* 2016;63(1):51–54.

CHAPTER 5

1. http://www.who.int/topics/health_policy/en/
2. Very loosely adapted from Edmunds M, Peddicord D, Bates DW. Clinical informatics policy and regulations. In: Finnell JT, Dixon B, et al. *Clinical Informatics Study Guide.* New York, NY: Springer; 2016:47–66.
3. https://www.hhs.gov/hipaa/for-professionals/security/laws-regulations/index.html
4. https://www.healthit.gov/sites/default/files/hitech_act_excerpt_from_arra_with_index.pdf
5. https://oig.hhs.gov/compliance/physician-education/01laws.asp
6. Safe harbor is a mechanism in a statue or regulation that designates certain procedures or conduct to specifically not violate the statue or regulation. It is used to avoid ambiguity or to define special cases where the law is not violated.
7. https://www.ftc.gov/tips-advice/competition-guidance/guide-antitrust-laws/antitrust-laws
8. https://www.fda.gov/RegulatoryInformation/LawsEnforcedbyFDA/SignificantAmendmentstotheFDCAct/FDASIA/default.htm
9. Slight SP, Bates DW. A risk-based regulatory framework for health IT: recommendations of the FDASIA Working Group. *J Am Med Inform Assoc.* 2014;21(e2):e181–e184. http://dx.doi.org/10.1136/amiajnl-2014-002638
10. https://www.healthcare.gov/where-can-i-read-the-affordable-care-act/
11. https://www.fda.gov/regulatoryinformation/lawsenforcedbyfda/significantamendmentstothefdcact/21stcenturycuresact/default.htm
12. https://www.kff.org/medicare/fact-sheet/medicare-advantage/
13. https://www.cms.gov/Medicare/Health-Plans/MedicareAdvtgSpecRateStats/Risk-Adjustors.html
14. *Fed Regist.* 2000;65(106):34988.
15. Ibid.
16. HITECH was part of a much broader economic recovery law that sought to stimulate the economy through massive and rapid government expenditures. It was not part of later healthcare reform legislation. The rush to pass this economic legislation may explain in part the hasty prose and the urgent demand for rapid (and often unrealistic) implementation.
17. https://www.federalregister.gov/uploads/2011/01/the_rulemaking_process.pdf

CHAPTER 6

1. Donaldson MS, Corrigan JM, eds. *To Err Is Human: Building a Safer Health System.* Washington, DC: Institute of Medicine; 2000.

2. https://www.ncbi.nlm.nih.gov/books/NBK53481/#
3. https://medicine.umich.edu/sites/default/files/2014_12_08-Friedman-IOM%20 LHS.pdf
4. An antibiogram is a listing of expected antibiotic sensitivities and resistances for specific bacteria of specific infections in the designated facility. This is based on the known sensitivities for similar previous infections in the facility.

CHAPTER 7

1. IMO is an abbreviation for Intelligent Medical Objects, a private US company that creates and licenses medical vocabularies commonly used in EHRs. SNOMED CT is a collection of terms and definitions with codes created by the UK-based nonprofit SNOMED International, which otherwise is termed IHTSDO, the International Health Terminology Standards Development Organization.
2. Type 1 diabetes would be series E10. These series have numbers after the E10 and E11 to indicate specific features of the diabetes.
3. Rightmost place is 1 + third from right is 4 + fourth from right is 8 = 13.
4. Other types, such as array and tree, are not discussed here because the concepts of data representation are addressed by the foundational three considered in this chapter.
5. For example, some complex data might be arranged in a list that is decoded by the database engine, whereas the same data from another facility might represent the data as a two-dimensional array.

CHAPTER 8

1. The sampling rate is the reciprocal of the sampling interval. $1/0.004 = 250$. Units are samples per second.
2. This is the DRAM type of RAM. There is another type called SRAM, which is more complicated and more expensive, composed of a series of transistors comprising a flip-flop circuit, a circuit that can have two states.
3. Coordinated Universal Time. The abbreviation UTC was a compromise imposed by the United Nations between the English speakers, who wanted the abbreviation to be CUT, and French speakers, who wanted TUC for *temps universel coordonné*. So, neither got their way.
4. https://en.wikipedia.org/wiki/Lists_of_programming_languages

CHAPTER 9

1. The PACS is mainly for radiology, cardiology, gastroenterology, pulmonary, pathology, and other clinical images.
2. The RIS is responsible for coordinating orders, results, and billing for radiology services.
3. Microwave relay towers were commonly used, especially in the 1980s. They are still used for some point-to-point communications. They are used much less because of the cost effectiveness and greater ease of securing satellite transmissions.
4. *Virtual desktop* can also refer to local desktop configurations. One type is where the desktop is larger than the actual display screen. Alternatively, both Microsoft Windows and Mac OSX provide the capability of creating multiple virtual desktops; we may use one for office applications, one for research tasks, one for educational materials, and another for personal tasks.

5. Flash memory has limitations in use for storage. Among these is the mechanism to erase and write data, where erasure is often a block at a time. Also, flash memory has a finite number of read/write cycles before it deteriorates, termed *memory wear*.

6. Internet Explorer (IE) is more than a browser but rather an integral part of the Microsoft Windows operating system. Some applications have been written that use functions of a particular IE version. Servers with updated IE might not support a legacy app. Virtual server architecture allows the specific operating system and IE versions and configurations to be running for that specific purpose.

7. There is also a hybrid, paravirtual machine (PVM), for which most of the computing runs on the virtual machine; however, the PVM passes some resource-intensive tasks to the host server itself. In this case, the guest instance asks for permission to run select tasks on the host and the host responds. This avoids some of the degradation in performance on resource-intensive tasks.

8. eXtensible Markup Language (XML) is a standard format for documents that achieves much of its power by allowing for markup, or inserting of annotations in documents, which can be tags and instructions. Therefore, XML documents can contain complex data structures, not just prose.

CHAPTER 10

1. *Transactional* means information recorded from single transactions.
2. The acronym ACID was created by German computer scientists Andreas Reuter and Theo Härder in 1983, building on the work of American computer scientist James Gray, who listed ACD but not I.
3. The name for the *Hadoop* framework used for data lakes comes from the name of the toy elephant of the son of data scientist Doug Cutting, former chairman of the board of the Apache Software Foundation.
4. https://www.healthit.gov/topic/safety/safer-guides

CHAPTER 11

1. This is not always true in clinical medicine. Some events are dependent on previous events, and these influences are unable to be modeled well by the Markov models. For example, in women who are *BRCA1* or *BRCA2* positive, having one cancer (ovary or breast) increases the likelihood of having another cancer, in comparison to patients with the gene defect but without having a history of cancer.
2. From https://en.wikipedia.org/wiki/Logic_gate

CHAPTER 12

1. https://www.hhs.gov/about/strategic-plan/overview/index.html
2. Bush M, Lederer AL, Li X, Palmisano J, Rao S. The alignment of information systems with organizational objectives and strategies in health care. *Int J Med Inform.* 2009;78(7):446–456.
3. https://www.beckershospitalreview.com/strategic-planning/the-only-five-strategic-plan-objectives-youll-ever-need.html

CHAPTER 13

1. The value equation is foundational in business practice. Michael Porter from Harvard Business School has discussed this in detail, and the formula has other permutations discussed by numerous experts.
2. https://en.wikipedia.org/wiki/Parkinson%27s_law
3. http://www.changetoolkit.org.uk/change-curve/

CHAPTER 14

1. https://dashboard.healthit.gov/quickstats/quickstats.php
2. Miyasaki JM, Rheaume C, Gulya L, et al. Qualitative study of burnout, career satisfaction, and well-being among US neurologists in 2016. *Neurology*. 2017;89(16):1730–1738.
3. https://healthit.ahrq.gov/sites/default/files/docs/citation/09-10-0091-2-EF.pdf
4. Krousel-Wood M, McCoy AB, Ahia C, et al. Implementing electronic health records (EHRs): health care provider perceptions before and after transition from a local basic EHR to a commercial comprehensive EHR. *J Am Med Inform Assoc*. 2018;25(6):618–626. doi:10.1093/jamia/ocx094
5. According to ONC, as of 2016, at least 22% of provider offices were still using paper. The number may be as high as 28%.
6. Montague E, Asan O. Physician interactions with electronic health records in primary care. *Health Syst (Basingstoke)*. 2012;1(2):96–103.

CHAPTER 16

1. Burke J. *Health Analytics*. Cary, NC: SAS Institute; 2013.
2. The discussion of SQL in Chapter 10 may be of particular interest to those who anticipate participation in analytics.

CHAPTER 17

1. Baseman JG, Revere D, Painter I, Toyoji M, Thiede H, Duchin J. Public health communications and alert fatigue. *BMC Health Serv Res*. 2013;13:295. doi:10.1186/1472-6963-13-295
2. Lehmann CU, Conner KG, Cox JM. Preventing provider errors: online total parenteral nutrition calculator. *Pediatrics*. 2004;113(4):748–753.
3. Lehmann CU, Kim GR, Gujral R, Veltri MA, Clark JS, Miller MR. Decreasing errors in pediatric continuous intravenous infusions. *Pediatr Crit Care Med*. 2006;7(3):225–230.
4. Alrifai MW, Mulherin DP, Weinberg ST, Wang L, Lehmann CU. Parenteral protein decision support system improves protein delivery in preterm infants: a randomized clinical trial. *JPEN J Parenter Enteral Nutr*. 2018;42(1):219–224. doi:10.1002/jpen.1034. Epub 2017 Nov 3.
5. Lehmann CU, Conner KG, Cox JM. Preventing provider errors: online total parenteral nutrition calculator. *Pediatrics*. 2004;113(4):748–753.
6. Adelman JS, Kalkut GE, Schechter CB, et al. Understanding and preventing wrong-patient electronic orders: a randomized controlled trial. *J Am Med Inform Assoc*. 2013;20(2):305–310. doi:10.1136/amiajnl-2012-001055. Epub 2012 Jun 29.

7. Stenner SP, Chakravarthy R, Johnson KB, et al. ePrescribing: reducing costs through in-class therapeutic interchange. *Appl Clin Inform.* 2016;7(4):1168–1181.
8. Sick AC, Lehmann CU, Tamma PD, Lee CK, Agwu AL. Sustained savings from a longitudinal cost analysis of an internet-based preapproval antimicrobial stewardship program. *Infect Control Hosp Epidemiol.* 2013;34(6):573–580. doi:10.1086/670625. Epub 2013 Apr 18
9. Agwu AL, Lee CK, Jain SK, et al. A World Wide Web-based antimicrobial stewardship program improves efficiency, communication, and user satisfaction and reduces cost in a tertiary care pediatric medical center. *Clin Infect Dis.* 2008;47(6):747–753. doi:10.1086/591133
10. https://www.beckershospitalreview.com/healthcare-information-technology/the-centers-for-medicare-and-medicaid-services-five-rights-of-clinical-decision-support-what-s-really-required-for-effective-decision-support.html
11. Bates DW, Kuperman GJ, Wang S, et al. Ten commandments for effective clinical decision support: making the practice of evidence-based medicine a reality. *J Am Med Inform Assoc.* 2003;10(6):523–530. Epub 2003 Aug 4.
12. https://healthit.ahrq.gov/ahrq-funded-projects/current-health-it-priorities/clinical-decision-support-cds/chapter-1-approaching-clinical-decision/section-2-overview-cds-five-rights
13. https://www.fda.gov/downloads/medicaldevices/deviceregulationandguidance/guidancedocuments/ucm587819.pdf
14. Kesselheim AS, Cresswell K, Phansalkar S, Bates DW, Sheikh A. Clinical decision support systems could be modified to reduce "alert fatigue" while still minimizing the risk of litigation. *Health Aff.* 2011;30:2310–2317.

CHAPTER 18

1. https://privacyruleandresearch.nih.gov/pr_06.asp
2. https://www.hipaa.com/hipaa-protected-health-information-what-does-phi-include/
3. https://privacyruleandresearch.nih.gov/pr_07.asp
4. https://biotech.law.lsu.edu/map/WhenCanPHIBeReleasedwithoutAuthorization.html
5. https://www.hhs.gov/hipaa/for-professionals/security/laws-regulations/index.html
6. https://www.hhs.gov/hipaa/for-professionals/privacy/laws-regulations/index.html
7. https://aspe.hhs.gov/report/health-insurance-portability-and-accountability-act-1996
8. At one of our hospitals, proposed new access rules would have made patients' records unavailable from anywhere other than the patients' nursing units. This is an example of a decision sounding logical to nonclinical staff but having potential adverse consequences for patient care.
9. https://www.hhs.gov/hipaa/for-professionals/breach-notification/breach-reporting/index.html

CHAPTER 19

1. https://hbr.org/2012/10/data-scientist-the-sexiest-job-of-the-21st-century

CHAPTER 20

1. Haux R, Howe J, Marschollek M, Plischke M, Wolf KH. Health-enabling technologies for pervasive health care: on services and ICT architecture paradigms. *Inform Health Soc Care.* 2008;33(2):77–89.
2. For example, subtherapeutic doses of antibiotics may induce resistance in organisms, whereas a full-strength dose might eradicate the infection altogether.
3. Wang Y, Lai F, Vespa P. Enabling technologies facilitate new healthcare delivery models for acute stroke. *Stroke.* 2010;41(6):1076–1078.

CHAPTER 21

1. Terhune C. Health care in America: An employment bonanza and a runaway-cost crisis. *Kaiser Health News.* April 24, 2017. http://khn.org/news/health-care-in-america-an-employment-bonanza-and-a-runaway-cost-crisis/
2. Fernandopulle R, Patel N. How the electronic health record did not measure up to the demands of our medical home practice. *Health Aff.* 2010;29(4):622–628. http://content.healthaffairs.org/content/29/4/622.abstract

CHAPTER 22

1. Palmieri JJ, Stern TA. Lies in the doctor-patient relationship. *Prim Care Companion J Clin Psychiatry.* 2009;11(4):163–168.
2. https://www.ahrq.gov/professionals/quality-patient-safety/patient-family-engagement/index.html
3. https://www.hhs.gov/hipaa/for-professionals/faq/570/does-hipaa-permit-health-care-providers-to-use-email-to-discuss-health-issues-with-patients/index.html
4. Baldwin JL, Singh H, Sittig DF, Giardina TD. Patient portals and health apps: Pitfalls, promises, and what one might learn from the other. *Healthc (Amst).* 2017;5(3):81–85. https://www.ncbi.nlm.nih.gov/pubmed/27720139
5. Horvath M, Levy J, L'Engle P, Carlson B, Ahmad A, Ferranti J. Impact of health portal enrollment with email reminders on adherence to clinic appointments: a pilot study. *J Med Internet Res.* 2011;13(2):e41.
6. Ammenwerth E, Schnell-Inderst P, Hoerbst A. The impact of electronic patient portals on patient care: a systematic review of controlled trials. *J Med Internet Res.* 2012;14(6):e162.
7. https://www.healthit.gov/topic/health-it-initiatives/telemedicine-and-telehealth
8. Martin JC, Avant RF, Bowman MA, et al. Future of Family Medicine Project Leadership Committee. The future of family medicine: a collaborative project of the family medicine community. *Ann Fam Med.* 2004;2(Suppl 1):S3–S32.
9. https://www.aafp.org/dam/AAFP/documents/practice_management/pcmh/initiatives/PCMHJoint.pdf
10. https://www.ncqa.org/programs/health-care-providers-practices/patient-centered-medical-home-pcmh/

CHAPTER 23

1. https://www.gartner.com/newsroom/id/3598917

2. https://verily.com/projects/
3. https://www.apple.com/ios/home/accessories/
4. https://www.apple.com/newsroom/2018/06/apple-opens-health-records-api-to-developers/

CHAPTER 24

1. Gosiewski T, Ludwig-Galezowska AH, Huminska K, et al. Comprehensive detection and identification of bacterial DNA in the blood of patients with sepsis and healthy volunteers using next-generation sequencing method—the observation of DNAemia. *Eur J Clin Microbiol Infect Dis.* 2017;36(2):329–336.
2. https://www.cancer.gov/about-cancer/causes-prevention/genetics/brca-fact-sheet
3. https://www.nccn.org/professionals/physician_gls/default.aspx
4. Dean L. In: Pratt V, McLeod H, Rubinstein W, Dean L, Malheiro A, eds. *Medical Genetics Summaries* [Internet]. Bethesda, MD: National Center for Biotechnology Information; 2012. [Updated April 18, 2018]
5. Vassy JL, Stone A, Callaghan JT, et al.; VHA Clinical Pharmacogenetics Subcommittee. Pharmacogenetic testing in the Veterans Health Administration (VHA): policy recommendations from the VHA Clinical Pharmacogenetics Subcommittee. *Genet Med.* 2018 Jun 1. doi:10.1038/s41436-018-0057-x
6. Score developed by the American Society of Anesthesiologists for assessing the preoperative health of the patient. Documentation of this value is often required, so a discrete field can be created in the EHR for recording this score.
7. APACHE II = Acute Physiology and Chronic Health Evaluation II (for ICU severity of illness); NIHSS = National Institutes of Health Stroke Scale (for acute stroke evaluation); SAPS = Scale for Assessment of Positive Symptoms (for schizophrenia).
8. Feblowitz J, Takhar SS, Ward MJ, Ribeira R, Landman AB. A custom-developed emergency department provider electronic documentation system reduces operational efficiency. *Ann Emerg Med.* 2017;70(5):674–682.e1.
9. Kannampallil TG, Manning JD, Chestek DW, et al. Effect of number of open charts on intercepted wrong-patient medication orders in an emergency department. *J Am Med Inform Assoc.* 2018;25(6):739–743.
10. Lim MC, Boland MV, McCannel CA, et al. Adoption of electronic health records and perceptions of financial and clinical outcomes among ophthalmologists in the United States. *JAMA Ophthalmol.* 2018;136(2):164–170.
11. Park JSY, Sharma RA, Poulis B, Noble J. Barriers to electronic medical record implementation: a comparison between ophthalmology and other surgical specialties in Canada. *Can J Ophthalmol.* 2017;52(5):503–507.
12. Dufendach KR, Eichenberger JA, McPheeters ML, et al. *Core Functionality in Pediatric Electronic Health Records.* Washington, DC: Agency for Healthcare Research and Quality; April 2015. Report No. 15-EHC014-EF.
13. Wald JS, Haque SN, Rizk S, et al. Enhancing health IT functionality for children: the 2015 Children's EHR format. *Pediatrics.* 2018;141(4). pii: e20163894.
14. Bryson SP. Patient-centred, administration friendly medicines for children—an evaluation of children's preferences and how they impact medication adherence. *Int J Pharm.* 2014;469(2):257–259.
15. Han YY, Carcillo JA, Venkataraman ST, et al. Unexpected increased mortality after implementation of a commercially sold computerized physician order entry system. *Pediatrics.* 2005;116(6):1506–1512. Erratum in: *Pediatrics.* 2006;117(2):594.

16. Ammenwerth E, Talmon J, Ash JS, et al. Impact of CPOE on mortality rates—contradictory findings, important messages. *Methods Inf Med.* 2006;45(6):586–593.

17. Del Beccaro MA, Jeffries HE, Eisenberg MA, Harry ED. Computerized provider order entry implementation: no association with increased mortality rates in an intensive care unit. *Pediatrics.* 2006;118(1):290–295.

18. Whalen K, Lynch E, Moawad I, John T, Lozowski D, Cummings BM. Transition to a new electronic health record and pediatric medication safety: lessons learned in pediatrics within a large academic health system. *J Am Med Inform Assoc.* 2018;25(7):848–854. doi:10.1093/jamia/ocy034

19. Ozkaynak M, Wu DTY, Hannah K, Dayan PS, Mistry RD. Examining workflow in a pediatric emergency department to develop a clinical decision support for an antimicrobial stewardship program. *Appl Clin Inform.* 2018;9(2):248–260.

20. Sundberg M, Perron CO, Kimia A, et al. A method to identify pediatric high-risk diagnoses missed in the emergency department. *Diagnosis (Berl).* 2018;5(2):63–69. doi:10.1515/dx-2018-0005

21. Deakyne Davies SJ, Grundmeier RW, Campos DA, et al; Pediatric Emergency Care Applied Research Network. The Pediatric Emergency Care Applied Research Network Registry: a multicenter electronic health record registry of pediatric emergency care. *Appl Clin Inform.* 2018;9(2):366–376.

22. Rea CJ, Wenren LM, Tran KD, et al. Shared care: using an electronic consult form to facilitate primary care provider-specialty care coordination. *Acad Pediatr.* 2018;18(7):797–804.

Chapter 25

1. Smith M, Saunders R, Stuckhardt L, et al., eds. *Best Care at Lower Cost: The Path to Continuously Learning Health Care in America.* Washington, DC: Institute of Medicine; 2013.

2. Landon BE, Keating NL, Barnett ML. Variation in patient-sharing networks of physicians across the United States. *JAMA.* 2012;308(3):265–273. http://dx.doi.org/10.1001/jama.2012.7615

3. Cohen J. Epic introduces 3-part functionality for data collaboration. *Becker's Health IT & CIO Report.* January 30, 2018. https://www.beckershospitalreview.com/ehrs/epic-introduces-3-part-functionality-for-data-collaboration.html

4. Mandl KD, Kohane IS. Time for a patient-driven health information economy? *N Engl J Med.* 2016;374(3):205–208. https://www.nejm.org/doi/full/10.1056/NEJMp1512142

5. https://www.fda.gov/regulatoryinformation/lawsenforcedbyfda/significantamendmentstothefdcact/21stcenturycuresact/default.htm

6. https://www.congress.gov/114/plaws/publ255/PLAW-114publ255.pdf

7. Office of the National Coordinator for Health Information Technology. Understand information blocking. In: *HealthIT Playbook.* Washington, DC: ONC; Section 2.4. https://www.healthit.gov/playbook/certified-health-it/#section-2-4. Last updated February 28, 2018.

8. Dolin RH, Alschuler L. Approaching semantic interoperability in Health Level Seven. *J Am Med Inform Assoc.* 2011;18(1):99–103. http://jamia.oxfordjournals.org/content/jaminfo/18/1/99.full.pdf

9. https://www.healthit.gov/playbook/health-information-exchange/

10. HIMSS. What is interoperability? 2013. http://www.himss.org/library/interoperability-standards/what-is. Accessed June 1, 2016.
11. Substitutable is a term used in object-oriented programming to refer to the ability of objects derived from parent objects to substitute for the parent object.
12. Mandel JC, Kreda DA, Mandl KD, et al. Smart on FHIR: a standards-based, interoperable apps platform for electronic health records. *J Am Med Inform Assoc.* 2016;23(5):899–908. http://dx.doi.org/10.1093/jamia/ocv189
13. https://smarthealthit.org/
14. Dolin RH, Alschuler L, Beebe C, et al. The HL7 Clinical Document Architecture. *J Am Med Inform Assoc.* 2001;8(6):552–569. http://jamia.oxfordjournals.org/jaminfo/8/6/552.full.pdf

CHAPTER 26

1. Barrett M, Combs V, Su JG, et al. Air Louisville: addressing asthma with technology, crowdsourcing, cross-sector collaboration, and policy. *Health Aff.* 2018;37(4):525–534. https://doi.org/10.1377/hlthaff.2017.1315

CHAPTER 27

1. Vreeman DJ, Finnell JT, Overhage JM. A rationale for parsimonious laboratory term mapping by frequency. *AMIA Annu Symp Proc.* 2007;2007:771–775. https://www.ncbi.nlm.nih.gov/pmc/articles/PMC2655785/

CHAPTER 28

1. Velentgas P, Cole JA, Mo J, Sikes CR, Walker AM. Severe vascular events in migraine patients. *Headache.* 2004;44(7):642–651.
2. Howard J, Clark EC, Friedman A, et al. Electronic health record impact on work burden in small, unaffiliated, community-based primary care practices. *J Gen Intern Med.* 2013;28(1):107–113.

CHAPTER 29

1. https://en.wikipedia.org/wiki/List_of_medical_and_health_informatics_journals
2. https://www.healthit.gov/topic/onc-programs/workforce-development-programs

CPSIA information can be obtained
at www.ICGtesting.com
Printed in the USA
BVHW071836120922
646819BV00007B/142